MORECAMBE BAY HOSPITALS NHS TRUST

£24.99

Fundamentals of Mental Health Nursing

Edited by

Victoria Clarke and Andrew Walsh

Birmingham City University

D1335690

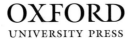

OXFORD
UNIVERSITY PRESS

OXFORD

UNIVERSITY PRESS

Great Clarendon Street, Oxford OX26DP

Oxford University Press is a department of the University of Oxford.
It furthers the University's objective of excellence in research, scholarship,
and education by publishing worldwide in

Oxford New York

Auckland Cape Town Dar es Salaam Hong Kong Karachi
Kuala Lumpur Madrid Melbourne Mexico City Nairobi
New Delhi Shanghai Taipei Toronto

With offices in

Argentina Austria Brazil Chile Czech Republic France Greece
Guatemala Hungary Italy Japan Poland Portugal Singapore
South Korea Switzerland Thailand Turkey Ukraine Vietnam

Oxford is a registered trade mark of Oxford University Press
in the UK and in certain other countries

Published in the United States
by Oxford University Press Inc., New York

© Oxford University Press 2009

The moral rights of the authors have been asserted
Database right Oxford University Press (maker)

First published 2009

All rights reserved. No part of this publication may be reproduced,
stored in a retrieval system, or transmitted, in any form or by any means,
without the prior permission in writing of Oxford University Press,
or as expressly permitted by law, or under terms agreed with the appropriate
reprographics rights organization. Enquiries concerning reproduction
outside the scope of the above should be sent to the Rights Department,
Oxford University Press, at the address above

You must not circulate this book in any other binding or cover
and you must impose the same condition on any acquirer

British Library Cataloguing in Publication Data
Data available

Library of Congress Cataloging in Publication Data
Data available

Typeset by SPI Publisher Services
Printed in Great Britain
on acid-free paper by
Ashford Colour Press Ltd, Gosport, Hampshire

978-0-19-954774-6

1 3 5 7 9 10 8 6 4 2

616.89
CLA

Oxford University Press makes no representation, express or implied, that the drug
dosages in this book are correct. Readers must therefore always check the product
information and clinical procedures with the most up-to-date published product
information and data sheets provided by the manufacturers and the most recent codes of
conduct and safety regulations. The authors and the publishers do not accept responsibility
or legal liability for any errors in the text or for the misuse or misapplication of material in
this work. Except where otherwise stated, drug dosages and recommendations are for the
non-pregnent adult who is not breast-feeding.

This book is dedicated to all those who have ever experienced mental health problems as well as to all those who have ever tried to help them.
Thanks to our family, friends, and colleagues for their hard work and support.
Special thanks to Angela, Luke, Annie, and to Mom, who was a mental health nurse before me.

Preface

We should like to welcome you to this textbook, which is written primarily by mental health nurses and is intended as an introductory text for students studying to become mental health nurses. At a time when mental health services are undergoing great transformation, this book will help to prepare mental health nurse students to work in flexible and effective ways, specifically working in partnership with service users. You will notice that we have asked service users to comment throughout and have also included a cast of fictional service users whose stories appear in the pages of this book as well as on the website that accompanies this book.

Many of the areas we have tried to cover in this book are hotly contested and debated. Commonly shared definitions of what constitutes 'mental health' are not possible to identify and neither is it clear where psychiatry and scientific approaches apply to understanding as opposed to more psycho-social approaches. The contributors to this book do not share a common approach and beliefs, and it would be dishonest of us to pretend otherwise. During your education you will be exposed to a wide range of ideas, and we would respectfully suggest that your task is to critically engage with these, and to talk to (and above all – listen to) service users and fellow professionals.

In putting this book together we have spoken with student nurses, newly qualified staff, and experienced staff. The clear message we heard was that you will only succeed in your education with a thorough knowledge of theoretical foundations alongside a consideration of how this theory translates into actual practice. This is why the theoretical aspects of this book are presented alongside realistic accounts of fictional service users. We have tasked contributors to this book to consider how the aspects of care they are discussing might look in the context of these fictional characters. In each case, the theoretical elements discussed have been translated into sample care plans – we leave it to you to judge how well this has been managed. We have not insisted that every contributor sticks rigidly to a particular care planning format and you will find different interpretations of how care plans should be completed throughout the book. We hope and believe that this diversity of approach reflects the reality of mental health nursing practice. You will find that you agree with some of the material in these pages and disagree with other elements. We would encourage you in this; the ability to critically assess such material is an essential characteristic of a mental health nurse.

A brief tour

Chapter 1, entitled 'Becoming a mental health nurse student', is intended to help you to understand both what will be expected of you as a student nurse as well as what you can expect from those whose job it is to guide and support you through your education.

Chapter 2 outlines approaches and skills adopted by mental health nurses in seeking to work with people experiencing mental health problems.

Chapter 3 – while mental health legislation is covered as it arises throughout the book, this chapter attempts to address more directly this important aspect of mental health working. Note that when we started to write we were aware that the legislation of the 1983 English Mental Health Act was in the process (at times controversially so) of being reframed. By the time we had finished the main process of writing the book, the 1983 law had been replaced by the new (2007) Mental Health Act. We are also aware that this book will be read across many other countries and that it is important to try and reflect the mental health law as enacted in these territories. We must stress, however, that we make no claims to provide anything other than a brief introduction and a raised awareness of this complex area.

Chapters 4 to 9 are practice based and generally provide an introduction to the areas and subjects that will be encountered by students during their education. The contributors have tried to ensure that they focused upon essential areas of knowledge required by mental health nurses. As you will discover, mental health nurses work in such a wide range of settings that it would not be possible for a single textbook to cover every possibly relevant area. Rather, it is hoped that this book will play its part in helping you to develop a foundation of knowledge for your future career – a basis to be developed by your studies and practice experiences.

In **Chapter 10** the focus moves towards helping you to find your first qualified mental health nursing post. As part of this we cover what employers are looking for, how to apply for jobs, and how to succeed at interview. We go on to make suggestions about how you might progress in your career. The book ends as it started, with contributions from mental health service users who share their opinions as to what makes a good mental health nurse.

In writing this book we have been privileged to work in collaboration with a range of service users and colleagues. We would like to take this opportunity to express our grateful thanks to these people. As editors we hope that this book reflects the diversity of modern practice and is a really useful tool for you, and we wish you every success in your studies.

Victoria Clarke and Andrew Walsh

How to use this book

Fundamentals of Mental Health Nursing has been developed to bring mental health nursing to life through the use of specific features and learning tools. This brief tour shows you how to get the most out of this textbook package.

Service user comments

> **♣ Service user's comment**
>
> Is it usual practice for people to be interviewed in unfamiliar, perhaps rather clinical and unwelcoming surroundings? This caused distress, adding to Albert's difficulty in giving answers to questions.
>
> Whilst the interviewer had a very friendly and sympathetic attitude, sometimes the interview seemed more like a test than an exploratory conversation. Is it good to ask certain kinds of questions that the person is clearly going to have difficulty with, e.g.
>
> find words they've forgotten, a good idea? It was noticeable that Albert hadn't forgotten the actions to go with what he was trying to explain, e.g. the wheel of a car. So, as in other areas of mental and emotional distress, is it equally important to pay attention to non-verbal communication?
>
> One of the things this clip highlighted for me – as well as the other clips – was how difficult it can be for practitioners to elicit information to help them make an assessment of what is actually going on, e.g. trying to find out about the betting shop and what Albert's

Throughout the book real service users offer their insights and perspectives on a range of key issues and on the fictional care episodes in chapters 4 – 9. This vital input will help readers to understand and deliver person-centred care.

Clinical scenarios

> **Clinical scenario: Anthony**
>
> In this chapter you will meet 'Anthony' and his brother 'David' following Anthony's referral to mental health services. You will find it useful to read the scenario first and then access the brief films that show both Anthony and his brother talking about the situation.
>
> ### Anthony's story
>
> Anthony is a 45-year-old man who lives alone in a rented
>
> little neglected. Anthony often appears to be hearing voices although he denies this; on occasions he hints to the practice nurse that the Internet is making it difficult to control him.
>
> Anthony has never worked and spends his time either alone in his flat or in the local library where he goes and spends most of his mornings, although recently he has been complaining that blurred vision is making it difficult to read the newspapers there. Anthony is quite overweight, smokes very heavily, and eats a diet that consists mostly of 'junk' food; he often complains of feeling hungry and gets

Practice based chapters (4–9) address the needs of a diverse range of fictional service users and explain how key nursing knowledge and skills are applied in practice. Each chapter introduces the reader to one or more clinical cases which are explored in depth so that readers can transfer these skills to their own practice.

Videos

> ▶ http://www.oxfordtextbooks.co.uk/orc/clarke
> and choose the video link.
> After watching the film you will also find it helpful to undertake Online quiz 2.

When you see the video icon, the clinical scenario is accompanied by a video of the fictional service user, mimicking real life presentations in practice. The videos are hosted online on a free accompanying website and the authors will prompt you to watch them at key points in the text. Accessing and watching the videos is very straightforward and instructions are included overleaf.

Student activity

> **Student activity 2**
> View the video of Joyce and her boyfriend Mark meeting with Simon. Make notes on anything you find significant. Do you think the short-term goals have been met?

These encourage you to consider issues particular to each case and to develop your nursing skills. These can also include prompts to watch the videos and/or undertake an online activity.

Assessment plan

> **♣ Assessment**
>
> Today, mental health nurses are much less likely to focus on assessment based on medical diagnosis, tending now towards a more person-centred approach
>
> ple's problems in living but also their strengths. Here it is stressed that it is important when assessing to consider the impact on the individual. The use of diagnosis to inform assessment and care is impractical. We know of people who suffer the same illness but who react to it in totally differing ways. The use of signs
>
> blow to the head is related to you and can not be assumed to have the same impact on another person. Therefore the use of the diagnosis that Joyce has bipolar affective disorder will not give us the whole picture about the nature of her crisis or its impact on her.
>
> Having seen the video of the first assessment, you will already have begun the process of assessing Joyce. It is important though that the assessment process is supported by knowledge. As previously stated, we must avoid jumping to conclusions. For example when Joyce swears loudly at the nurse, is this symptomatic of disinhibition or just the result of Joyce being angry at

This highlights core issues and skills for the nursing assessment that readers can begin to use in their own practice.

Care plan

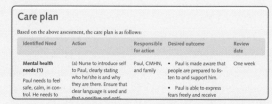

> **Care plan**
>
> Based on the above assessment, the care plan is as follows:
>
> | Identified Need | Action | Responsible for action | Desired outcome | Review date |
> |---|---|---|---|---|
> | **Mental health needs (1)** Paul needs to feel safe, calm, in control. He needs to | (a) Nurse to introduce self to Paul, clearly stating who he/she is and why they are there. Ensure that clear language is used and that a positive and opti- | Paul, CMHN, and family | • Paul is made aware that people are prepared to listen to and support him. • Paul is able to express fears freely and receive | One week |

Each fictional service user has a care plan which is clearly written and laid out to illustrate the approach and rationale for nursing care so that students can develop their own skills in this arena.

Pharmacist's view

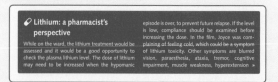

> **✎ Lithium: a pharmacist's perspective**
>
> While on the ward, the lithium treatment would be assessed and it would be a good opportunity to check the plasma lithium level. The dose of lithium may need to be increased when the hypomanic
>
> episode is over, to prevent future relapse. If the level is low, compliance should be examined before increasing the dose. In the film, Joyce was complaining of feeling cold, which could be a symptom of lithium toxicity. Other symptoms are blurred vision, paraesthesia, ataxia, tremor, cognitive impairment, muscle weakness, hyperextension »

Where relevant, pharmacists explain and explore issues of medication, side effects, dosages, concordance, and advice for management.

Discussion points

> ● Discussion point: Social Inclusion
>
> We really debated whether it was appropriate and realistic to include the community mental health nurse in meeting the residents in Anthony's community to raise their awareness of mental health issues. One major concern was the issue of whether this strategy could compromise Anthony's confidentiality. We agreed that any such approach must be carried out with sensitivity to Anthony's rights and wishes at all times. One of the options we considered was that a CPN uninvolved with Anthony's direct care should take on the responsibility for promoting social
>
> health nurses in any circumstances, due to their caseload pressures and requirements from their employing trusts to be involved in the delivery of service user care, not education of local communities.
>
> We also discussed whether this is actually part of the community mental health nurse's role, or whether it should be referred to a social worker as an aspect of social care, not health. Eventually we agreed to disagree. There are clear policy guidelines and very specific drivers that indicate that the Department of Health and a range of gov-

Key issues in care plans and in chapter text are often explored in further detail, particularly where there are important debates around a topic.

Assignments and developing your knowledge further

> ⚡ Useful web links
>
> ❷ Sources of help and advice
>
> ◌ References

Each chapter finishes with directions to our online resource centre where quizzes and other activities can help you develop your skills further. Directions to useful websites and further reading are given in addition to the references employed by the authors.

Glossary terms

> • In cluster A, which they refer to as the odd/eccentric cluster, they identify three types of disorder: paranoid; schizoid; and schizotypal.
> • In cluster B, the dramatic/erratic cluster, there are four types: antisocial; borderline; histrionic; and

Technical terms particular to mental health nursing are highlighted in colour in the text and then explained in the glossary at the end of the text.

How to use the online resource centre

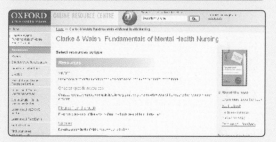

This textbook is accompanied by a free online resource centre (website) that provides students and lecturers with interactive resources, including the videos for each clinical scenario. You can access the online resource centre from any computer with internet access and so you will find it helpful to save the web address in to your 'favourites' at the earliest opportunity:

www.oxfordtextbooks.co.uk/orc/clarke

Videos of fictional service users

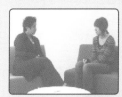

Each clinical scenario is accompanied by a short film of the fictional service user to mimic real life presentations to mental health nursing services. Where you see the video icon 📹 in the chapter text, you should watch the accompanying video of the fictional service user at your earliest convenience. These can be watched as many times as you like so you can you observe different user needs and issues and practice a variety of nursing skills in each viewing.

To access the videos, visit the home page for the online resource centre and click on 'videos'. You will see that the videos are listed according to the fictional service users name AND chapter number.

You will need Windows Media Player to watch the videos. Simply click on the link and the video will start playing. For some video clips you may find it helpful to use headphones, particularly if in the university library or a noisy environment.

Chapter specific resources: quizzes, extra scenarios and activities

Each chapter is supported by a range of online resources written by the authors to help readers apply and develop their skills around the issues discussed in the chapter.

Chapter 1 and 10 include helpful student-centred activities such as accounts of nursing students' experiences beginning a mental health nursing course (Chapter 1) and a blank CV template (Chapter 10).

The remaining chapters have very helpful quizzes, activities, and scenarios covering fundamental nursing areas such as nursings kills and mental health law, as well as clinical practice related issues.

Acknowledgements

We would like to thank the following:

Birmingham City University pre-registration mental health nursing students.

Birmingham City University CETL, especially Stuart Brand, Luke Millard, and Rachel Moule.

Birmingham City University CELT SALT project – Filming, editing, and advice, Niall Mackenzie, Mark Hetherington, Guillaume Piot, Dario Faniglione, and Professor Alan Staley.

Actors in films: Robert Ball, Lauren Bate, Zena Brennan, Leasa Clarke, Emma Cooper, Juliet Cooper, Paul Forrest, Charles Fulford, Janet Grant, Angela Green, Chrissy Griffiths, Simon Hetherington, Daniel Hawthorne, Glendon Jackson, Gerry Lucas.

Mental health nurses: Tony Barlow, Doug Scrivens, Denise Steeves.

Sarah Holland and 'Mrs Bibi'.

Geraldine Jeffers and Marionne Cronin at OUP and everyone who reviewed the draft manuscript.

Aneesa Adam at Birmingham City University.

Mr Man's wife, for pemission to use an extract from her blog in Chapter 3.

The editors would like to acknowledge the contribution made by Dave Brookes who first developed some of the scenarios used in this book.

Contents

Detailed Contents

Contributors

Frances Byrne RNMH, PG Cert (Education)

Frances currently works for Birmingham and Solihull Mental Health Trust as senior nurse for Health Care Education and Quality. Frances has worked in mental health for 23 years within the health service and voluntary sector.

Jim Chapman RNMH, PG Cert (Education), MA, RNT

Jim is a senior lecturer in the Clinical Skills Division, Faculty of Health, Birmingham City University. He has previous clinical experience in acute and community mental health care, and currently teaches on a range of pre- and post-registration nursing courses.

Cheryl Chessum RNMH, RNLD, Bsc (Hons), PG Cert (Education)

Cheryl is a lecturer/practitioner in mental health with over 20 years' experience of working with adults in a community setting. Her main focus of teaching experience is at post-registration level in the role of Branch Leader for BSc (Hons) Community Mental Health Nursing – Specialist Practitioner Award.

Nicola Clarke MSc General Psychiatry, PG Cert (Education), Cert Reality Therapy, Bsc (Hons) Mental Health, RNMH

Nicola is a senior lecturer at Birmingham City University. She has worked in the field of substance use for over ten years for the NHS and in private practice. Nicola has also worked as a commissioning manager designing and commissioning services in the field of substance misuse. Nicola now teaches pre- and post-registration mental health nurses.

Victoria Clarke RNMH, RCNT, RNT, Cert Ed (FE/HE), BeD (Hons), MA

Victoria has worked as a mental health nurse for 26 years and within nurse education for the last 17 years. Victoria's current post is Head of Division/Director of Quality (Mental Health) at Birmingham City University.

Glyn Coventry RNMH, BSc (Hons), MA (Gerontology), PG Cert (Education)

Glyn was formerly senior lecturer in Mental Health Studies and Head of Mental Health Division at Birmingham City University. He is currently semi-retired and working as a freelance mental health lecturer and education consultant. He has worked in mental health clinical and educational settings for over 30 years.

Karen Cross RNMH, BSC (Hons), PG Cert (Education), PG Dip (education)

Karen is a registered mental health nurse with over 20 years' experience. Karen is now working as a senior lecturer at Birmingham City University, working within the department of practice learning and teaching pre-registration mental health nurses and nurse assessors.

Sandy Fitzgibbon PhD, MSc, FAHE, RNMH, CPN, CAMH

Sandy is a senior lecturer at the City of Birmingham University and has worked in mental health since 1972. She commenced working with children, young people, and their families in CAMHS in 1980.

Catharine Jenkins BA (Hons), RNMH, Dip N, MSc, PG Dip Education, PG Cert (Education)

Catharine is a senior nurse lecturer at Birmingham City University who teaches older peoples' mental health and diversity issues. She has many years experience as a community mental health nurse, specializing in trans-cultural nursing of older people.

Marion Johnson ONC Med Lab Sciences, RNMH, LPE, ENB 998, BSc (Hons), PG Cert (Education), MSc

Marion is a senior lecturer in Mental Health Nursing and the Mental Health Branch coordinator for the BSc Course at Birmingham City University.

Marjorie Lloyd RNMH, SCMH, LPE, MSc, BSc, Dip N

Marjorie is a senior lecturer at the Glynd University in Wrexham, North Wales. Marjorie has worked in mental health care for 20 years, from inpatient to community and as a lecturer practitioner. Marjorie has been a full-time lecturer for the last five years and is researching service user and carer involvement and empowerment.

Linda Playford MA, BSc (Hons), RMNH, CPN Cert

Linda is a registered mental health nurse who has worked for the past six years as nurse consultant for older people's services at Birmingham and Solihull Mental Health Trust. Her career has spanned over 20 years, working within both inpatient and community mental health team settings.

Chris Smith RNMH, Dip HE, ENB 998

Chris has worked for 30 years in mental health nursing in both Yorkshire and the West Midlands, and more recently as a community mental health nurse in psychiatric liaison.

Simon Steeves RNMH, LPE, Dip Dth, PG Cert

Simon has been an acute psychiatric nurse for over 35 years. As a senior lecturer at Birmingham City University, he is involved in pre- and post-registration teaching. His main interests are law, specifically mental health law (with some years as a magistrate), psychodynamics, and drama therapy.

Victoria Taylor RNMH, MTheol, MA, MA, Dip HE

Victoria worked as a mental health nurse in the NHS for ten years in a variety of settings before becoming a senior lecturer at Birmingham City University.

Pam Virdi RNMH, MEd Psychodynamic counselling, Diploma in Anatomy, Advanced Diploma of Mental Health Studies (Child and Adolescent Pathway), Physiology and Therapeutic Massage – (College of Natural Health 1999), PG Cert (Education), Certificate in Hypnotherapy and Psychotherapy

Pam has worked in mental health settings for 27 years. For the last 17 years she has been a lecturer/practitioner in eating disorders. She currently works at the Birmingham Eating Disorder Service and is an honorary lecturer at Birmingham City University. Pam is also trained in psychodynamic therapy, interpersonal psychotherapy, CBT hypnotherapy, massage therapy, and EMDR (eye movement desensitization and reprocessing).

Andrew Walsh RNMH, LPE, Bsc (Hons), PG Dip (Health Development), PG Dip (Education), PG Cert (Education)

Andrew is a senior lecturer at Birmingham City University where he teaches pre-registration mental health nurses. He previously spent over 20 years working in a variety of mental health care settings.

Chapter 1
On becoming a student mental health nurse
Victoria Clarke, Frances Byrne, Karen Cross, Andrew Walsh

Learning outcomes

After reading this chapter you should be able to:

- Identify the four aspects of professions.
- Summarize what a nurse is.
- Give examples of nurses' personal values and beliefs.
- Understand what values and beliefs are.
- Demonstrate increasing self-awareness.
- Demonstrate increasing awareness of professional behaviour within both university and clinical placements.
- Identify and develop increasing understanding of models used in mental health nursing.
- Recognize the importance of maintaining professional boundaries in service user relationships.

Introduction

This chapter is all about helping you to understand what mental health nursing is. To this end, we will consider what you must know and do when you first meet people with mental health problems. We will introduce a personal account from a mental health service user early in the chapter in order to help you begin to understand what working with people with mental health problems is like and what service users want from mental health nurses. In an effort to help you become familiar with what mental health nursing is, we will explore the following issues: what is a profession; what is nursing; what beliefs and values inform nursing; why is it important for mental health nurses to be self-aware; and what do mental health nurses need to know? In the final part of this chapter we explore the nature of boundaries in professional relationships and the implications of this for practice as a mental health nurse.

Before you read any further we would encourage you to recognize that mental health service users are, quite rightly, the real experts in their care and needs. It is vitally important that you listen and really attend to what they are saying to you. We have asked a service user, Deborah Living, to represent for you some of the important issues that she would like mental health nurses to be aware of, and Deborah is going to tell you part of her own life story.

> ### 👤 Personal account of mental health services by Deborah Living
>
> I consider myself to be a survivor…not just a survivor of mental health difficulties but also a survivor of mental health services.
>
> I feel I am a survivor because I have reclaimed my life after more than ten years of mental health diagnoses and treatments: diagnoses from clinical depression to cyclothymia (described as a 'milder' form of manic depression); antidepressants and mood stabilisers from prozac to lithium; and »

» interventions from counselling to psychiatry, through ECT to being an inpatient.

It took me over a decade and a 12-month stay in a residential therapeutic community to stop the 'revolving door' approach within the mental health service, whereby I would gain short-term stability only to relapse yet again.

In order to provide the effective intervention and support that has proved to be vital to the reclamation of my life, the practitioners who helped me embodied a particular approach to mental health treatment.

I believe the key underlying ethos in my effective treatment was that mental health practitioners applied 'joined-up thinking'. They sought to make connections between events in my past to the situations and symptoms that were apparent in my present. They helped me make active links between experiences in my adult life, adolescence, and childhood so that I could see the patterns in my own behaviour. They approached me as a whole person and sought to treat the whole person, rather than purely dealing with whatever symptom I was presenting at the time. I feel this not only hastened my recovery but also made it more meaningful; all too often mental health professionals will treat whatever is being presented to them at the time, whether it is depression or drug use, stress or self-harm. Much more is to be gained when a holistic approach is taken to the individual, and the mental health practitioners who helped me were able to see past what I appeared to be presenting with and sought to discover the root cause.

The mental health professionals that I responded to best actively listened to me and took me seriously. They approached me in a way that sought to acknowledge and understand my own internal world, and gave it as much credibility as the external world. Rather than telling me that my belief systems and behavioural patterns were 'wrong' or 'bad' (whether explicitly, or implicitly by prescribing medication), these practitioners fully engaged with me and my way of thinking and acting. More than just non-judgemental understanding, which is in itself rare, it was an approach that seemed to be more akin to them meeting me as one individual human being to another.

So as to facilitate such an approach, the mental health professionals who worked with me maintained clear and explicitly defined boundaries with regards to disclosure of their own personal details and issues. By having firm boundaries, and a contained environment for interactions, they were able to give of themselves as complete individuals and interacted with me as people, rather than hiding behind the label of 'professional'.

These elements of their approach allowed me to build up my trust in them, and in the long term what has proven to be trust in people in general. Once a level of trust had been achieved I was able to work with them on a much more meaningful level; I was able to accept direct, open, challenging feedback and gradually my thought patterns and behaviours began to change. This approach also aided my own growth and development, moving me from a negative, over-reliant relationship with mental health practitioners towards self-actualization and empowerment.

Having had over ten years' experience of being a mental health service user, my view is that the system can, in certain circumstances, 'support' an individual to remain as they are, offering a range of often ineffective solutions such as medication and short-term interventions that do very little to help the individual in the long term. Often it has felt as if my relationship with the mental health service has been one of dysfunctional parenting, and that ultimately the best approach was one that sought to help me detach from this and become independent. As difficult as this was, it was in the context of a contained, supportive structure which all those involved in my care worked to uphold.

Fundamental elements of the ethos and approach that were upheld and have been beneficial to me in the long term are:

- An emphasis on emotional support over medication.

- Encouragement to verbalize thoughts and feelings rather than 'act them out' physically.

- An understanding of the clear consequences of acting out thoughts and feelings.

- The acknowledgement of self-harm as being any behaviour that is destructive to the individual, and being treated seriously as such.

- Self-ownership of issues.

- An emphasis on developing awareness of personal risks and assuming responsibility for them and their management.

- Peer support (groups, friends) rather than an over-reliance on health professionals.

- Challenging, direct, honest interactions in a contained framework.

»

The role of art/art therapy:

- A constructive form of self-expression as an alternative to self-destructive 'acting out' behaviours.
- A tangible form by which the individual self is made manifest, and thus an aid for communicating conscious and subconscious issues for which there may be no words, or that the creator feels otherwise inhibited by.
- An expression of deep emotions formed at a pre-verbal age, coupled with the power of group work whereby others can vocalize their own thoughts and feelings in relation to the images.
- The potential to share the creative process within a group as a form of 'play' and social therapy.

Box 1.1 The role of art therapy

» As part of my care and treatment I also benefited greatly from the use of art and art therapy. For me, art therapy provided a constructive form of self-expression and an alternative to self-destructive behaviours, allowing me to 'act out' my thoughts and feelings creatively rather than channel them into destructive or self-destructive actions.

Creative work was approached as thoughts and feelings made manifest. Through this my conscious and subconscious issues were given a tangible form that could be connected with, related to, and discussed. This was particularly helpful when the art was an expression of deep emotions formed at a pre-verbal age for which I had no words. It was also a helpful tool in aiding me to introduce thoughts, feelings, and issues to others when I felt too inhibited to speak out directly. As well as art therapists I was also helped by other mental health practitioners who facilitated group creative activities and encouraged me to take part in them as a form of 'play' and social therapy.

Through the effective intervention, care, and support I received I have achieved the following results:

- I have a clearer understanding of my fundamental needs.
- I am more able to ask for what I need.

- I am aware of my risks and am able to undertake personal risk management.
- I am able to access care and support in a more direct and constructive way.
- I have been free of prescribed medication for more than two years.
- I have been able to build a life that, with support, is sustainable, personally fulfilling, and productive.

I was fortunate enough to come into contact with a team of mental health service professionals, from nurses to psychologists, who saw their role as to empower me to live my life to my full potential as a unique individual. They did not see me as having 'an illness' they needed to 'cure'. Their approach was in sharp contrast to what I feel was the bad, indifferent, or misguided treatment I had previously encountered over ten years. My hope is that this approach becomes the norm in mental health services, rather than a rarity.

Due to the help I have received I have now rebuilt my life, which I dedicate to change and development, and am now involved with various projects to do with the arts and media within the field of mental health.

Deborah Living, June 2007

What is a profession?

As a student nurse you need to understand what a profession is and what nursing is. This will give you an overview before we focus on the specifics of mental health nursing.

A profession is recognized by having:

- A body of specialized knowledge and practice.
- A professional association.
- A process of certification or licensing (University of Texas at Arlington 1998).
- An ethical code.

However, there is significant contention over whether nursing meets all of the criteria to be considered a profession. Some people would argue that it is an emerging profession that meets many, but not all, of the established criteria. There is disagreement over whether nurses fully control their own work or have an exclusive body of knowledge; some argue that while nursing knowledge may have originated in other disciplines, it is applied to nursing in a unique fashion that confirms nursing's professional status (Hood and Leddy 2006). In the UK and in many other countries, nursing is regularly referred to as a profession; however, this does vary from country to country.

Therefore, to work in a profession or be a professional you will need to have a high standard of knowledge and skills that are distinct to your profession. These are underpinned by a set of ethics and values that clearly define the boundaries of your practice.

Specialized knowledge

As a mental health nurse you will continually develop specialized knowledge. In the UK, the Nursing and Midwifery Council (NMC) acts as the professional regulatory body and their proficiency statements identify a basic level of knowledge and skills for students (NMC 2004). Mental health nurses also have special responsibilities under mental health law Codes of Practice, which inform the implementation of this law and government legislation. This varies from country to country. We refer to specific examples taken from English law in later chapters; however, we have also included some additional perspectives on mental health law in Chapter 3 and on the website link to this textbook.

Student activity 1

Follow the NMC web link below and read through the Nursing and Midwifery Council proficiency statements for student nurses (NMC 2004). Briefly identify what you think each statement means. You will become increasingly familiar with these as you work through your clinical placements.

 http://www.nmc-uk.org/

then choose 'Nursing' from the menu and choose 'Relevant Publications'. The standards are available for download.

Working to achieve your proficiencies throughout your course to safe, effective and proficient levels will ensure that you are fit for practice, purpose, and award; in other words, fit to qualify.

The professional association and the process of certification

The NMC is the UK's professional nursing association and it is required to establish and maintain a register of qualified nurses and midwives. Without an active NMC registration (licensing) you will not be able to practise as a qualified nurse in the UK.

The ethical code

You will spend half of the course at university and half in placements in a variety of settings. You are expected to act professionally and adhere to professional codes at all times. In the UK, these are found in *The Code: Standards of conduct, performance and ethics for nurses and midwives* (NMC 2008). The code is a list of expectations and standards for nurses, intended to tell us what to do and what the public can expect from us; it also helps us to define the boundaries of our practice and relationships with service users.

The key features for nurses and midwives are to:

- Ensure people in your care are able to trust you with their health and well-being.
- Put people first and treat them as individuals whilst respecting their dignity.
- Protect and support the health of individuals, patients, and clients.
- Protect and support the health of the wider community.
- Act in a way that justifies the trust and confidence the public have in you.
- Uphold and enhance the good reputation of the professions.

(NMC 2008)

It is vital that nurses remain familiar with this document, so please ensure that you regularly visit the website (the address is included under 'Useful web links' in the reference list at the end of this chapter).

But what does all of this mean in terms of your own behaviour as a student nurse?

> **Student activity 2**
> *Go online and try the interactive quiz on the code of conduct.*

@ www.oxfordtextbooks.co.uk/orc/clarke

and choose the online resources for Chapter 1.

Professional behaviour is a concept that provides nurses with a way of managing their actions. It should include, as the University of Victoria (2000) identifies:

- **Responsibility**: Managing your own progress and being prepared for classes, practice or assignments.
- **Commitment to quality**: Aiming for your optimum level. Taking pride in all aspects of your work.

- **Integrity**: A professional will always follow through on commitments they have made; they will avoid conflicts of interest or bias.
- **Respect for others**: Respect and courtesy are fundamental parts of being a professional. Professionals show respect in all of their communication, written, verbal, and non-verbal, with everyone, regardless of their personal feelings. They show respect for others' opinions, listening and providing feedback when asked. Regardless of the person's status, they are attentive and polite.

It is combining the requirements of a profession with the necessary values, professional behaviour, and boundaries that makes nursing a profession and thus makes each one of us a professional. Perhaps the following quote is worth noting as well: 'The job doesn't make you a professional, your attitude does' (Norton 2007).

What is a nurse?

The Royal College of Nursing (RCN) found that while they could not provide a complete definition of nursing, they were able to establish a set of characteristics of nursing (Royal College of Nursing 2002). These are summarized below:

1) **A particular purpose**: This being to promote the health, well-being, and development of an individual along with prevention of illness, disease, or disability. Additionally it is a nurse's role to minimize distress and provide education and advice in order for patients to understand not only their illness but also their treatment and its likely outcomes.

2) **A particular mode of intervention**: Nursing is a process that includes assessment of needs, delivery of therapeutic interventions, and care. Nurses aim to empower individuals, helping them to achieve, maintain, or recover their independence.

3) **A particular domain**: This is about recognizing the importance of individual responses.

4) **A particular focus**: This is seeing the individual holistically, i.e. seeing the person as a whole.

5) **A particular value base**: As nurses we share key common values such as respect for human life; this is explored later in this chapter.

6) **A commitment to partnership**: Nurses work in collaboration with all members of the multidisciplinary team, including the client and their carers.

A professional nurse isn't something that you can just be, it takes time and practice. You also need a great deal of self-awareness and an understanding of your own values and beliefs. In the next part of the chapter you are encouraged to explore your own values and beliefs, particularly in relation to mental health nursing, and also to develop your self-awareness. One useful way to prepare for starting in your branch is to consider what your hopes, fears, and expectations are (see p. 6). You may also find it helpful to undertake the following activity and then read accounts of other students' hopes, fears, and expectations at this stage of training.

> **Student activity 3**
> *Start off by making a list of what your life has given you so far that you could use as a student nurse. Focus on your personal resources and skills – what are you good at, what support have you got available to you already, what healthy strategies have you got for managing your stress and anxiety?*
> *Now take a look at comments from other student nurses online at:*

@ www.oxfordtextbooks.co.uk/orc/clarke

and choose the online resources for this chapter.

Identify in the rectangle the things that you most fear may happen to you during your nursing education and the things you are least worried about.

Most

Least

Identify in the rectangle the things that you most hope to achieve while on your student nurse course and the things that you are least concerned with achieving.

Most

Least

Identify in the rectangle the things that you most and least expect to get out of your student nurse course.

Most

Least

It is useful to speak to your mental health nurse student colleagues, your personal tutor, or your course lecturers about these issues and to keep a record of your first thoughts in your portfolio. This will provide you with an opportunity to reflect on what you have achieved at the end of the course. It is important to maintain your portfolio as evidence of your learning; as a professional you will have a life-long responsibility to keep learning and to keep evidence of this for your professional registration (NMC 2005).

Many mental health nursing students express the same concerns about working in mental health services as members of the general population do and there are many myths and stereotypes surrounding people with mental health problems. It is useful for you to consider what your own personal beliefs and values are concerning people with mental health problems, and what exactly you think a mental health nurse does.

What are beliefs and values?

A simple definition of these terms would include the following:

- Values are principles or standards (e.g. valuing human life).
- A belief is the acceptance of the truth of something (e.g. the sun will rise tomorrow).

Your values and beliefs will determine how you respond to situations and people.

To help you understand the idea of values and beliefs, it may be worth thinking about them as your own personal code of practice. You will find that they differ from person to person. You may also find it useful to consider the *10 Essential Shared Capabilities for Mental Health* (National Institute for Mental Health in England/Sainsbury Centre for Mental Health Joint Workforce Support Unit/National Health Service University 2004), which are seen as central to mental

Achievement	Friendships	Physical challenge	Advancement and promotion	Growth
Integrity		Cooperation	Responsibility and accountability	Quality
Pleasure	Affection (love and caring)	Helping others	Having a family	
Privacy	Adventure	Challenging problems		Change and variety
Close relationships	Independence	Influencing others	Inner harmony	Religion
Country	Recognition/ Status	Intellectual status	Job security	Community
Creativity	Truth	Fast living	Money	Ethical practice
Working alone		Self-respect	Knowledge	The environment
Competition	Freedom	Honesty		Power and authority

Box 1.2 Values exercise

1.
2.
3.
4.
5.

Box 1.3 Your top five values

health professional practice and were developed in partnership with mental health service users.

The following exercise is designed to help you reach a better understanding of your most significant values.

First step: What I value most …

From the following list of values (both work-related and personal), circle the ten that are most important to you (feel free to add any of your own values that are not included in the blank spaces). You can also find these boxes online and you can save them on your computer, print them off, and include them in your portfolio.

 www.oxfordtextbooks.co.uk/orc/clarke

and choose the online resources for this chapter.

Second step:

Once you have identified ten values, choose your top five – think about which five you would be able to give up …

Now, list your top five values in order of priority:

What are beliefs?

When hearing the word 'schizophrenia', what do you first think of and where does this image come from? What about when you hear the words 'mentally ill'? Have you noticed any differences in what your fellow students from the adult, child, and learning disabilities branch think?

How are our beliefs formed?

Our beliefs are formed through our experiences and reflections, exposure to events, or through blind acceptance of what others tell us. For example, our beliefs about mental health/illness could arise from personal experience of mental distress, along with influences from the media, culture, and community. The more people we come into contact with who have mental health problems and the more we read about them, the broader our understanding will become. And the more we reflect upon our values and beliefs, the more self-aware we become.

Why is self-awareness important?

If we are aware of our own values and beliefs, the task of becoming self-aware is much easier. 'Becoming self-aware is a conscious process in which we consider our understanding of ourselves' (Jack and Smith 2007). Self-awareness is an essential characteristic in being an effective mental health nurse. It is an ongoing process, and is crucial when the 'self' is used as a tool; this means that we purposely use our communication skills, emotional availability, and physical selves in helping a person. Self-awareness is made up of three components: affective (emotional); behavioural (actions); and cognitive (thoughts).

It is important that you become aware of how you think and feel about situations at work, as this affects your behaviour. If you feel negative towards people who use drugs or alcohol, you may avoid dealing with these people when in placement or it may affect the way you interact with them. If you are aware of your thoughts and feelings, you are more likely to manage your emotions and be able to act professionally. This does not mean you will always feel comfortable in difficult or new situations, but the more self-aware you are, the easier it will be to accept your anxieties and concerns.

Student activity 4

Reflect on an occasion in placement when your feelings may have influenced your thoughts and behaviour.

How did you feel? How did you behave? On reflection, would you react differently now?

Evidence shows that mental health service users and their carers want mental health workers who are self-aware to care for them, so that the health workers' own problems and issues do not intrude into client interactions (Institute of Health and Care Development 1998). As student mental health nurses, it is important that you develop as much knowledge about yourself as you do about others, as this will increase your effectiveness in communicating with others. We will be asking you to do more specific work on self-awareness in Chapter 2.

How do mental health nurses organize their work?

Through examining our own values and beliefs, we begin to recognize that we are trying to understand complex systems such as human behaviour, thoughts, and feelings. In such situations, a model can be a useful tool for mental health nurses. A model offers

an explanation or representation that helps us understand how humans function, why they can stop functioning, and what the role of the nurse is in relation to this. A model provides us with a framework for deciding what we mean by such concepts as thoughts, feelings, health, illness, and nursing. In nursing, a model is a way to show what we as nurses should be doing; the idea is that it will help nurses understand what they are doing, or should be doing, and why they are doing it. Essentially, therefore, the model shows what knowledge needs to underpin nurses' practice.

What do mental health nurses do?

In thinking about what models influence mental health nursing today, it may be useful to consider how best to explain to a new student with very little experience of working within mental health what mental health nurses do. New students often find it very difficult to actually grasp the purpose and nature of mental health nursing. It's useful to think about what you have seen mental health nurses do in practice; you may have seen a person visited at home and given an injection of medication, and when carrying out this procedure the nurse spoke to the person about how they were feeling. This is common to all types of nursing and we often refer to this work as *procedural*, or concerned with completing a specific task.

The injection of medication administered in the above example would have been prescribed by a psychiatrist, meaning the biological or medical model approach is being used. The medical model emphasizes a possible malfunction in the biological systems of the body. For example, if you break a bone, a doctor is likely to 'set' the bone and fix it in place with a cast in order to allow it time to heal. In this context, and very simplistically put, if a person has a mental health problem, someone working from the medical model would see this as a malfunction in the way that the brain works. The medical model suggests that chemicals within the brain may hit too many receptors or become depleted. Medication used in psychiatry tries to remedy the malfunction and get the balance of chemicals in the brain correct.

There is considerable evidence to support this approach; however, most people working in mental health services recognize that humans are not just made up of biological systems. We are also influenced by both our social context (our relationships, families, environment, purposeful activity) and our psychological make-up (the way we as individuals think and feel). In mental health nursing we recognize the need to use a holistic approach to care; one that is made up of biological, social, and psychological perspectives. This is often referred to as a bio-psycho-social model.

You may have seen nurses meet with people with mental health problems in a different way to the procedural example described earlier. For example, a nurse might meet with a young woman in distress, and it emerges that this woman is feeling very low in mood. This could be seen as a psychological problem, and would require the use of a psychological model. The nurse would talk to the woman about her problems and together they would look at how to manage or resolve the difficulties over time. This aspect of the mental health nurse's role is seen as *therapeutic*; it is working in a way that seeks to benefit the mental health service user.

During her talk with the nurse, it also emerges that the woman in our example, who is in her early twenties, has just had a child and now has three children under the age of four. She feels unable to cope, and she is frightened that she may hurt her children. This gives her problem a social perspective. Mental health nurses may involve social services if children are at risk. A nurse using the social model in their practice would consider the social implications of this woman's difficulties; for example, what family support is available, and how her class, age, gender, culture, and ethnicity impact on her situation. It is worth noting here that mental health professionals may decide an admission to a mental health unit is in the woman's best interests and in the best interests of her family. This highlights another aspect of the mental health nurse's role: providing custodial care. In this case, the woman is required to receive care within a specified environment.

It is clear that mental health nurses carry out procedures, work therapeutically, and may provide custodial care within their practice. The way they practise is informed by the holistic approach or the bio-psycho-social model, which has value and relevance in mental health nursing. To demonstrate this, consider again the example of the young woman referred to earlier. Having just had a child, her hormone balance may have been disrupted and so there could be a biological basis for her problems. Similarly, her feelings of being low in mood highlight a need to address her psychological state, and of course adjusting to three very young children adds significant pressure to a person's social circumstances.

A further, emerging model of practice is the recovery approach. It is fair to say that there are really four significant approaches that influence mental health service provision and mental health nursing in the UK today: the biological or medical model, the psychological model, the social model, and the recovery approach. However, please note that there are also different and relevant approaches within these models.

In order to help you develop a better understanding of these four models, we have asked proponents of these approaches to provide a brief introduction to each model and describe its relevance to mental health nursing practice. Some of the writers have addressed questions of particular relevance to student mental health nurses; others have also offered a brief overview of the model. You will find that some of the authors also refer to other models informing practice and you will notice that the psychological model includes a range of approaches (see Chapter 5 for some specific examples).

Biological model: why is biology relevant to mental health nurses?

By Pat James – physiologist

An understanding of the structure and function of the human body should be central to the education of all health care professionals. While maintaining the needs of a client as an individual, we must not forget that ultimately health depends on the functioning of complex biological structures. Central to the study of physiology is the concept of 'homeostasis': the maintenance of a constant internal environment. Observations on a client such as blood pressure, body temperature, and fluid balance can be monitored as these provide us with information about a person's internal environment. Although they fluctuate, they should always remain within a desired range to maintain 'health'.

The body has many signalling systems, both neural and hormonal, which work together to maintain this balance. Deviation from the normal range brings about a corrective response. These responses are predictable, and with a sound physiological knowledge, the health care professional should be able to look for, change, and predict what might happen next and what, if any, intervention is required. In a clinical situation a rapid response to change could be lifesaving.

This underpinning physiological knowledge is as important to mental health nurses as to any other branch. Unlike earlier scientists, we now realise that the mind and body function in conjunction with each other to maintain health. Consider an anxious, stressed client. Their physiological responses to anxiety will lead to changes in other body systems, for example circulatory changes (increased pulse), and visual changes (accommodation of lens for distant vision). This is all part of a deeply seated fight or flight response controlled by the hypothalamus. An understanding of the physiological mechanisms involved can contribute to more holistic client care (see also Chapter 8 for further discussion of the effects of anxiety).

Health statistics suggest that:

- 34.6 per cent of men and 28.3 per cent of women in the United Kingdom have hypertension (British Heart Foundation 2005).
- 2.2 million people in the United Kingdom have diabetes (Diabetes UK 2006).
- One in four people in the United Kingdom will, in the course of a year, have some type of mental health issue (Office for National Statistics 2001).

Considering these figures it is highly probable that someone presenting with a mental health issue will also have other underlying pathologies. For a mental health nurse to optimize the quality of care, a sound physiological understanding of all body systems is paramount (see also Chapter 4).

Medication commonly prescribed for people with mental health issues often has side effects. For example, lithium-based prescriptions will have implications for renal function due to lithium's structural similarity to sodium.

In conclusion, as mental health student nurses progress from dependent to independent decision-makers an understanding of physiology and pharmacology is central to effective and holistic client care.

Psychological models: why is psychology relevant to mental health nurses?

By Pam Morley and Devinder Rana

While psychology is one of the younger branches of science, its fundamental importance in informing mental health nursing practice has long been recognized (Marks *et al.* 2005). There is no single definition of psychology, but to focus on an interpersonal perspective (a key element of mental health nursing), the definition given by Walker *et al.* (2004) states:

> Psychology is the study of human behaviour, thought processes and emotions.

Psychology offers a number of perspectives on these areas that assist mental health nurses to develop greater understanding of people in their care and of themselves. Also, rather than concentrating solely on ill health, psychology can be useful in facilitating concepts about the attainment of well-being.

The most relevant areas are cognition, behaviourism, humanism (including Carl Roger's work), psychodynamic approaches (see Chapter 5 for details), communication and interpersonal relationships, and values/beliefs and attitudes. Some of the knowledge underpinning these areas has been gathered into two spheres, namely health psychology and clinical psychology. Michie and Abraham (2004) state that a crucial component of effective care is the development of an understanding of not only the patient's behaviour, but also that of the health professional. We will go on to discuss some examples of how particular fields of knowledge can be linked to practice.

Cognitive psychology attempts to define and understand the processes used in thinking, e.g. memory, decision-making, perception, and learning. Understanding how thinking processes occur can assist nurses to utilize effective strategies with, for example, a service user suffering from dementia to enable them to retain information for as long as possible. Another example is the experience of hallucinations or delusions. Again, understanding the best way of communicating with someone who is experiencing 'voices' will promote more effective nursing care (see also Chapter 8 for further discussion of these terms).

Nurses who understand how unhelpful behaviour may be learned and maintained will be best placed to help someone to develop alternatives. This might include teaching someone how to use relaxation to combat anxiety, or negotiating a behavioural contract with someone who regularly self-harms. An alternative point is that nurses' behaviour will be scrutinized by service users and visitors, who may draw conclusions about the individual nurse. Therefore, an awareness of how one's behaviour appears to others can play a central role in encouraging positive attitudes from others.

Another major concept is that of attitude and stereotyping. Nurses need to know how attitudes are

formed and how they can be influenced in order to promote useful attitudes towards maintaining healthy lifestyles. Also, awareness of one's own attitudes and beliefs, and how one might stereotype an individual, is crucial for the nurse. This then leads on to the topic of interpersonal interaction. This is particularly meaningful for mental health nurses, as interacting with service users is how we do our job. Communication is a vast area, and one that cannot be covered effectively here; however, much of the knowledge of communication theory, counselling skills, and psychotherapy derives from psychology. It is perhaps the greatest way that one individual can influence another, and a robust insight into this area will enable mental health nurses to ensure that their influence is helpful, ethical, and as effective as possible. In this way, nurses can engage in therapeutic use of self to offer the best service possible to people in need of their care.

Sociological model: why is sociology relevant to mental health nurses?

By Elaine Denny

In relation to a sociological understanding of human function, why is it important for mental health nursing students to have a knowledge and awareness of this approach? Sociology provides us with insights into society, and into social interactions. In doing so it encourages us to develop a 'sociological imagination'; that is, to take a fresh look at things that we tend to take for granted, to be open to different interpretations. Using a sociological approach may provide us with new insights and explanations of everyday life, including the way we experience health and illness, and the way we interact with health professionals.

One way in which it does this is to demonstrate a link between 'personal troubles' and 'public issues'; to look beyond the individual as being responsible or to blame for their problems or position in society and to consider the structures of society that influence or even determine events. Sociology teaches us that the structures of society are a powerful force in shaping the world. In particular, sociologists have considered the structures of diversity or inequality, such as socio-economic class, gender, age, ethnicity, and disability, as having a strong influence on various aspects of life and life chances. Differences throughout society in the amount of power we can exercise, our health, and our life expectancy are all influenced by these factors.

Let us consider an example. Among the government's health targets are aims to reduce the levels of smoking in society. In order to do this, health education and initiatives such as offering free nicotine patches have been started. Such strategies target individuals, and imply that the solution is in their hands and that refusal to comply is some sort of personal failing. However, sociological research that has looked at smoking among lone mothers (one of the largest single groups of smokers) has found that they are well aware of the health risks of smoking, but see the activity not in isolation, but within the context of their lives. For women living in poverty (as many lone mothers do) smoking is the one way they can manage the stress of having sole responsibility for children, and of trying to survive on a low income. Smoking is the one thing that they do for themselves. By considering this issue not as a 'personal trouble' but as a 'public issue', influenced by poverty and gender, different explanations of the activity can be found. You can view mental health problems from the same perspective – not as an individual pathology or personal failing, but as the result of a complex set of social determinants.

Sociology encourages critical thinking about issues that may at first seem 'common sense'. It requires a consideration that moves beyond the obvious to the complexity of a situation in order to develop a deeper understanding and to offer explanations.

How does this inform mental health nursing and practice? Along with other fundamental disciplines such as psychology and physiology, it is a tool in the armoury for delivering holistic care.

Sociology can contribute to mental health nursing by providing:

- A different perspective on mental health and illness from the dominant biomedical model.
- Insights into inter-professional relationships in mental health care.
- Analysis of mental health nursing as an occupation.
- A critical perspective of the role of medicine in health care.
- Determinants of current health policy.
- The organization of health care and care settings.

The recovery approach: why is the recovery approach relevant to mental health nurses?

The recovery approach is an emerging model of practice. This approach is driven and defined by mental health service users who are undertaking their own strategies to live positively and fully, despite the somewhat disabling impact of an ongoing mental health problem. Mental health nurses need to incorporate this approach into their practice. The National Institute for Mental Health in England (2004) states that recovery includes the following:

- A return to a state of wellness.
- Achievement of a quality of life acceptable to the person.
- A process or period of recovering.
- A process of gaining or restoring something (e.g. one's sobriety).

- An act of obtaining usable resources from apparently unusable sources.
- Recovering an optimum quality and satisfaction with life in disconnected circumstances.

It goes on to describe the goals for mental health service users in recovery as follows: 'to realize personal potential; function at their optimal level and use and/or provide support outside mental health services' (National Institute for Mental Health in England 2004). For examples of the implementation of the recovery model, take a look at Chapter 6. This approach places the mental health service user central to practice and recognizes their expertise. For mental health nurses it is therefore essential that in using this approach they work in a collaborative partnership with service users.

How mental health nurses use models in their practice

In mental health nursing we have developed our own models of practice, which pay heed to the particulars of the bio-psycho-social model. Mental health nurses adopt a problem-solving approach to the implementation of these models, which is called the *nursing process*. It is a useful tool to help mental health nurses work in a structured, logical, and coherent way. The elements of the nursing process are illustrated in Figure 1.1 and there is more detail provided in Chapter 2.

Mental health nurses use this problem-solving strategy in the implementation of models of practice. In the next section we have provided more information on the tidal model (Barker 1998) as an example of a specifically recovery-focused approach. This model has also received national acknowledgement and is a popular model used in many mental health services, so there is a chance that you will see it used in your clinical placements. It is worth noting the influence that Hildegard Peplau (1998) had on Barker in his tidal model work, and also her contribution in detailing the role and practice of mental health nurses from as early as the 1950s. The importance of the mental health nurse-patient relationship is stressed by Felicity Stockwell, a respected former mental health nurse and nurse educator:

> When I completed my training in 1959, I went as a ward sister to a ward for the acutely mentally ill, situated in a general hospital. It was an exciting time. The new Mental Health Act was about to be passed, and there was news of various hospitals or units putting new ideas into practice.
>
> The psychiatrists in the ward where I worked were in complete accord with the way of nursing that I had been taught. Their belief was that there would be a physical means of treatment for all mental illnesses one day, and with the arrival of antidepressant and anxiolytic drugs, they thought that a nursing input would become unnecessary.
>
> I came to realize that it was only because of the nursing input that any of the treatments were effective at all. Pills sent by post will not do any good at all. Physical treatments for mental illness, given where the patient has trust in the doctor and where hope is given, will allay some symptoms, but the help given to re-engage with social life and find some contentment only comes from the nursing contribution.

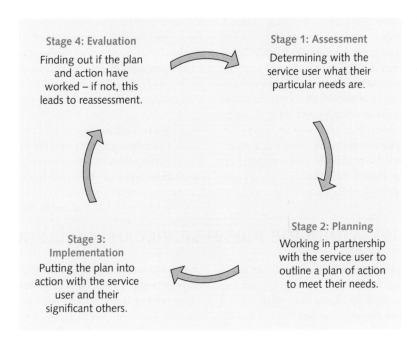

Stage 4: Evaluation
Finding out if the plan and action have worked – if not, this leads to reassessment.

Stage 1: Assessment
Determining with the service user what their particular needs are.

Stage 3: Implementation
Putting the plan into action with the service user and their significant others.

Stage 2: Planning
Working in partnership with the service user to outline a plan of action to meet their needs.

Figure 1.1 The Nursing Process: a problem-solving cycle (Yura and Walsh 1967, adapted by Clarke 2008)

You can read the rest of Felicity's contribution online:

 www.oxfordtextbooks.co.uk/orc/clarke

and choose the online resources for this chapter.

Both Peplau and Barker focus on the importance of the relationship between the mental health nurse and the service user in promoting recovery, and this is a recurring theme within this textbook.

The mental health nurse and service user: a unique collaboration

Peplau (1998) is often described as the mother of mental health nursing. Her model of nursing places a strong emphasis on the interpersonal nature of nursing and the importance of health promotion. She describes individuals as 'systems' that are comprised of physiological, psychological, and social aspects. For an individual to experience health, there has to be a balance between all of these aspects. The role of the mental health nurse in assisting this equilibrium or balance is manifold and is based on trust. Peplau felt that mental health nursing worked in two ways: educative and therapeutic. The ability of the mental health nurse to combine these aspects encourages the client to develop their own problem-solving skills. The role of the nurse incorporates teaching, counselling, being a resource, and helping the service user to assume responsibility for meeting their goals. Most importantly, the nurse and service user work together in resolving issues. Barker (2001) also promotes collaborative working and stresses the importance of mental health nurses developing and using interpersonal skills.

The tidal model developed by Barker is a philosophical approach to a service user's recovery. It promotes person-centred care that focuses on self-management and recovery. Barker notes that all of us experience challenges through our life and it is no different for individuals who experience mental health difficulties. However, to experience mental health problems within the mental health system can be disempowering and can limit the individual's ability to function at their best. Through skilful assessment and intervention using one's 'self', the mental health nurse focuses on working in partnership to address what needs to be done now in order to aid people in living full and meaningful lives.

The tidal model focuses on an individual's needs as they perceive them. In order to do this we have to listen to what is going on currently and what has gone on previously for that person in all aspects of their life. Seeing the whole person, and not just symptoms or a service user, is vital. The strategy for this is to focus on the service user's story or narrative. Barker (2001) suggests that the only constant is change. The tidal model emphasizes ways to help service users recognize what changes are going on for them and how they can affect these changes to gain a positive result. For mental health nurses, using this model means starting from a position of believing that real and meaningful recovery is possible; of course change will happen, but ultimately the person knows what's best for them and they have the ability to make the changes they desire.

We cannot close this section on models of practice without referring you to the work of Tom Kitwood and person-centred care (Kitwood 1997, Baldwin and Capstick 2007) but we don't elaborate further here as there are excellent examples of the use of this approach in Chapter 7. We are keen to encourage you to be open to working with a range of different models in your clinical practice and we have only raised your awareness of some of the more popular ones.

Student activity 5
Read through and review the materials on models and take some time to consider your own preferences and why you prefer a certain approach.

Boundaries within the nurse–service user relationship

Hopefully what you have read and worked through so far in this chapter has helped you to recognize the need for you to work in partnership with mental health service users. However, we feel that it is important to acknowledge that as student nurses you can be placed into distressing circumstances with people, and that in an attempt to offer help you may inadvertently overstep appropriate professional boundaries. There is often a fine balance between working effectively in partnership with a service user and yet at the same time keeping a boundaried relationship with them.

Student activity 6

We would like you to take a little time here to consider what form your friendships take – think about a close relationship you have, perhaps with a sister or brother. What would you discuss with or do for that person? Also consider what you do to attract people. Are you funny? Do you wear very fashionable clothes? Are you a good listener? Spend about five minutes jotting down your responses. Now consider that list and compare and contrast this to what might be appropriate, effective, and legal in relationships with service users.

As student nurses it is important to consider how you choose to present yourself within the practice context. What would you like mental health service users to think of you when they meet you? You also need to be aware of issues around your personal safety and the safety of others. In any new relationship we are uncertain about how a person will respond to our communication, and people with mental health problems may do so in very unpredictable ways. In clinical practice your mentor and assessor are there to support and guide you in working through these issues and developing effective communication skills. It is also important that you discuss how you are feeling with them; it is absolutely normal to be nervous in any new job or new situation, especially when you are learning how to act. You can develop emotional protection by sharing your thoughts and feelings with your mentor and assessor, and this can help to ensure that your personal boundaries, safety, and resilience are maintained.

As mental health nurses we are extremely privileged to be part of an individual's journey to recovery. For service users, this often involves disclosure of extremely personal information and feelings, information that perhaps would usually be reserved for those closest to us. The NMC (2008) makes it clear that as nurses we are responsible for safeguarding the interests of service users at all times. It is important to remember that everyone who comes into nursing care is vulnerable in some way; not being able to function in their usual way makes them so. As mental health nurses working with possibly very vulnerable service users, our ability to have power over, influence, abuse, neglect, and harm them is considerable.

The NMC (2002: 4) is clear about the nurse–client relationship when they state:

> The only appropriate professional relationship between a client and a practitioner is one which focuses exclusively upon the needs of the client. Registered nurses and midwives should be aware of the potential for imbalance of power in this relationship.

What are professional boundaries?

A boundary can be defined as a line or mark that indicates the limit of something. But what is a professional boundary? In the case of mental health nursing, it is working with mental health service users while keeping the primary concern of the nurse's role (to prevent illness, promote health and recovery, and to protect from and alleviate suffering) absolutely in mind (Rich 2005). As the NMC (2008: 2) Code states, 'You must make the care of people your first concern.' They also offer very specific guidance on how to maintain clear professional boundaries:

> You must refuse any gifts, favours or hospitality that might be interpreted as an attempt to gain preferential treatment.
>
> You must not ask for or accept loans from anyone in your care or anyone close to them.
>
> You must establish and actively maintain clear sexual boundaries at all times with people in your care, their families and carers. (NMC 2008: 3)

Professional boundaries need to be built upon a foundation of trust, respect, and a responsible approach to power. As student nurses, when you become involved in a caring relationship you will constantly have to establish, restate, and renegotiate appropriate boundaries with service users. Take for example this simple question from a service user, 'Are you married, nurse?' Before you respond, consider why the service user is asking you this question. Does it harm your relationship to answer this? As you ask intimate questions all the time, shouldn't there be some reciprocal self-disclosure or sharing of information? Where will this take your communication if you answer this directly? Are you comfortable sharing this information? Does this breach professional boundaries? How can you respond in a way that maintains safe professional boundaries but doesn't offend the service user, i.e. a respectful, professional response? A possible response to this question could be, 'It seems from your question that you're interested in personal relationships and marriage. Is there something about your current relationships that's worrying you or that you wanted to talk about?' As you can see from this example, the response acknowledges the content of the question but focuses very much on the service user's situation, their possible worries and concerns, and encourages them to explore these further, without damaging your professional boundaries. Of course if you are wearing a ring, have known the service user for some time, and are comfortable sharing this information and skilled enough to use this general conversation to refocus on the service user, then it may well seem very dismissive not to share some personal information.

Developing a professional approach and maintaining your boundaries comfortably takes time and effort. Relationships with service users constantly change as the service user makes their journey to recovery, and so boundaries change too and need to be redefined. You need to revisit this regularly with your assessor in clinical practice and constantly work on establishing and maintaining effective and appropriate professional boundaries. Along with your clinical mentor, you may also have a practice placement facilitator/educator/manager working in your area, or possibly clinical link teams or your personal tutor, any of whom will always be happy to discuss any issues you may have within this area. It is important to restate that your relationship with service users should always focus on the needs of the client and not on those of the nurse or organization. The purpose of a therapeutic relationship is not to gain new friends or sexual partners. Personal relationships with vulnerable service users or ex-service users are not acceptable and risk becoming abusive.

When does a relationship become abusive?

Throughout this chapter we have had the opportunity to look at the role of the mental health nurse, the models that shape our practice, professionalism and what it means to be a professional, and the uniqueness of our relationships with service users and the boundaries of these. As part of our consideration of this relationship, we also have to address issues surrounding the abuse of it. It is important for you to remember when considering these issues that should you have any worries or concerns, support is always available to you via your mentor or clinical facilita-

tors, personal tutors, and student services.

The NMC (2002: 5) is clear in its definition of what constitutes abuse of this relationship:

> Abuse within the practitioner–client relationship is the result of the misuse of power or a betrayal of trust, respect or intimacy between the practitioner and the client, which the practitioner should know would cause physical or emotional harm to the client. Abuse takes many different forms and may be physical, psychological, verbal, sexual, financial/material or based upon neglect.

Failure to maintain appropriate boundaries, according to the Council for Healthcare Regulatory Excellence (2007), can lead to harm such as long-term psychological harm, major depressive disorders, post-traumatic stress disorder, and a failure to access health services when needed. Not only can harm be caused to the service user, but it can impair our judgement and damage the reputation of the health service. As the professional in this relationship, it is your responsibility, not the service user's, to establish and to maintain appropriate boundaries.

Professional responsibility in potentially abusive situations

It must be noted that not only are we accountable for our own actions, we are also accountable should we suspect or know that abuse in some form is taking place, and in order to promote the welfare of the client we are obligated to act. As a student nurse you must inform your assessor of your suspicions or concerns.

Student activity 7
Using the six categories of abuse identified by the NMC (physical, psychological, verbal, sexual, financial/material, and based upon neglect), it may be helpful for you to consider possible examples of abuse or neglect within the nurse–client relationship.

Should you feel attracted to a mental health service user, you should immediately ask for guidance from an appropriate colleague and should only spend time with this service user if accompanied by a qualified nurse who is aware of the situation. Furthermore, if it is a service user that is attracted to you and they have made this clear, it is your responsibility to address this issue. As a student you will need help in doing this; developing feelings for someone who is trying to help us is 'only human' and so this must be managed sensitively and in a way that doesn't damage the service user.

The NMC recognizes that in some cases when the professional relationship was minor or temporary it is not realistic to impose a total ban on future relationships. However, as a mental health nurse, given the vulnerability of clients in contact at any time, regardless of duration, it would always leave one to question whether the relationship was ever free from a power imbalance and whether you could honestly say that the client was not vulnerable at the point of contact. The onus is on you to prove that there was not an imbalance of power in your relationship; that the relationship began outside the clinical environment and that the service user was not vulnerable.

While abuse is difficult to comprehend in an environment that should be promoting care, neglect is even harder. The NMC (2002: 7) goes on to define neglect as '...the refusal or failure on the part of the registered nurse, midwife or health visitor to meet the essential care needs of a client.'

Remember what the NMC (2008) stated regarding the nurse–client relationship: its focus should always be on the needs of the client and the nurse should always safeguard the interests of the client.

> **Student activity 8**
> *Reconsider the list of examples you made for student activity 7, trying to think as a service user would. What are some examples that they may constitute abuse or neglect?*

Further information on the boundaries of our relationships can be found in *The Code: Standards of conduct, performance and ethics for nurses and midwives* (NMC 2008) and in *Practitioner–client relationships and the prevention of abuse* (NMC 2002). The NMC has summarized this information and provided detailed examples of cases where the fitness to practice of a nurse has been investigated; this is available on the web link for this chapter and will give you some clear indicators of unprofessional and unacceptable behaviour.

🌐 www.oxfordtextbooks.co.uk/orc/clarke

and choose the online resources for this chapter.

Before you move on, we would like you to go back to the beginning of this chapter and re-read Deborah's story. Reflect on what she says and consider what you would have needed to do in order to help support her, and what knowledge and skills you may need to work with other service users like her.

Evidence-based practice

This chapter introduces you to professional issues for student mental health nurses. As a member of a profession, you are required to develop a specific knowledge and skills base. It is expected that mental health nursing practice will be evidence based (Newell and Gournay 2000) and we have sought to refer to relevant supporting evidence throughout this textbook. Having considered some of the important issues and knowledge that mental health nurses need to be aware of, the second chapter of this textbook will focus on what skills you need to practise appropriately.

Finding information in mental health nursing

In the following sections, we have asked Senior Librarian Stephen Gough to provide you with the relevant information on how best you can access evidence to support your practice.

As part of your academic and professional development, and in clinical decision-making, you will need to access information. This can be from many different sources, as you will see from the references and suggested further reading at the end of each chapter in this book. As a student nurse you will be expected to demonstrate a breadth of reading drawn from all formats in which information is published. And as a qualified practitioner, to ensure that you are aware of the best practice and developments in the care you give, you will need to maintain the information-seeking habit developed as a student.

Published information can be found in three main resources: books, journals, and the Internet. None of these by itself can answer all of your questions, so by understanding the structure and means of accessing each, it is possible to target the most appropriate combination of resources to effectively meet your need.

The ability to do this is the first step in becoming information literate.

The resources
Books

Books come in a variety of formats, serve different functions, and are the place where knowledge is consolidated. The categories of books are shown in Table 1.1.

Journals

Journals are the best source of up-to-date information. Journals are the place where research is first published and professional issues first reported and discussed. There are three types of journal, each with a particular function, as described in Table 1.2.

The Internet

The Internet and World Wide Web is a major resource for information but needs to be used effectively to avoid either being overwhelmed or missing vital sources.

Basic preparation
To be able to search for information effectively you need to be able to:

- Define your search question.
- Select the keywords.
- Structure your search.
- Understand how to use the keywords in different databases.

Defining the search question
Put your question in the form of a sentence and only use definite terms. Do not say 'I want something on chlorpromazine', be definite: 'Is chlorpromazine an effective intervention in schizophrenia?'

Select the keywords
Selecting keywords is not always straightforward. In the above question the keywords are schizophrenia and chlorpromazine. Chlorpromazine is also known by the manufacturer names Largactil and Thorazine, both of which should therefore be included in a

Table 1.1   Categories of books

Format	Function	How to find
Readers	Give an overview of a subject area, each chapter written by an authority defining the current state of knowledge.	Library catalogue
Textbooks	Give a general overview of a subject to give an understanding of the key concepts.	Library catalogue
Reference books	Basic factual content, including dictionaries and formulary.	Library catalogue/search engines
Manuals	Similar to both reference books and textbooks. Manuals give information on performing a particular task or procedure.	Library catalogue
Official publications	Any publication produced by national government or governmental organizations such as the Department of Health.	Library catalogue/search engines
Clinical guidelines	The guidelines produced by, for example, the National Institute for Health and Clinical Excellence (NICE).	Library catalogue/search engines
Pamphlets, booklets, Trust policies	Valuable sources of patient information and local procedures.	Search engines

Table 1.2 Categories of journals

Primary	First place of publication of research. Authoritative referees review articles prior to publication.
Secondary	General publications aimed at practitioners. They summarize research from primary publications as well as reporting professional news.
Popular	These are aimed at the general public and interpret information from the primary and secondary journals.

search. Also, most databases and Internet search engines search for the exact sequence of letters that you type in the search box. If there is any variation in spelling (e.g. paediatric/pediatric) or in a name, the variation may be missed.

Structure your search

Do not use multiple terms in a single search. Put each term in separately and then use AND, OR, and NOT to make the right combinations. For the above question, the search structure would be:

1) schizophrenia

2) chlorpromazine OR Largactil OR Thorazine

3) 1) AND 2)

By using AND, you will find all the articles that mention both schizophrenia and chlorpromazine in the same article. Using OR will find all the articles that mention chlorpromazine or Largactil or Thorazine.

Entering the keywords individually enables you to go back in the search if, for example, you want articles that compare haloperidol with chlorpromazine in relation to schizophrenia. You would then have the additional lines in the search structure:

4) haloperidol

5) 3) AND 4)

Using NOT excludes a keyword from a search. Thus if you were looking for the use of haloperidol but not with schizophrenia, the search would be:

6) haloperidol NOT schizophrenia

AND, OR, and NOT are referred to as Boolean operators.

Understand how to use keywords in a database

Most databases (library catalogues, journal databases, the Internet) search using the sequence of letters typed in the search box. If there are synonyms or alternative spellings these must be used as search terms as well as your main keywords. CINAHL, Medline, and some other specialist journal databases use defined lists of terms called subject headings to overcome this. These act in the same way as a thesaurus and bring together all of the subject terms, suggest alternatives, and provide definitions for ambiguous terms With journal databases, look to see whether they use keywords or subject headings. Choose subject headings if they are offered.

Selecting databases

Library catalogue The library catalogue should be the first place to look for books. Use keyword searching to find titles related to your topic. Most healthcare libraries will collect major reports and other documents from the National Health Service and the Department of Health but most of these are also published on the Internet and can therefore be viewed and downloaded that way.

Journal databases Finding information in journal databases needs careful planning. Each database serves a different purpose, indexing articles appropriate to its overall purpose.

Which database (or combination of databases) is most likely to meet my information need?
To decide this you need to look at the subject coverage of the databases and at whom they are targeted. The five main journal databases for mental health practitioners are:

- CINAHL – aimed at nurses and the allied health professions.
- Medline – aimed at the medical professions, including psychiatry.
- ASSIA – covers the social sciences, including community care.

- Cochrane – a database of systematic reviews of research into clinical practice.
- PsycINFO – the largest database of psychology related material (from the American Psychological Association).

CINAHL and Medline both use subject headings for keyword searching. CINAHL subject heading definitions reflect the needs of the patient/client-focused professions. Medline uses medical subject headings (MeSH), which are based on the medical model or are disease-focused. Therefore, if you are looking for information on the care of a patient or client, use CINAHL. If you are looking for information on therapeutics or your search is disease-focused, use Medline.

The Cochrane Library is the best source of high-quality systematic reviews of the evidence used to inform practice. Systematic reviews assess the available research on a specific topic and draw a conclusion upon which best practice decisions can be based with confidence.

Understand how to use keywords on the Internet

The Internet is a vast resource. Searches should be structured with the same care as you would use when using journal databases. Most search engines will have an advanced search option, which should always be chosen as the features it offers makes searching considerably more precise.

The two key features for advanced searches are Boolean operators and domain searching. The advanced search screen in Google refers to Boolean operators as:

- with *all* the words – AND
- with *at least one* of the words – OR
- *without* the words – NOT

Standard Internet searches for more than one word will find pages where the individual words are mentioned. A search for *mental health* could find a page with the statement 'Mental activity while on holiday is bad for your *health*'. Search engines overcome this in the advanced search by using exact phrase searching.

In Google this is the search box labelled *this exact wording or phrase*.

A domain is the part of a web address after http://www. If you specify a domain the search will be confined to that domain. By specifying .dh.gov.uk, your search will find pages only from the Department of Health.

An advanced search for 'What has the Department of Health said about quality of life in the elderly?' would be structured as shown in Box 1.4.

Be cautious in your use of websites. It is better to use a primary source of information than an interpretation or summary. For example, the online Wikipedia article on Birmingham quotes statistics from the Birmingham City Council web pages, which are an extrapolation of data from the Office of National Statistics. If you use the Wikipedia article you are quoting third-hand information when the original source can easily be found and used.

Do not use unreferenced information presented as fact. Try to establish the original source of any factual information found, especially on pages with Internet domains that end with .com or .co.uk. Both of these are commercial organization addresses and are therefore unlikely to present information that may be detrimental to the company.

Remember:

1) Plan before you start to search. Map your search need, write a sentence or question that includes the key terms, and list alternative keywords.

2) Select the sources you need to search according to need. Books tend to give a broad view of a subject; journals publish the research and are focused on the particular.

3) For journals, select the database according to your need. If your focus is the care of a client, use CINAHL and/or ASSIA. For therapeutic interventions and supporting evidence, use Medline and/or Cochrane. A search may involve using more than one database.

4) On the Internet, target particular sources by using domain searching. Look for primary sources and

with the *exact phrase*	quality of life
with *at least one* of the words	elderly old aged elder older geriatric
domain	.dh.gov.uk

Box 1.4 Example of using keywords

critically analyse information found. Information presented as fact may not tell the whole truth.

5) Do not rely on one source for all your information.

Summary

Having read through this chapter, we hope that you have a grasp of the basic purpose and knowledge that begins to inform mental health nursing today. The chapter opens your journey to becoming a mental health nurse. It places particular emphasis on working in partnership with people with mental health problems and places the mental health service user centrally to the development of nursing knowledge and practice. The chapter outlines how you need to behave and develop personally in becoming a professional. The chapter also helps you to develop a basic understanding of what mental health nursing is and what mental health nurses do. This chapter also emphasizes the importance of evidence-based practice to mental health nursing.

In the next chapter we consider what mental health nurses do in practice and what the skills are that they use and that you will need to develop. We will also explore how these skills (in partnership with mental health service users) determine what nursing care is delivered.

References and other sources

References

Baldwin C and Capstick A, eds (2007). **Tom Kitwood on dementia: A reader and critical commentary**. Open University Press, Buckingham.

Barker P (1998). It's time to turn the tide. **Nursing Times**, 18(94), 70-2.

Barker P (2001). The tidal model: developing an empowering, person-centred approach to recovery within psychiatric and mental health nursing. **Journal of Psychiatric and Mental Health Nursing**, 8(3), 233-40.

British Heart Foundation (2005). [online] <http://www.bhf.org.uk/> accessed 09/08/2007.

Council for Healthcare Regulatory Excellence (2007). **Clear sexual boundaries between health professionals and patients: Guidance for health professionals**. 2nd Draft Consultation Paper (unpublished).

Derbyshire Multi-Agency Partnership, Sefton Recovery Group, Allott P, and Gardner D (2004). **Emerging best practices in mental health recovery**. UK Version 1 National Institute for Mental Health in England (available to download from the Sainsbury Centre for Mental Health website).

Diabetes UK (2006). [online] <http://www.diabetes.org.uk/> accessed 09/08/2007.

Hood L and Leddy S (2006). **Conceptual bases of professional nursing**. Lippincott Williams and Wilkins, Philadelphia.

Institute of Health and Care Development (1998). **Core competencies for mental health workers: A project commissioned by the NHS Executive North West Regional Office**. IHCD, Bristol.

Jack K and Smith A (2007). Promoting self awareness in nurses to improve nursing practice. **Nursing Standard**, 21(32), 47-52.

Kitwood T (1997) **Dementia reconsidered: the person comes first**. Open University Press, Buckingham.

Marks DF, Murray M, Evans B, Willig C, Sykes CM, and Woodall C (2005). **Health psychology: Theory, research and practice**. Sage, London.

Michie S and Abraham C (2004). **Health psychology in practice**. Blackwell Publishing, Oxford.

National Institute for Mental Health in England/ Sainsbury Centre for Mental Health Joint Workforce Support Unit/National Health Service University (2004). **The 10 essential shared capabilities for mental health**. Department of Health, London.

Newell R and Gournay K (2000). **Mental health nursing: an evidence based approach**. Churchill Livingstone, Edinburgh.

NMC (2002). **Practitioner-client relationships and the prevention of abuse**. NMC Publications, London.

NMC (2004). **Standards of proficiency for pre-registration nursing education**. NMC Publications, London.

NMC (2005). **The PREP handbook**. NMC Publications, London.

NMC (2008). **The Code: Standards of conduct, performance and ethics for nurses and midwives**. NMC Publications, London.

Norton (2007). **Career focus: What is professionalism?** [online] <http://www.glencoe.com/norton/online/ezine/display_article.phtml?id=182> accessed 26/04/2007.

Office for National Statistics (2001). [online] <http://www.statistics.gov.uk/> accessed 09/08/2007.

Peplau HE (1998). **Interpersonal relations in nursing**. Macmillan, London.

Rich KL (2005). Introduction to bioethics, nursing ethics and ethical decision making. In Butts J and Rich K, eds. **Nursing ethics: Across the curriculum and into practice**, pp. 39-79. Jones and Bartlett, London.

Royal College of Nursing (2002). **Defining nursing**. RCN, London.

University of Texas at Arlington (1998) **What is a profession?** [online] <http://ranger.uta.edu/carroll/cse4317/profession/tsld005.htm> accessed 25/03/2008.

University of Victoria Faculty of Engineering (2000). **Standards for professional behaviour** [online] <http://www.engr.uvic.ca/policy/professional-behaviour.html> accessed 26/04/2007.

Walker J, Payne S, Smith P, and Jarrett N (2004). **Psychology for nurses and the caring professions**, 2nd edition. Open University Press, Maidenhead.

Yura H and Walsh MB (1967). **The nursing process**. Appleton-Century-Crofts, Norwalk.

Online Resource Centre

You can find these on our website:

 www.oxfordtextbooks.co.uk/orc/clarke

Useful links

You may find it helpful to copy and paste these into your web browser and save them as Favourites or Bookmarks

National Institute for Mental Health in England
http://www.nimhe.csip.org.uk

Nursing and Midwifery Council
http://www.nmc-uk.org/

Sainsbury Centre
http://www.scmh.org.uk

MIND
http://www.mind.org.uk

Young Minds
http://www.youngminds.org.uk

Rethink
http://www.rethink.org

Sane
http://www.sane.org.uk

Posner R (2006). The power of personal values. [online] <http://www.gurusoftware.com/gurunet/ValuesCenter.htm> accessed 14/05/2007.

Departments of Health

UK: http://www.dh.gov.uk
England: http://www.dh.gov.en/
Isle of Man: http://www.gov.im/dhss/
Northern Ireland: http://www.dh.sspni.gov.uk; http://www.healthandcareni.co.uk/
Scotland: http://www.sehd.scot.nhs.uk

Wales: http://www.wales.nhs.uk/;
http://www.mentalhealthwales.net/uk

◯ Futher reading

Biology

Waugh A and Grant A (2006). **Ross and Wilson's anatomy and physiology in health and illness,** 10th edition. Churchill Livingstone, Edinburgh.

Psychology

Gross R and Kinnison (2007). **Psychology for nurses and allied health professionals: applying theory to practice.** Hodder Education, London.

Rana D and Upton D (2008). **Psychology for nursing.** Pearson, Harlow, Essex.

Sociology

Denny E and Earle S, eds (2005). **Sociology for nurses.** Polity, Cambridge.

Recovery

Repper J and Perkins R (2003) **Social inclusion and recovery: a model for mental health practice.** Balliere Tindall, Edinburgh.

Chapter 2
Fundamental skills of mental health nursing
Jim Chapman and Cheryl Chessum

Learning outcomes

This chapter will help you to learn:

- How to be 'with' people with mental distress based on a humanistic philosophy and approach.
- To develop your understanding of therapeutic relationship building using communication skills.
- How to apply some of these ideas to the cycle of the nursing process.

Introduction

A mental health nurse practises the skill and craft of their role in a variety of different settings to reflect the varied range of services provided in today's mental health services. Whatever the setting or nature of the mental health problem, a set of adaptable mental health nursing skills will be required to enable the nurse to facilitate the safe and effective care of the service user. This care is expected to be individually tailored to the needs of the service user, developed (with only occasional exceptions) collaboratively with the service user, and evaluated with the service user and key partners in care.

The principles of the nurse's practice have to be underpinned and informed by the policies and guidelines that shape contemporary and future services. In the UK, nurses must respond to the essential capabilities (Department of Health 2006a) and the Chief Nursing Officer's review of mental health nursing (Department of Health 2006b) in order to deliver a service that reflects the reform and quality improvements expected in modern mental health services. Practical skills have to be backed up by a strong knowledge base, with nurses knowing why they do what they do and being able to explain their actions whenever called upon to do so. Where possible and available, what mental health nurses do needs to be done on the basis of the most up-to-date evidence or guidance, which comes in many forms (Sainsbury Centre for Mental Health 2004, National Institute for Clinical Health and Excellence 2004a, Nursing and Midwifery Council 2008a and 2008b). As not all the scenarios that nurses encounter have a textbook answer, it is important that other complementary skills are developed to help them make decisions and deal with scenarios for which there is no clear and obvious answer available. These skills include:

- Reasoning using principles and frameworks to weigh up a situation, e.g. 'To adhere to the NMC Code of Conduct, what do I need to be aware of in this case?'
- Reflecting in or on practice (Schön 1987, Rolfe and Freshwater 2001, Johns 2004) to get a deeper understanding of situations and your own reactions and judgements, especially those values and attitudes you hold that may cause conflict with service users and significant others.
- Relating to the person's experience of distress by using empathy and self-awareness, in order to understand what might be happening and how you in turn may be reacting to the situation.
- Consulting with others, especially colleagues with more experience and expertise, for advice and support or to discuss issues in clinical supervision.

- **Communicating** 'not knowing' and including service users and carers in problem-solving conversations in difficult situations where possible.
- **Negotiating** safe or short-term strategies while pursuing the above options, including relying on occasion on intuition and what 'feels right'.

Many of these skills have formed the foundation of mental health nursing for a long time and have their origins in a number of disciplines and theoretical perspectives. The challenge for student nurses is to develop those skills and to understand why they are so critical in delivering respectful, inclusive care for the broad range of service users who present with so many forms of mental distress.

Involvement with mental health services is often a frightening and coercive experience for people, who not only have mental health problems to contend with but have also to negotiate a route through the bewildering range of services provided (Sainsbury Centre for Mental Health 2002). Contact with mental health nurses can often be one of the first points of contact if not the primary contact. This is an opportunity. If the first encounter is sensitive, respectful, and skilful then the perception of the whole service can be positively influenced. This can then lead to productive engagement whereby the service user can be helped to recover safely from their mental health problem, or to engage in a productive relationship enabling them to live more successfully with mental distress, and to see the mental health service staff as valued supporters and allies.

This chapter therefore aims to provide the reader with an overview of how the process of nursing care is organized and why it is organized in this way, with particular reference to the 'person-centredness' of care at all stages of the nurse–service user relationship, and as identified in The Ten Essential Shared Capabilities (ESCs) (Department of Health 2006a). The chapter also focuses upon the skills that the mental health nurse requires to do their job effectively, respectfully, and to the best of their ability.

The nursing process

Nursing theorists (see also Chapter 1) have made efforts to describe a model that represents the whole process of nursing care, from the first contact with the service user and the start of the assessment process through the different stages to the conclusion of the nursing care and the ending of the relationship with the service user. Each theory makes an effort to describe the role of the nurse based on a set of beliefs about how they view the service user and their role (e.g. holistically), and breaks the process of care into a number of stages or elements to guide the nurse through nursing the service user in a systematic way based on these beliefs and ideas.

A number of theories are analysed and summarized in textbooks that students may find helpful in exploring this subject further (for example George 2002, and see the list of further reading at the end of this chapter). These theories can help you develop and formulate your own understanding of the reasoning and thinking behind nursing actions and the steps or stages in care-giving.

A universal model used by most nurses is the *nursing process*. This systematic cycle of assessment, planning, implementing, and evaluating care for service users was an approach imported from America to the UK in the late 1970s and began to be universally adopted in the early 1980s. It was an attempt to improve the delivery of nursing care by making the process of care more explicit, logical, and based on identified need, as well as including the service user in the process of their care. It had two key ideas behind it:

1) To demonstrate the professional contribution of the nurse to service user care and the specific role of the nurse within this (at this time nurses were seeking to increase their professional standing amongst other health-care professionals and needed frameworks and methodologies to support this aim).

2) To support and demonstrate the practice of empowering and including the service user in

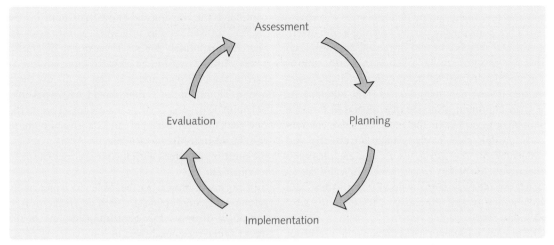

Figure 2.1 The central elements of the nursing process

decisions about their own care, during a time when the principle of 'consumerism' in the domains of health care and public services was a priority in health care reforms.

The development and structure of the nursing process (see also Chapter 1) as described by Habermann (2005) was adapted to provide a universal structure to the process of care as described in the Care Programme Approach (Department of Health 1990), which became a legal requirement from then on in adult mental health services. It is a standardized model of nursing and indeed of multidisciplinary care. Although it is now standardized as such, the nursing process developed from the work of nursing theorists.

The central elements of the nursing process are often represented in a diagrammatic way that shows the process is not linear but kinetic – flowing and cycling, moving backwards, forwards, and round the elements until care is concluded (see Figure 2.1).

The cycle is based on the premise that people are changed constantly by the external influences upon them. This changes them in various ways – their views and perceptions, their social experiences, their mood, their physical health – it could be said that every meeting with a service user is a reassessment in the face of such new experiences and information, though some aspects are more consistent and slow to change than others.

The key to putting the nursing process into practice effectively is the development, maintenance, and ending of therapeutic relationships with service users.

The therapeutic relationship and its relevance to the process of giving nursing care

When considering 'What is a therapeutic relationship?' there are many elements to consider. Aldridge (2006) explores the subject in some detail but acknowledges that brief definitions are scarce, as it is a complex and skilful aspect of practice. Usually key elements are that it is a purposeful human interaction that is goal directed, and these goals serve to meet the service user's best interests and needs (Bazley *et al.* 1973, Registered Nurses Association of Ontario 2002). One brief description (Barker and Buchanan-Barker 2005) is given below:

> Building a genuine human alliance that might begin to address the person's problems with living.

The elements of a therapeutic relationship in nursing practice relate strongly to the work of Carl Rogers (1951) and are examined in more detail below.

Without being able to *engage* the service user voluntarily and in a meaningful partnership, many opportunities can be lost, not least the chance to help the service user quickly and facilitate early intervention. This can then prevent further deterioration in mental state with all the associated risks in social, physical, psychological, and financial areas of a service user's life. Sometimes a person's mental health deteriorates and they become so distressed and disturbed that the opportunity for a voluntary partnership is lost, and the distressing (and possibly avoidable) compulsory involvement with services is the outcome. As it is an important principle that mental health care should be provided in the least restrictive environment possible, skills in engagement are essential and influential for the service user's and their family's experience. As the service user's mental health deteriorates it is often the family who bear the distress, fear, and burden of this experience (Arksey *et al.* 2002, Saunders 2003).

Engaging with service users begins the process of developing a therapeutic relationship. The duration of a therapeutic relationship is variable. It can be one meeting, or a relationship spanning several years. The notion of the therapeutic relationship is an enduring one, developing across the span of the twentieth century and integrated into many types of care-giving transactions. It remains a central tenet and an essential element of mental health nursing care today (Department of Health 2006a), promoting important values in working with service users.

The way you engage with service users will have been, and will continue to be, influenced by many things. Your own upbringing and life experiences will have influenced your beliefs, values, and behaviour. You are likely to take these into encounters with service users, families, and colleagues. Sometimes they will serve you well. Sometimes they might make you upset, judgemental, or lead you to make the wrong assumptions and cause potential problems in your professional relationships. It is not unusual to have these feelings but it is important to recognize them so that you can learn to keep an uncontaminated therapeutic relationship with the service user. A non-judgemental attitude is reflected in the person-centred approach; this underpins relationship building and is part of the expected capabilities of a contemporary mental health nurse.

Maintaining a therapeutic relationship is connected to the delivery and review of the care plan. However, for various reasons therapeutic relationships end and this has to be skilfully managed too. It is necessary to maintain professional boundaries throughout the relationship, as this should make it clear that it will not be permanent or a friendship. Having a therapeutic relationship with a service user that encourages dependency (i.e. they rely on you too much practically or emotionally) is unethical and contradicts the Nursing and Midwifery Council Code (2008a), as well as the principles of the Essential Shared Capabilities (ESCs) (Department of Health 2006a). Endings need to be prepared for in advance as part of the care plan and it is best to discuss them openly. Timing of this ending should, where possible, be mutually negotiated. If clear aims are set out in the care plan, their achievement can be a natural point to end the relationship. As a student, preparing to review the positive outcomes with the service user can help termination.

The nurse needs to be able to cope with, acknowledge, and empathize with any expression of emotional distress whilst remaining resolute in the intent to end the episode of care.

Carl Rogers and the humanistic approach

Carl Rogers (1902–1987) is widely accepted as being the father of 'service user-centred' therapy. When we refer to 'person-centredness' today, much of Rogers' (1951) work is reflected in this and has been adapted into the person-centred approach.

Rogers believed that psychological distress or difficulty was caused by a division between our 'true self' and our 'ideal self'. He suggested that each of us possesses an underlying true (or organismic) self, which is characterized by a basic human drive to grow, develop, and fulfil our potential, and it is that aspect of ourselves that is associated with our personal values, attitudes, and beliefs. We develop as humans when we try to adhere to these values and attitudes.

Rogers also suggested that we have an 'ideal self', which is characterized by 'conditions of worth'. We all have a need to feel worthy to other people and over time we adopt and internalize the standards and expectations of others. We must continue to meet these expectations in order to feel worthy and loved. Often the true self and the ideal self can be in conflict with one another, and it is this conflict that is the cause of psychological distress.

Student activity 1
Think of a time when you acted in accordance with the beliefs and standards of somebody else rather than your own beliefs – this can be from your time at work or from your personal life.
Why did you behave in this way?
How did it make you feel?

With this theory in mind, Rogers believed that it is the role of the helper to help the service user to resolve the conflict between these two aspects of the self, by creating a 'growth-promoting climate' where the service user can gain a deeper insight into their true selves. The growth-promoting climate was created by adopting three 'ways of being' in the helping relationship.

Genuineness or congruence

The person who is accepting of who they are is said to have a high degree of congruence or genuineness, and so the role of the helper in a person-centred environment is to encourage people to be more genuinely who they are, and to listen to their true selves.

Unconditional positive regard

Rogers believed the helper should have unconditional positive regard for the service user – that is, they should be non-judgemental towards the service user's character. Low self-regard, or low congruence, is the result of the service user's experience of being judged in the past, and measured by the expectations and standards of others. By displaying unconditional positive regard, the helper can see who the service user really is, not who they believe they should be, and can thereby allow the service user to value their true self.

Empathy

Empathy refers to an attempt to 'get inside' the service user's world and to experience their thoughts and feelings in that world as if they were our own. By reflecting on these thoughts and feelings to the service user, Rogers suggested that the service user could gain a better understanding of their own thoughts, and thereby gain a deeper understanding of their true self.

Using some of the ideas above, you can try and relate them to the experience of being 'assessed'.

> **Student activity 2**
> *Imagine you are going to see someone for a mental health assessment at your GP's suggestion. You have been feeling really low in mood for several months and it is getting worse. You are tearful, cannot sleep for more than three to four hours a night, cannot concentrate or relax, have no energy, and nothing you do gives you any enjoyment.*
> *You are really worried about going to see the mental health nurse at the community mental health centre, wondering what they will ask you and what they will think about you, if they can really help you or whether you are wasting their time.*
> *Now make a list of anything you can think of that would be helpful in this situation.*

Assessment

An assessment could be the first encounter a member of the public has with mental health services. This is therefore likely to be very influential in developing their views and formative opinions of mental health services, especially if they are fearful, distressed, and disturbed by their own mental health at the time.

When starting the process of assessment, there are many assessment frameworks. A bio-psycho-social approach can provide a structured framework for exploring aspects of a person's life that have *contributed to* mental distress or have been *affected by* mental distress (see Figure 2.2 and Chapter 1).

This framework can be complementary to trying to develop a holistic perspective of the service user; a way of looking at the person beyond the 'label' or 'diagnosis' and focusing on their concerns. The bio-psycho-social model does make the assumption that there can be an underlying biological basis for the mental distress known as 'illness' or 'disorder', but

other factors such as psychological and social factors are potentially implicated in the development and maintenance of mental distress. Not all service users or practitioners accept the premise that there is a biological basis for mental distress. Diagnoses such as schizophrenia are contentious (see Chapter 8). However, belief in the biomedical model is strongly held in Western approaches to psychiatry and the reality is that in a multidisciplinary team, these views are likely to prevail and have to be accommodated alongside other models including psychological and nursing (Neuman 1995, Peplau 1988, Barker and Buchanan-Barker 2005), whose philosophical position is sometimes different.

Within the assessment framework are concerns very specific to mental health services and nursing, namely risk assessment (see also Chapter 5) and decision-making about what interventions will help and in what order these need to be addressed. This helps

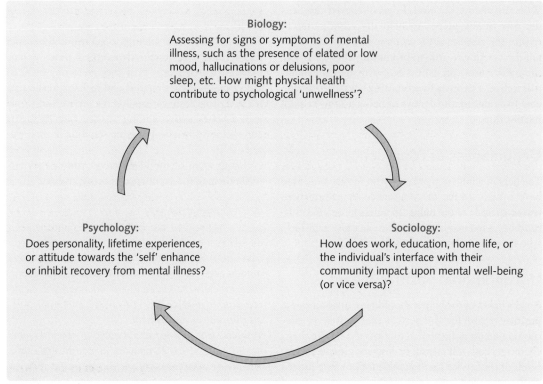

Figure 2.2 The bio-psycho-social approach in assessment

to develop planning and prioritizing skills for nursing actions as well as safeguarding the service user where risk may be present.

A mental health assessment, sometimes undertaken by a nurse, has a specific focus:

- To determine if there is some supporting information/evidence of mental distress or problems by gathering relevant information from as many sources as is ethically and legally acceptable within a practical time frame, and working within Nursing and Midwifery Council (2008a) stipulated guidelines.

- To identify the impact the mental distress has on the service user and others.

- To determine the risks associated with this mental distress – immediate, short term, medium term, or longer term.

- To identify factors or triggers for the distress, including those amenable to intervention in resolving the problem.

- To understand the service user's perspective about their distress and their concerns and priorities.

- To understand how much the service user'

perspective about their distress correlates with that held by professionals, family members, and significant others.

- To determine whether the service user has the capacity to recognize deterioration in their own mental state and capacity to make decisions about their own care.

- To understand what service users themselves brings to the experience of mental distress – for example coping styles, past and recent life events, strengths and abilities, current patterns of behaviour.

- To identify what the service user finds helpful and unhelpful, especially if they have had similar difficulties in the past.

- To help make decisions, in negotiation with the service user, about what to do in their best interests, especially the safety of themselves and others, without any unnecessary infringement on their liberty.

The format for the assessment is usually a face-to-face interview, a verbal interaction between the service user and the nurse. There is a structure or plan guiding the areas to cover in the gathering of information.

This concept of 'whole' predates the medical model, which, viewed critically, can be seen to deconstruct the individual person into small parts/cells. Consequently, medical treatment aims to deal with these disordered parts. The bio-psycho-social model, on the other hand, views people as a whole system with all the elements interacting. Restoration of health requires interventions that take account of the whole system and help restore its balance. This has promoted an interest in non-medical solutions to mental distress, including complimentary therapies, self-help, psychological/talking therapies, and recovery approaches. Generally people prefer to see themselves as a more complex whole and the bio-psycho-social approach incorporates a systems approach to mental distress, from cell biology within people to the interaction of people with their larger community and even the biosphere.

The elements of the bio-psycho-social model are usually complementary to elements of different nursing models.

Assessment as a narrative approach to the service user's story of their journey/experiences

This approach has developed over the last 30 years and comes from a family of approaches based on systems theory (Von Bertalanffy 1972). It has slowly been moving into mainstream practice, particularly since there has been the gradual development of the service user movement and efforts to make the voice of the service user central to the caring process, as well as influencing how mental health services are reformed and devised.

One way of viewing the assessment process is as 'listening to the service user's story'. The journey of assessment uses skilled communication and conversation techniques to guide the person in telling their story from their experience and perception. The role of the helper, who may be a nurse, is to set the conditions to enable this, while feeling emotionally safe to do so. It requires supporting and listening to the service user, enabling them to share their information in a congruent, logical manner, respecting their relationship and reactions to what is going on without interpreting or undervaluing their concerns. Another aspect is managing any time boundaries without

rushing or disrespecting the service user by closing them down or ending the interaction thoughtlessly. You may also need to get permission to take a few notes to help you remember details accurately, without alarming people.

As the UK's population continues to grow, assessment skills need to incorporate a respect for diversity in order to facilitate fair access to services. The use of interpreters, formal or informal, can be a frequent and important part of care depending on the local population. Using and being familiar with information in different languages and formats, and having access to information on and learning about the service user's cultural identity or diversity needs and related values, beliefs, and preferences, will be essential to respecting diversity and delivering quality care.

Using communication skills during the assessment process

These are central to the gathering of useful information when undertaking a comprehensive mental health assessment. The setting for the assessment is potentially very varied, e.g. they may take place homes, clinics, GP practices, hostels, prisons, police cells, or courts.

Student activity 3
On placement or during a related experience, speak to a mental health professional.
Ask them to share with you:
1) The most unusual location where they have conducted a mental health assessment.
2) The challenges to practice this posed.
3) The skills and techniques they employed to overcome the challenges.
You can reflect on your own learning from the above conversations by writing a reflective journal piece for your own portfolio of learning, but remember to anonymize your writing for confidentiality purposes.

We all communicate, but the fact that we refer to communication 'skills' suggests that the methods and techniques of communicating with others are deliberately practised, developed, and used mindfully for a purpose. In this section, communication skills are considered specifically. Many communication skills used in assessment are transferable skills and can be applied to other care-giving and teamworking experiences, and as such will be replicated throughout your practice.

Use Table 2.1 on p.32 to identify the type of skills and abilities you may need most to communicate in this way.

> **Student activity 4**
> *Imagine you are in practice as a mental health nurse. Think about all the potential ways you may have to communicate with service users or about service users.*
> *Each different method may pose different communication challenges.*
>
> *Use Table 2.1 on p.32 to identify the type of skills and abilities you may need most to communicate in this way.*
>
> *You may wish to try this alone or try out this exercise with other people to get a bigger perspective of all the possibilities in practice and a more enjoyable shared learning experience.*

Listening

Listening is a core skill in the process of assessment, where you are trying to gather useful information about a person and their situation in relation to their current mental health status. An assessment is a purposeful activity, usually aiding the process of decision-making and helping to determine priorities about need, as well as informing your professional judgement of what to do/how to act in response to the information. Listening well requires close/intense concentration, and visibly demonstrating to the service user that you are doing just that. This is so they get the communication cues to continue to engage with

you and to share the relevant information to help you in your task of assessment. Listening well and letting people know you are doing it is a precursor to the development of trust between people in a potentially therapeutic encounter.

Showing that you are ready to listen to somebody is a skill that can be learned and enhanced with practice. Egan (2006) uses the acronym SOLER to help remind us of some of the non-verbal skills that the nurse can use to demonstrate attentiveness, or active listening.

1) S – Sit square on.
2) O – Use an open posture.
3) L – Lean slightly forward.
4) E – Make eye contact.
5) R – Relax.

Sit square on

By this, Egan means having opposing chairs at an angle of 90° to one another. If two people are face on, this can sometimes be interpreted as intimidating. A square on position is much more informal and relaxed and more useful for a therapeutic conversation.

Consideration should also be given to the type of chairs that are used. It is more beneficial to use chairs that are of a similar type and height in order to reduce any suggestion of power that the patient might feel the health care professional holds.

If sitting down is difficult or not possible, a square on position can be maintained while standing, by

Table 2.1 Skills and abilities required to communicate

Method of communication identified	Skills and abilities required for this method
Writing an assessment report to a GP	
Being assertive with a colleague	
Multidisciplinary team meetings	
Telephone calls	
Emails	
Breaking unwelcome news to somebody	
Face-to-face communication	
Writing an electronic care plan	

observing the 90° rule. However, try to avoid standing over someone who is sitting or lying down, as this can also be intimidating.

When sitting squarely, it is important to maintain a comfortable distance between yourself and the service user. If you are too close, again this can feel intimidating. Too far away, and the personal, one-to-one nature of the discussion becomes lost. There are cultural differences in what constitutes a comfortable interpersonal distance, which are covered in the section on proximity further on in this chapter.

Open posture

An open posture is important to demonstrate that you are being receptive to communication. While sitting down, you should try to avoid sitting with legs crossed and arms folded as this may convey disinterest and defensiveness. However, crossing your legs at the ankles still feels quite open, as does loosely clasping your hands together. This also helps you to relax.

Lean slightly forward

Leaning forward conveys interest in the message that you are hearing, as though you are saying 'I'm ready to listen.'

Make eye contact

Generally speaking, people make eye contact more when they are listening than when they are talking. When listening, people make eye contact about 70 per cent of the time, and it is useful to try and emulate this level of eye contact when listening therapeutically. Breaking eye contact or looking away from someone can convey disinterest in what is being said. A very high level of eye contact, though, can sometimes be misinterpreted as staring and can be intimidating or uncomfortable.

There are a whole host of difficulties associated with eye contact. Some people are naturally uncomfortable with looking at others, and in many cultures it is considered to be rude if you make eye contact with older people or with people from the opposite gender. You may need to discuss with the service user what they find acceptable.

Relax

It is quite difficult to try to perform all of the above skills and relax at the same time! Bear in mind that

the acronym outlined here should act as an *aide memoir*. Try to think about using these skills not all at the same time, but during the course of an interaction. Above all, though, try to retain a relaxed posture. Doing this often helps the other skills come naturally.

Student activity 5
Have a look at the two online activities for Chapter Two entitled 'Communication Skills' – 'Office' and 'Hospital ward'.

http://www.oxfordtextbooks.co.uk/orc/clarke

and choose the online resources for this chapter.

Student activity 6
Tune out: Try to recall a situation where you were concerned or distressed about something and wanted to communicate this to someone and for them to really listen to you.
However, it became clear to you that they failed miserably to achieve this skill. List everything they did that demonstrated how they failed on this occasion.
Do a supplementary list of anything you could do to show 'not listening' – be creative. Do this as a pair or in a small group if you have the chance.

Of course, communicating with somebody is not just about listening to them. Communication is a two way process that involves listening, processing information, and responding appropriately. As well as the SOLER principles, we use a whole range of other verbal and non-verbal responses to help a therapeutic conversation to develop.

Verbal communication
Open and closed questions

Closed questions usually elicit a one word response such as 'yes' or 'no'. They are particularly helpful when trying to gather statistical information about a subject, but are not good at establishing the way one feels:

e.g. 'Have you had a wash today, Mr Smith?'

Open questions are non-restrictive in terms of the response. They are more useful when trying to ascertain people's feelings about a subject, and allow people to express things in more detail:

e.g. 'How have you been since we last met?'

The value of open questions is that the questioner makes no assumptions about the person they are communicating with, and they also encourage the receiver to respond with more than just a 'yes' or 'no' answer.

Leading questions

Leading questions are those questions that force somebody to give a desired response. In a therapeutic setting these are not an effective means of communicating, as it takes away people's choice:

e.g. 'You'd like to have your lunch now, wouldn't you?'

Clarifying

For therapeutic communication to be effective, it is important for all parties involved to understand the same message. Sometimes, clarification can be used to establish clear meaning and eradicate any ambiguities. This is particularly important when meanings of words may be misunderstood or misinterpreted:

e.g. 'Now let me see if I've understood you correctly.'

Paraphrasing and reflecting

Paraphrasing and reflecting both involve the repeating of a message back to the sender to demonstrate that it has been understood. To paraphrase, a message is simply echoed back:

e.g. Patient: 'I'm scared about my operation today.'

Nurse: 'So you're nervous because you have to go for your operation?'

A reflective response conveys some understanding of feeling, and would be accompanied by a change in voice tone or other non-verbal form of communication, which is congruous with the message:

e.g. Patient: 'I'm scared about my operation today.'

Nurse makes eye contact and sits beside the patient.
Nurse: 'You feel nervous because you have to go to theatre.'

> ### Student activity 7
> *Watch somebody speaking for a while, say on a TV programme (a political programme is a good example), then close your eyes for a while and continue to listen.*
> *Notice how your senses adapt to the way you are receiving the message.*
> *Do you understand less or more of what is being said?*

Paralinguistic communication

The different ways in which we moderate our speech can be defined as 'paralinguistic communication'. Intonation, pitch, volume, rhythm, tone of voice, and timing can be considered as paralinguistic forms of communication.

Williams (2002) considers grunts, 'ums', and 'ahs' as forms of paralinguistic communication, and defines them as *conversational oil*. These sounds are important during telephone conversations, for example, when the message receiver cannot see your face and you need to communicate that you are following the thread of the conversation. They act as verbal prompts to encourage the flow of conversation.

Other forms of paralinguistic communication include yawning, coughing, tutting, laughing, and groaning.

Other forms of non-verbal communication skill
Silence

The use of silence is a tremendously powerful method of therapeutic communication. Arnold and Boggs (2003) believe that silence serves a number of purposes within the nursing environment. It allows the individual and the nurse time to think about what has just been said. It also serves to validate what has been said – a pause before moving on lets the individual know that their message has been understood. Sundeen *et al.* (1998) believe that silence non-verbally communicates the nurse's acceptance of the individual.

Silence is important for individuals, as sometimes it takes time for people to internalize and understand something (often something quite profound) that they have perhaps just thought about for the first time. The skill for the nurse is first of all to feel comfortable with silence, and secondly to convey to the individual a readiness to continue to receive information when the individual wishes to continue.

Gestures

Gestures can be used to elaborate a point (illustrators), such as pointing; or can be used to replace speech (emblems), such as a thumbs up sign. They are also used to express closeness in relationships. Groups of friends will often mirror or copy one another's gestures. Gestures are used universally, and many gestures are the same around the world. However, many are open to cultural misinterpretation.

Some examples (from Axtell, 1998):

Shaking hands as a greeting

In Western culture, a firm handshake is the expected formal way of greeting somebody. In the Middle East, this would signify aggression, so a gentle handshake is more appropriate. In India, a slight bow with hands in a prayer position is the most common form of greeting, whilst in Japan, a bow is also used, but without the use of hands.

Thumbs up

In Britain, this signifies 'good luck' or 'well done', but it can mean 'up yours' in Australia.

Student activity 8

Spend five minutes having a conversation with someone while you sit on your hands.
How does this feel?
Do you think that you can convey your message as effectively?

Touch

Touch is the most basic form of communication. It is important for the nurse to show respect for individuals' space by not getting very close or touching them without first seeking their permission or at least notifying them, as feeling crowded or being grabbed is most uncomfortable for anyone. In addition, lower your stature by occasionally sitting or bending in an individual's presence. This can have a beneficial effect on individuals' morale and speaks to individuals in ways that invite their response.

The tactile system is the first sensory system to develop and is essential for the development of:

- Emotional and social development.
- Learning about the body.
- Motor skills.
- Object recognition.
- Cognitive development and communication.

Some individuals experience difficulties with touch because of:

- Institutionalization (self-care needs are the main priority and lack of activities means that the individual becomes withdrawn and/or engages in self-stimulatory behaviours).

- Negative experiences of touch (abuse, rough handling).
- Their developmental level.
- Their tactile defensiveness – a condition where heightened sensitivity to tactile input causes the individual to respond with excessive withdrawal to touch and tactile experiences (Hill 1995).

Facial expression

Universally, according to Ekman (2004), there are seven main facial expressions, which we use to display surprise, fear, sadness, joy, disgust, anger, and interest. Facial expressions are used to reinforce the verbal message, or to confirm understanding on the part of the listener.

Proximity

According to Hall (1966), in Western culture, most interpersonal communication occurs at between 45 centimetres (18 inches) and 120 centimetres (4 feet). Communication that occurs within 45 centimetres is considered to be intimate communication. This has particular relevance to the nurse and other health professionals, as we often have to invade people's intimate space.

Again, space and proximity vary between cultures. In Japan, for example, people prefer a greater distance for interpersonal communication to occur, whereas in Latin American countries, less distance is needed.

Student activity 9

Note that when you look at the online films for the other chapters there are several examples of mental health nurses talking to service users. To what extent do you think that these mental health nurses are displaying these communication skills? Which nurses are displaying good skills and which display poor skills? You may wish to look at the following videos as an example:

📹 http://www.oxfordtextbooks.co.uk/orc/clarke

and choose the video link for Chapter 5, Simon the nurse and Joyce.

📹 http://www.oxfordtextbooks.co.uk/orc/clarke

and choose the video link for Chapter 8, Cathy the nurse and Mrs Bibi.

📹 http://www.oxfordtextbooks.co.uk/orc/clarke

and choose the video link for Chapter 9, Pam the nurse and Sarah.

Assessment tools

Assessment tools are just that, something to help the process of gathering information in a systematic, organized way so it is possible to interpret and come up with some formulation of what the person with mental distress needs or has difficulty with at the present time. Formal or structured tools are many and varied. Some have been developed from research and have been tested to see if they gather the information intended in a reliable, consistent way within the population for which they have been designed, for example the Camberwell Assessment of Need scale (Phelan *et al.* 1995).

There are standardized rating scales used to indicate the likelihood of a specific problem, e.g. mood disorder being present or suicidal intent, such as the Beck Depression Inventory (Beck 1961) and Beck Hopelessness Scale (Beck *et al.* 1974).

It is also helpful to know something about the accuracy of the scale and what it will and will not give information about. It is not surprising then that standardized scales are used in conjunction with other assessment methods such as interviews and observation. Some scales also have social and cultural limitations. For people with literacy problems and learning difficulties, scales or forms requiring them to read and write may prove useless and embarrassing.

Concepts and ideas in some scales may not translate well in certain cultures – 'mental illness', 'feeling depressed', or 'self' may be unacceptable or not understood. Likewise the scales may not have been translated at all or could even have been inaccurately translated into other languages. This can affect the achievement of consistency and confuse the person about what is being asked.

Scales often rely on people giving truthful and accurate answers, and for many reasons people may not want or be able to do this. Therefore they need to be used in conjunction with interviewing and observation methods.

Assessment tools – a word of caution

Using these research-based scales can be very helpful and insightful but there are important considerations for the practitioner to bear in mind. Training in the correct use and interpretation of scales is usually necessary. The reason for this is that results may then need to be followed up by certain actions for which the practitioner is then accountable. Also, research-based scales are 'intellectual property' – they belong to the person(s) whose hard work in researching the area is recognized. Permission to use the scales sometimes comes via a licence, usually purchased for a specified period of time by the employer, conferring the right to use the scale for the purpose it was intended and in the manner intended. In addition, if used alone scales may not be accurate enough to rely on.

Assessment tools can be subdivided into broad groups:

- **Global** – snapshot or overall views.

- **Observational** – completed from watching the person's behaviour or behaviour patterns over time by people, often nurses, who spend prolonged periods of time in the person's company. These scales are useful when people with mental distress are very disturbed or uncommunicative.

- **Questionnaires** – self-completed or directed/asked by a nurse. These can be very general in nature or may ask questions that relate to a specific concern or identified problem area.

- **Structured** – used to guide the mental health worker about specific areas to cover in the assessment or can even be carefully phrased or scripted questions. Some structured formats are devised locally to be used across an organization like a mental health trust and are both assessment forms and Care Programme Approach documents combined. They can set down a guide to areas the organization expects will be considered in assessment, as well as being a good guide for a novice practitioner who has not yet learned to carry a well-developed and structured format in their head.

Risk assessment and management

Since the implementation of the Care Programme Approach it has been mandatory for people referred to specialist mental health services to have a health and social care assessment, and this has to incorporate a risk assessment. A risk assessment process concerns itself with identifying the likelihood of an undesirable event(s) occurring to the detriment of the affected person or others in their community, close or distant (see also Chapter 5). It also considers the severity of such an event and its likely impact on the service user and other parties. The four key areas of risk are harm to self, harm to others, self-neglect, and vulnerability. Since the publication of the *National Service Framework for Mental Health* (Department of Health 1999) there has been major investment in developing guidance for the frameworks and tools used in the assessment and management of risk. The policy and related guidelines, as well as recommended tools, have been based on the best research evidence from large-scale studies such as *Safety first: five year report of the national confidential inquiry into suicide and homicide by people with mental illness* (Department of Health 2001). The findings from this report informed the *National Strategy for Suicide Prevention* (Department of Health 2002) and this has resulted in reducing the trend in suicide rates as a population approach to suicide prevention (National Institute for Mental Health in England 2006).

Negative, sensationalist media reporting continues to influence public perceptions of the 'mentally ill', particularly that they need to be protected from people with mental disorders as well as the 'patient' being protected from themselves. Public protection is seen as paramount, even when accurate assessment of positive risk has been statistically poor, and the level of fear of violence and homicide by strangers is not reflected in the actual crime statistics. For example, a study by the University of Manchester (2006) found that there were approximately 52 homicides by strangers per year in England and Wales (based on figures for the years 1998–2003).

To inform practice the National Institute for Health and Clinical Excellence (NICE) has developed several clinical guidelines, once again evidence based, related to various areas of risk management (see for example NICE Clinical Guideline 16, National Institute for Clinical Health and Excellence 2004c, and NICE Clinical Guideline 25, National Institute for Clinical Health and Excellence 2005). Where risk is assessed as being too great to be managed in the community, service users can be offered an informal admission to an inpatient setting, or sometimes detention under mental health legislation can be used. The Mental Health Act 2007 will be discussed in Chapter 3 and considers the implications for the role of the mental health nurse.

Skills in risk assessment require up-to-date knowledge of policy and relevant literature alongside the interpersonal skills needed to engage and maintain a therapeutic relationship with the service user and significant others. However, as well as this, a strong degree of objectivity is required to maintain safety. Drawing on information from other sources – e.g. past and current records and people who know the service user – in order to corroborate information and give a more detailed perspective is sometimes essential if the nature of the risk warrants it. For students, the following are critical:

- Having the opportunity to observe.
- Participating in and practising clinical interviews incorporating risk assessment questions.
- Use of appropriate tools (once related training in their use has been completed).
- Involvement with team discussions to formulate and plan interventions and make shared decisions with service users and carers.

The above are required to gain necessary experience and to ensure safe practice and decision-making for all, as well as remaining supported by a team of experienced practitioners.

Once again the process is cyclical and a current risk assessment is only a snapshot. It can change in the face of the loss of protective factors or presence of known risk escalators such as increased use of drugs and alcohol or certain losses like key relationships or cessation of medication.

Positive risk taking vs risk minimization

In practice there is a difficult balance to be struck in promoting safety and encouraging autonomy. This can be seen as the conflict between over-controlling people or encouraging positive risk taking. However, promoting safety and positive risk taking are part of the essential capabilities (ESC 9) of mental health workers, so skills development in this area of practice is essential. The idea is to promote personal growth, to allow people to take collaborative, negotiated risks and make their own choices, and to put in place a safety plan in case there are undesirable changes or problems.

However, there are many barriers to taking positive risks. One is the potential for serious outcomes like suicide and homicide, and coping with the consequences of decisions when there is a 'duty of care'. Conflicting opinions or views on the nature, intensity, and severity of the risk posed between different professional and lay people can be hard to manage, and support and sharing such practice issues are once again crucial.

The techniques of risk assessment are a combination of many elements:

- Interviewing skills (one-to-one with service user) – feeling able to ask for very detailed information about risk areas in a reflexive way depending on what is revealed.

- Observational skills – about mental state including mood and temperament, self-care and physical status, intuitive concerns – some of which might contradict what the service user says about the degree of risk.

- Use of tools and training frameworks to guide the process of assessment, e.g. STORM (Green and Gask 2005) or GriST (Buckingham 2007), that have been specially developed to aid the practitioner in undertaking systematic risk assessments. Both are detailed and reviewed alongside others in the Department of Health document *Best Practice in Managing Risk* (Department of Health 2007).

- Collating information from multiple sources – e.g. service user, family, carers, GP records, past incidences, other agencies – including dealing with information sharing protocols (police, social services, probation, schools/colleges, prison services).

- Education on factors increasing risk and protective factors reducing risk for service users. Factors vary depending on the area of risk, e.g. suicide factors are different to factors indicating risk of harm to others.

- Training and supervision when undertaking risk assessments and planning with service users.

Training in risk assessment is a mandatory three year requirement for employees in mental health Trusts in England, as a result of past concerns about the variable quality and inconsistency in risk assessment processes and documentation.

Care planning: the principles

To plan care 'with' someone can be linked to humanism, as identified by Corey (2004).

As a student it is useful for you to consider the following:

- Self-awareness – strive to know yourself.

- The idea that you have personal freedom but that with this comes responsibility for your actions.

- That your identity is individual, even when in relationships with others.

- That you engage in a search for the meaning behind your human experiences.

- That in taking responsibility for your own life you may experience some challenging emotions.

- That to know the significance of being alive you have to be aware of the reality of death.

Adopting a humanistic approach to care planning would lead you to plans that were:

- Person-centred – placing the person, their intrinsic worth as a human being, and their preferences (where safe to do so) at the centre of the caring and care planning process.

- Based on an individualized plan reflecting the person's unique identity.

- Self-determined – where possible and depending on mental state, planning should be in accordance with the expressed and felt needs of the individual (Barker 2004).

- Identifying people's expressed needs and strengths, focusing on ability rather than disability and weaknesses, and using these to promote recovery.

The purpose of making a plan and putting it into action is to try and achieve the improvements, changes, or outcomes agreed with the service user at the assessment and information-gathering stages. It is necessary to clearly identify a service user's needs, problems, strengths, and resources, and how these affect the service user (and possibly others), in order to set up a clear, meaningful plan of action. The needs and problems will almost certainly change, possibly many times, throughout the episode of care and the care plan will need to reflect these changes.

Care planning has to incorporate the need for regular physical health assessments and screening, at a minimum of 12-monthly intervals for service users with a severe mental health problem or on an enhanced Care Programme Approach (CPA). People with mental health problems have higher rates of poor health and illness (Department of Health 2006c). Nurses are well placed to facilitate these health checks and will have to comply with Trust policies in ensuring these take place. Nurses are also able to pay attention to any signs of deterioration in a service user's physical health as well as mental health, and to offer routine health observations like blood pressure checks to service users as part of a care plan (see Chapter 4).

Depending on the service user's mental state, there may be many challenges to devising a care plan everyone agrees to – service user, family/carers, and professionals. In order to understand what the differences in perspectives may be, try the following exercise alone or with a small group of people.

Student activity 10

Part A

Using your clinical experience to date or sharing this with colleagues, identify as many barriers as you can to there being a complete agreement, and the sorts of areas/ issues likely to cause dissent.

Part B

What efforts can you and other multidisciplinary team members make to try and develop a person-centred care plan with a person who is compulsorily detained?

This chapter has emphasized the importance of completing a care plan 'with' somebody, collaboratively, and consistent with the person-centred approach. However, it is possible to write or develop a care plan 'about' someone without adhering to these principles.

Student activity 11

 http://www.oxfordtextbooks.co.uk/orc/clarke

Take a look at the online exercises for Chapter 2 on care planning to explore the differences between the two approaches in more detail.

In practice, Care Programme Approach documentation, including care plans, is likely to vary not only from Trust to Trust, but also from team to team. However, in essence the stages should all relate to the care process identified earlier. See Care plans 2.1 and 2.2 for examples.

Further barriers to developing a care plan *with* someone may need to be acknowledged and the service user may not have the ability to participate at different levels. Consideration may need to be given to how much mental health problems can make it difficult for a service user to take an interest in the development of the care plan. Negative symptoms of schizophrenia or severe depression and poor insight or agreement on the presence of a mental illness can affect participation. The maximum effort to try and involve the person is important if the expectations of

how contemporary mental health nurses practise are to be realized. Literacy levels and language skills can be a barrier, as can expectations of what a care plan will or will not achieve. Previous long-term experiences of institutional mental health care can render service users severely disempowered and 'voiceless' or overly compliant, and it would then be easy to 'do to' rather than 'with'.

Care planning for relapse

Identifying the earliest potential signs of relapse and what actions are best taken if this should happen is another opportunity for collaborative working with service users and families. Often the service user and relatives know the pattern of relapse and early signs really well. Once people have begun to make progress in their recovery, this is an ideal time to sit with them and their family or carers to map out what happens and discuss a preferred and realistic course of action if a relapse does occur.

The rationale for relapse management with early intervention includes:

- Keeping people safe and well.
- Minimizing distress and disruption caused by avoidable relapses.
- Facilitating open and honest dialogue concerning patterns of relapse and triggers (e.g. increased substance misuse, altered sleep pattern).
- Helping people take some control and have choices over their care and illness.
- Supporting carers and listening and responding to their expertise.
- Reducing carer burden and stress wherever possible.
- Keeping care-giving going in the least restrictive manner.
- Making responsibilities clear and explicit to avoid confusion leading to crisis.
- It is documented and shared with key people as guidance so everyone has the information to act as a supporting team.
- It suggests everyone in the system is acting as a team and in partnership, reducing reliance on one person.

Each person's pattern of relapse is unique to them, and is sometimes described as a 'relapse signature'. Therefore, it is particularly essential that relapse work is collaborative and individually tailored to each

(Continued on p. 45)

Care plan 2.1

Service User Need/Problem	Goals	Care Plan
1. I respond to voices (command auditory hallucinations) by following their instructions when I feel unable to cope with the strength of the pressure the voices exert on me. It means that I can be vulnerable to cutting myself on my arms, thighs, and chest with a knife or burning my body with lighted cigarettes. At my worst I have tried to strangle myself because the voices said I'd be better off dead.	**Short-term goals** To reduce the risk of acting on the voices and hurting myself seriously by seeking early support from people I trust and who I think understand my problems. **Long-term goals** To recover from my early experiences and manage my voices so they have less power over me and I can resist acting on them using different things to help me.	To keep a copy of my early warning signs and action plan near me so I can remind others and myself what can be done to help when I am having these experiences. My GP has one too. To try and live my life in ways that place me under less stress, as it is when I get very stressed or distressed that the voices emerge (they go away for periods of time). The more stressed I feel the more powerful the voices are in my head and they always say terrible things about me and try to persuade me to harm myself as I am worthless. Although I don't like being on medication, my doctor has found one that does weaken the voices and makes me less anxious without lots of side effects. I take a low dose of this and we have agreed I can increase it whenever things get worse with the voices if I ring and tell her. She will support me in this decision and says I can be in control with support. I will try telling my support worker and care coordinator rather than keep it to myself, which I've done before and I ended up in hospital as things got worse. I find that going out and doing things like shopping, going to new places, and seeing new things distracts me and helps me cope. Doing crafts helps me too and so does being with friends who I can just be myself with. I know that if none of the medical and support things help I can agree to the support from a crisis team rather than go into hospital, as I prefer my own home. My care coordinator is trying to find a hearing voices group for me but has given me an internet site for people with the same

Service User Need/Problem	Goals	Care Plan
		experience in the meantime, as it might help to know what other people go through and how they cope. When I feel stronger I might be ready to try some counselling for the abuse, but I'm not yet. **Rationale:** *Complies with Standards 1 and 7 of the National Service Framework for Mental Health (Department of Health 1999).* *NICE guideline – Self Harm (National Institute for Clinical Health and Excellence 2004c)* *Safety First Report (Department of Health 2001)* *National Strategy for Suicide Prevention (Department of Health 2002)* *CNO review (Department of Health 2006b) – recovery based, person-centred practice*
2. I sometimes severely restrict my food and drink intake when I think I am overweight and ugly. This also happens when I get preoccupied with my previous experiences of childhood sexual abuse and I feel unhappy with my body being like a grown woman.	**Short-term goals** To maintain a regular daily diet of foods I enjoy as well as drink at least 2 litres of drinks a day. To prevent admission to hospital with dehydration as I was before, when I had to go on a drip. **Long-term goals** To break the cycle of bingeing and starving over many years, which makes me ill and has put me in hospital, disrupting my life and career and worrying my family. To like me as I am.	To plan my meals and make sure I shop for things I like to eat every few days. I like to have meals in company so this helps me and I can arrange to go out to eat with friends. I don't weigh myself as it worries me too much. I learned some CBT strategies to help me challenge my thoughts and ideas about starving myself when I was in hospital, so if I try to remember these and use them it can help. I will tell my care coordinator and get help to use my strategies to keep my eating going when I am struggling. I have a specialist doctor who will see me as an outpatient if I need it, so I must learn to ask for help early so the starvation does not get a grip. When I am hungry I know I get more anxious and low so it gets into a vicious circle easily. Only as a last resort will I have some medication to calm me if it gets really bad and I can't handle it.

Service User Need/Problem	Goals	Care Plan
		Rationale: *Complies with duty of care requirements.* *Nursing and Midwifery Council (2008)* *NICE (2004b) – Eating Disorders*

3. I have done things for people in the past to keep them happy or because they have been able to frighten me with what they would do if I did not do what they asked.	**Short-term goals**
	To recognize when this is going on and do something to prevent me acting in ways I regret or that leave me feeling used.
	
	Long-term goals
	Get more assertive and stand up for myself, not letting people who are bad for me get too close too quickly.
	Judge people better.
		When I have a gut feeling or know that really people are trying to control me I want to share it with people I can talk it through with to help me make the right decisions for me. I can tell my care coordinator, my friend Lily, or my support worker Jodie, who have told me that's what they are there for.
		    I must open up and try not to bottle things up and then act without thinking if it's going to hurt me. I must see my support people regularly.
		    I am going to give an assertiveness course a go and buy a book recommended to me on standing up for myself.
		    I will have the chance to do these things and feel OK with them.

4. I want to reduce my four types of medication to two so I am only taking what I need to cope with everyday life. It makes me feel like I am unable to think clearly and am relying on it.	**Short-term goals**
	To come off diazepam and zopiclone by Christmas.
	
	Long-term goals
	To come off all medication on a regular basis. I might be willing to take some for short periods now and again if I really struggle to cope.
		To work with my psychiatrist on a withdrawal plan to support me in this aim.
		    To use other things to help me relax, like gardening, aromatherapy, and preparing carefully for bed so I can sleep well without medication.
		    See my support workers regularly and share my concerns and worries.
		    Use a relaxation tape or listen to certain CDs I find relaxing.
		    Plan my day so I don't do too much and have time to relax and to eat properly, and time for myself.

Service User Need/Problem	Goals	Care Plan
5. I want to go on a college course so I can retrain to do a job that I like and can do my own hours to suit my stress levels. I want to earn wages and not be relying on benefits in the future.	**Short-term goals** To find out where the local colleges are and ask them to send me information to look at. To work on other things in the plan so I can be well enough to go and cope with a course. **Long-term goals** Get trained in an alternative therapy and find work. Fit in and have the same sort of life as other people my age.	Keep hopeful about the future and realistic about what I can take on. I don't think I can fill my time too much. Read about different therapies so I can get an idea of what I might be interested in at college. I will find out with help from my care coordinator what help I might get with course costs. I can attend short courses for six weeks to start with if I want to. **Rationale:** *CPA Requirements (Department of Health 1990) to consider the education and employment needs of clients in the care plan.* *Social inclusion complies with Standard 1 of the National Service Framework for mental health (Department of Health 1999).*

Care plan 2.2

Service User Need/Problem	Goals	Care Plan
Risk of self-harm and suicide.	**Short-term goals** To prevent Tania hurting herself by cutting or burning or trying to commit suicide. **Long-term goals** For Tania not to commit suicide.	CPN to monitor mental state with weekly visits at home. CPN to check client is compliant with prescribed medication. Ask family to supervise medication. To educate Tania and her family about borderline personality disorder and how she will have to live with this condition as a long-term mental health problem. CPN to report any concerns to RMO and arrange urgent medical review. Refer to personality disorder service for assessment. Ask family to report any concerns as soon as they notice them.

Service User Need/Problem	Goals	Care Plan
		If risk increases ask for crisis team assessment; may need to go into hospital. Give crisis number to Tania and her family. Do Beck's Hopelessness Scale at regular intervals on Tania.
To stay within a normal weight limit and eat a healthy diet.	**Short-term goals** For Tania to eat properly. **Long-term goals** For Tania to recover from her eating disorder.	To keep regular outpatient appointments with eating disorder service. To give Tania a leaflet on healthy eating and weigh her on home visits. Encourage Tania to tell staff when she has stopped eating and drinking properly. Ask the family to report any changes. Remind Tania to challenge negative thinking about her food and refer to psychology if she is not coping. Refer to dietician as extra help with eating normally.
To deal with polypharmacy, as Tania has kept getting more prescribed drugs over the years and she complains of being 'drugged up'.	**Short-term goals** To come off tranquilizers in the day and at night. **Long-term goals** To reduce all psychiatric medication.	Speak with Tania about coming off some of her drugs and tell her why she will benefit from this change. Give literature on side effects to support intervention. Speak with doctor prior to outpatient appointment and review about reducing medication. Place on waiting list for anxiety management group. Refer to physiotherapist for relaxation classes. Check medication to make sure she is not taking more than prescribed amount.
To get Tania usefully occupied in the day and back to work.	**Short-term goals** To increase Tania's motivation to re-educate herself. **Long-term goals** Get Tania off benefits back into meaningful employment to distract her from her problems.	Send for adult education booklets and college prospectuses to give to Tania at next visit. Tell her the government is keen to get people off benefits and

Service User Need/Problem	Goals	Care Plan
		back to work and will probably help her with course fees
		Ask Tania what sort of work or retraining she would like to do.
		Be supportive and tell her not to take too much on to start with and that you will go with her to enrol if it would help.
		Explain how a valued work role is socially inclusive so she will feel more a part of society by returning to work.

service user. Good practice dictates that such a signature will only be useful if the mental health worker has invested time in sitting down with the service user and significant others to develop this document. In turn, this fosters a sense of ownership on behalf of the service user, and empowers them to seek help at the earliest signs of relapse.

Implementation of the care plan in the process of care-giving

This stage represents putting into action the activities agreed upon with the service user in the planning stage to assist with meeting the needs identified. It may also mean trying out the agreed activities to resolve the problems identified. As the care plan requires a clear indication of who is doing what, it is expected that this has been discussed and agreed as realistic and manageable.

Poor practice that is likely to fail the service user and cause tensions and problems with the care plan being implemented occurs when individuals are mandated, in their absence and without discussion, to contribute to a care plan. This risks a lack of ownership for their role; expectations may be unrealistic and misunderstood. Here again communication, teamworking, and collaboration can be a key factor in successful implementation of the care plan. To try to ensure action is progressive for the service user, it is important that time frames are agreed for actions to be completed either in part or fully, with a monitoring or review date set in place, either formally (around

a meeting) or informally (a phone call or brief conversation face-to-face). This helps to keep momentum going and allows early intervention if it is becoming clear that an aspect of the plan needs to be revised as it is not achieving its aims.

These elements are often described or taught as SMART goals, an acronym for Specific, Measurable, Achievable, Realistic, and Timely. Not all aspects of the care plan can be subjected to SMART principles as some aspects of human distress can be difficult to quantify, but this is not to be taken as a reason for being vague and inactive in the implementation of one's own elements or responsibilities within a care plan.

Once 'on duty' during a working day or shift, all actions carried out by a nurse are nursing actions and potentially the delivery of a part of the care plan currently in place. While there are named individuals of varying disciplines identified on the care plan, all staff have a collective duty of care in their general actions and interactions with all service users. As such, every purposeful action with or on behalf of a client is the implied implementation of the care plan. Such actions could include:

- Time management and prioritizing of use of time.
- Advocacy skills – using a person-centred knowledge of the client on their behalf with other agencies and individuals, either by being a supporting voice, or a challenging one on occasion.
- Technical clinical skills – undertaking procedures, for example blood pressure monitoring, injection techniques, or manual handling.
- Talking clinical skills – for example using structured approaches commonly termed talking

therapies, information sharing, or even problem-solving techniques.

- Communication skills of all types as identified earlier in the chapter.

- Interpersonal skills – often used specifically as teamworking skills, liaising, sharing, and discussing all aspects and issues related to the service user. This can benefit the service user directly and also help facilitate others' involvement in their care-giving by sharing helpful and relevant information related to the service user.

- Administration skills – from the completing of documentation in a literate manner and adhering to standards of record keeping to recording in a person-centred context to make the care plan personal. You may need to organize and chair meetings like reviews, ensuring contributions are balanced and include emphatically the voice of the service user and carer(s). You may have to ensure the dissemination of documentation to a number of different parties with the consent of the service user being formally obtained. These skills are particularly relevant when it comes to the evaluation of care (see the next section).

By reviewing the skills of the nurse needed in implementing care plans it is possible to identify personal characteristics of the nurse that will aid in being effective in this part of the nursing process. It means doing what is agreed; therefore commitment, reliability, and consistency will aid the implementation of the care plan and support the team and service user in achieving goals, resolving problems, and responding to difficulties. Valuing and respecting the roles and contributions of service users and others is vital.

The care delivery and planning process does not happen in isolation, nor is it the responsibility of one person alone. Many people can be part of its development and delivery. At a local level, staff resources and support are important. Colleagues need to cooperate with each other in the process. The duties associated with the development and delivery of a care plan can be very time-consuming, so workload levels are an issue, and time as a resource needs to be available in order to be effective and to build in quality to the process. Where there are staff shortages and absences this can prove problematic and a barrier to care delivery.

Team leadership and case management and review, as well as clinical supervision, are related to supporting the nursing process and multidisciplinary care delivery. Problems can arise from shortages of key personnel or long waiting lists for specialized services, resulting in unmet needs or ongoing tensions in the system of effective care delivery. Clearly identifying these in documentation and using a reporting system for these gaps in resources can aid others in the process of clinical governance and service planning and development, as well as discharging your responsibilities to the service user (see also Chapter 10).

The Care Programme Approach underpinning the nursing process has a legislative framework that confers individual and organizational responsibilities. It is important to be familiar with the expectations and boundaries of these. Often care-giving and how well it is performed rely on this process as an indicator of quality and of whether care has been given to an acceptable standard. The inclusive approach to care is audited using the measure of care plans being signed and service users being aware of the care plan and having a copy of their own. In the delivery of care all policies and procedures of the employing Trust remain a requirement of care. Likewise there may be other legislative frameworks that continue to apply to the care of the service user, regardless of the content of the care plan, that influence the practice of the nurse. Examples include the Mental Health Act (2007), The Children Act (1989), and the Mental Capacity Act (2005), as well as the wide range of NMC guidelines and standards.

Evaluation of care-giving

Evaluating care is about establishing whether or not the interventions we have put into place with service users have worked, and if not, what needs to be done differently. Have the resources that have been used been used appropriately, and can something else more suitable be accessed and utilized? Evaluation of care should be a collaborative process whereby a care plan can be looked at critically and, if necessary, the nursing process cycle recommenced, adjusting, amending, and refining the plan of care where necessary.

Establishing improvements (or deterioration) in someone's health status can be achieved in both subjective and objective ways. Subjectively, service users will frequently feedback as to whether or not they are 'feeling better' (or worse), and objectively this will be complemented by the mental health professionals' opinions as to whether there have been improvements in health, combined with an opinion as to the overall success of the care plan.

Evaluation can be seen from both formal and informal perspectives. Formally, following the guidance of the Care Programme Approach, every service user should have their care plan evaluated at CPA review meetings. Each review meeting should formally record the date of the subsequent meeting. It is the job of the care coordinator, in discussion with others, to determine how frequently CPA reviews should take place, with such reviews commonly occurring every 3–6 months for those people under an enhanced care plan, and every 12 months for those people in receipt of a standard care plan. CPA reviews should be attended by all professionals involved in the service user's care, and should not be regarded as proper reviews of care unless the service user is present at such a meeting. CPA reviews are often attended by family members (if consent is given by the service user) and the service user's GP is usually invited as well. The CPA review is an opportunity for everybody to discuss the success (or otherwise) of the care plan, so that decisions can be made about whether there is a continuing need for certain elements of the plan, or what changes need to be made.

Such a process ensures quality, where everybody in receipt of mental health care is having their care evaluated at regular intervals. However, this process is not without its problems. The relative infrequency of the reviews only tends to provide a snapshot of where someone is 'at' in their lives. For instance, if a review takes place only every six months, a person's mental health may have fluctuated quite a lot during that period. It's therefore important that the review takes into account the whole period since the previous meeting. Furthermore, such reviews can be daunting for service users, so it is vital that the service user either feels confident enough to be able to discuss their care, or has a suitable advocate at the meeting to express the service user's views on their behalf.

In between CPA reviews, and as with assessment, the evaluation of care takes place on a much more informal level. In fact, some kind of evaluation takes place at every meeting between a service user and a health professional. Every interaction involves an assessment and evaluation of that person's mental state (the two go hand in hand, really) and will leave the health professional able to decide whether somebody is better or worse than they were when they last met. Ultimately, the accuracy of this informal evaluation will depend upon the interpersonal skills of the professional – how well they asked questions, how well they listened, how much the service user felt able to trust the professional, how well they observed the environment or surroundings. Such informal evaluations will frequently lead to small changes in the care plan, but may sometimes also call for further discussion amongst those involved in the service user's care.

Student activity 12

The following vignette contains all the elements of the nursing process. Can you identify where each of the elements (assessment, planning, implementation, evaluation) are taking place?

Joan's nurse visits Joan at home as part of a routine fortnightly visit. Joan has had a sustained period of low mood and poor sleep following the death of her husband a year ago. Recently, Joan has felt significant improvements in her health, feeling brighter in mood and sensing that her sleep is returning to normal. At this visit, though, Joan reports that she has had two or three restless nights, and has found herself becoming tearful as the anniversary of her husband's death comes round. The nurse probes Joan's sleeping pattern further, and finds that she has been sleeping during the day because she has felt so exhausted. The nurse therefore advises Joan to try and stay awake during the daytime, no matter how tired she feels, and teaches her some simple relaxation techniques to unwind at the end of the day.

Back at the office, the nurse updates Joan's care plan to include the interventions she has just introduced to Joan, and makes a note to bring this up at the next team meeting.

The skills of evaluation

Interpersonal skills are crucial in accurately evaluating the care that someone is receiving. Informal evaluation requires skills such as:

- Asking good, relevant questions.
- Listening well.
- Being able to develop a rapport.
- Being able to reflect and summarize.

For formal evaluation processes, such as in the CPA review meetings, the health professional, as care coordinator, needs to rely on other sets of skills in order for evaluation to be successful. Firstly, good organizational skills are useful, because the setting up of such meetings often falls to the care coordinator. He or she therefore needs to be mindful of when the next meeting is due, inviting relevant people to that meeting, booking an appropriate room (considering size, privacy, comfort, etc.), and allowing enough time.

Secondly, leadership skills are useful during the meeting itself. Again, it often falls to the care coordinator to chair such meetings, so skills such as good timekeeping, keeping to an agenda, allowing everyone to have their say, not allowing anyone to dominate the meeting, ensuring a relaxed atmosphere, and making people feel welcome are all important skills to have.

Finally, the care coordinator may find themselves in a position of advocacy, especially if the service user feels unable to express themselves fully in such a formal situation. Therefore it may be pertinent to meet with the service user beforehand to establish their views on how things are progressing and what, if anything, needs to be changed or given further

attention. The care coordinator should also take into consideration the opinions of relevant family members and carers within the formal review process. Very often they concur with the views of service users, but sometimes they may well conflict (e.g. the service user feels that they no longer want to take a particular medication that the carer feels is beneficial), so conflict resolution skills may also be a useful skill to possess.

> **Student activity 13**
> *Some points for further consideration and reflection, when you are next in placement:*
> *Some service users find formal CPA reviews an uncomfortable experience.*
> *What can we do to make such reviews as easy as possible for the people we care for?*
> *What should we do if a service user decides that they would not like to be involved in their CPA review?*

Summary

In summary, this chapter has set out to introduce you to some essential skills and aspects of mental health nursing. The ideas and principles covered here are intended to form the basis for your interactions with people with mental health problems. You will see that

in the following chapters, examples are given of how these mental health nursing interactions might work in practice, but first, in Chapter Three, we consider the implications of mental health law.

References and other sources

References

Aldridge J (2006). The therapeutic relationship. In M Jukes and J Aldridge, eds. **Person-centred practices: A therapeutic perspective**, pp. 24–43. Quay Books, Wiltshire.

Arksey H, O'Malley L, Baldwin S, Harris J, Mason A, and Golder S (2002). **Literature review report: Services to support carers of people with mental health problems.** National Co-ordinating Centre for NHS Service Delivery and Organisation, London.

Arnold E and Boggs KU (2003). **Interpersonal relationships: Professional communication skills for nurses.** Elsevier Science, Missouri.

Axtell RE (1998). **Gestures: The do's and taboos of body language around the world.** Wiley, New York.

Barker PJ (2004). **Assessment in psychiatric and mental health nursing: In search of the whole person,** 2nd edition. Nelson Thornes, Cheltenham.

Barker P and Buchanan-Barker P (2005). **The tidal model: A guide for mental health professionals.** Routledge, London and New York.

Bazley M, Cakman N, Kyle J, and Thomas L. (1973). **The nurse and the psychiatric patient.** Heinemann, Auckland.

Beck AT, Ward CH, Mendelson M, Mock J, and Erbaugh J (1961). An inventory for measuring depression. **Archives of General Psychiatry, 4,** 561–71.

Beck AT, Weissman A, Lester D, and Trexler L (1974). The measurement of pessimism: the Hopelessness Scale. **Journal of Consulting and Clinical psychology, 942,** 861–65.

Bertalanffy L Von (1972). **General systems theory.** Penguin, Harmondsworth.

Buckingham CD (2007). Improving mental health risk assessment using web-based decision support. **Health Care Risk Report, 13**(3), 17–18. See also [online] http://www.galassify.org/grist>.

The Children Act (1989). **The Stationery office,** London.

Corey (2004). **The theory and practice of counselling and psychotherapy,** 6th edition. Wadsworth Pacific Grove, CA.

Department of Health (1990). **The care programme approach for people with a mental illness referred to specialist psychiatric services.** Joint Health/Social Services Circular HC (90)23/LASSL(90)11. HMSO, London.

Department of Health (1999). **The National Service Framework for mental health: Modern standards and service models.** DH, London.

Department of Health (2001). **Safety first: Five year report of the national confidential inquiry into suicide and homicide by people with a mental illness.** DH, London.

Department of Health (2002). **The national strategy for suicide prevention**. DH, London.

Department of Health (2006a). **The 10 essential shared capabilities: A framework for the whole of the mental health workforce.** DH, London.

Department of Health (2006b). **From values to action: The Chief Nursing Officer's review of mental health nursing.** DH, London.

Department of Health (2006c). **Our health, our care, our say.** DH, London.

Department of Health (2007). **Best practice in managing risk.** DH, London.

Egan GE (2006). **The skilled helper – a problem-management and opportunity development approach to helping**, 8th edition. Brooks Cole, Pacific Grove, CA.

Ekman P (2004). **Emotions revealed: Understanding faces and feelings.** Phoenix, New York.

George JB (2002). **Nursing theories: The base for professional nursing practice.** Prentice Hall, Englewood Clifs, NJ.

Green G and Gask L (2005). **The development, research and implementation of STORM (Skills-based Training on Risk Management). Primary Care Mental Health, 3**(3), 207–13.

Habermann M (2005). **The nursing process: A global concept.** Churchill Livingstone, London.

Hall ET (1966). **The hidden dimension.** Doubleday, New York.

Hill G (1995). **The Multi-sensory Action Pack.** Social Education Centre, Stallington Hall, Blithe Bridge, Stoke on Trent, Staffs.

Johns C (2004). **Becoming a reflective practitioner,** 2nd edition. Blackwell, Oxford.

Mental Capacity Act (2005). The Stationery Office, London.

Mental Health Act (2007). The Stationery Office, London.

National Institute for Clinical Health and Excellence (2004a). **Depression: Management of depression in primary and secondary care.** NICE, London.

National Institute for Clinical Health and Excellence (2004b). **Eating disorders: Core interventions in the treatment and management of anorexia nervosa, bulimia nervosa and related eating disorders.** Clinical Guideline 9, NICE, London.

National Institute for Clinical Health and Excellence (2004c). **Self Harm – The short term physical and psychological management and secondary prevention of self harm in primary and secondary care.** Clinical Guideline 16, NICE, London.

National Institute for Clinical Health and Excellence (2005). **Violence: The short-term management of disturbed/violent behaviour in in-patient psychiatric settings and emergency departments.** Clinical Guideline 25, NICE, London.

National Institute for Mental Health in England (2006). **National suicide prevention report on annual progress 2006.** NIMHE (in association with Care Services Improvement Partnership).

Neumen B (1995). **The Neuman systems model,** 3rd edition. Appleton and Lange, Norwalk, CT.

Nursing and Midwifery Council (2008a). **Standards of conduct, performance and ethics for nurses and midwives.** NMC, London.

Nursing and Midwifery Council (2008b). **Standards for medicines management.** NMC, London.

Peplau HE (1988). **Interpersonal relations in nursing.** Springer, New York (original 1952, by GP Putnam's Sons, New York).

Phelan M, Slade M, Thornicroft G et al. (1995). The Camberwell Assessment of Need: the validity and reliability of an instrument to assess the needs of people with severe mental illness. **British Journal of Psychiatry, 167,** 589–95.

Registered Nurses Association of Ontario (2002). **Establishing therapeutic relationships.** Registered Nurses Association of Ontario, Toronto.

Rogers CR (1951). **Client centred therapy - its current practices, implications and theory.** Houghton, Mifflin, Boston.

Rolfe G and Freshwater D (2001). **Critical reflection for nursing and the helping professions: A user's guide.** Palgrave Macmillan, New York.

The Sainsbury Centre for Mental Health (2002). **Breaking the circles of fear: A review of the relationship between mental health services and African and Caribbean communities.** Sainsbury Centre for Mental Health, London.

The Sainsbury Centre for Mental Health (2004). **The Capable Practitioner Framework: A framework and list of the practitioner capabilities required to implement the National Service Framework for mental health.** Sainsbury Centre for Mental Health, London.

Saunders JC (2003). Families living with severe mental illness: A literature review. **Issues in Mental Health Nursing, 24**(2), 175–98.

Schön D (1987). **Educating the reflective practitioner.** Jossey-Bass, San Francisco.

Sundeen SJ, Stuart GW, Rankin ED, and Cohen SP (1998). **Nurse-client interaction: Implementing the nursing process.** Mosby, St. Louis.

University of Manchester (2006). **Avoidable death: Five year report of the National Confidential Inquiry into suicide and homicide by people with mental illness.** University of Manchester, Manchester.

Williams D (2002). **Communication skills in practice: A practical guide for health professionals.** Jessica Kingsley, London.

Online Resource Centre

If you have not already done so, look at the online resources for this chapter

http://www.oxfordtextbooks.co.uk/src/clarke

Further reading

Barker P (1998). Psychiatric nursing. **In AC Butterworth, J Faugier and P Burnard, eds. Clinical supervision and mentorship in nursing,** pp. 66-80. Stanley Thornes, Cheltenham.

Barker P (2000). The Tidal Model: The lived experience in person-centred mental health care. **Nursing Philosophy, 2(3)**, 213-23.

Bowlby J (1997). **Attachment and Loss Volume 1.** Pimlico, London (originally published 1969 by Hogarth Press, London).

Callaghan P, Playle J, Cooper L (2009). **Mental health nursing skills.** Oxford University Press, Oxford.

Digby A (1985). **Madness, morality and medicine: A study of the York Retreat 1796-1914.** Cambridge University Press, Cambridge.

Engel GL (1980). The clinical application of the biopsychosocial model. **American Journal of Psychiatry, 67**(5), 535-44.

Erikson EH (1977). **Childhood and Society.** Paladin, London (originally published 1950 by Norton, New York).

Newman C (2005). Too close for comfort: Defining boundary issues in the professional-client relationship. **Rehab and Community Care Medicine,** Spring, 7-9.

Papero D (1990). **Bowen family systems theory.** Allyn and Bacon, Boston.

Pilgrim D (2005). **Key concepts in mental health.** Sage, London.

Social Exclusion Unit (2004). **Mental health and social exclusion.** Office of the Deputy Prime Minister, London.

Chapter 3
Mental health law

Andrew Walsh, Simon Steeves, Victoria Clarke

Learning outcomes

After reading this chapter you should be able to:

- Describe the main characteristics of mental health law across a range of different countries.
- Give examples of how mental health law might influence the care and treatment of some of the characters who are in this book.
- Demonstrate an awareness of the relevant mental health law in your practice.

Introduction

This book has been written to reflect modern ideas about what constitutes good mental health nursing care, and you will see that values such as partnership working within the framework of a therapeutic relationship have been deliberately stressed. However, the role of the mental health nurse has always required some involvement in what is essentially custodial care. It is necessary for us as mental health nurses to try to balance the demands of these two seemingly paradoxical elements of the role of a mental health nurse.

This chapter is intended to introduce you to some aspects of mental health law. We have partly based this upon the law as it currently applies in England and Wales but you will notice that we have also tried to include some material from an international perspective.

Mental health law

The history of the profession of mental health nursing is inextricably bound up with the story of the rise and fall of the asylum and with institutionalized models of care. It was only following the Macmillan commission, which was set up to investigate allegations of abuse at Prestwich Hospital in 1924, that the term 'psychiatric nurse' (which later evolved to mental health nurse, Department of Health 1994) became a commonly used description (Coppock and Hopton 2000). Prior to this time, people working in institutions for the mentally disordered were more often referred to as 'attendants' or 'keepers' (Nolan 1998), and as these names imply, their roles were mostly custodial or supervisory in nature. Mental health nursing has moved away from this limited model of providing 'care' but is still unusual amongst other health care

professions in that its members continue to be involved in compulsory detention (even though the main responsibility for this rests with the medical profession; Rogers and Pilgrim 2001).

In England and Wales the 1983 Mental Health Act and its 2007 update is currently the legislation directing compulsory treatment of people with mental disorder. In common with legislation in most countries, this Mental Health Act aims to achieve a balance between the rights of the individual mental health patient to be treated and protected and the perceived need to protect others. The extent to which this balance has been achieved or not really depends upon who you ask; the 2007 update to the Mental Health Act had a stormy passage through parliament and is still the subject of some disagreement.

Read these two statements about the Mental Health Act amendment, firstly from the Government and then from the Mental Health Alliance, which is a coalition of organizations working in the area of mental health (you might also access the websites of both these bodies – see the web link references at the end of this chapter). Throughout your mental health nurse education you will see that many of the ideas encountered are contested and cause controversy. As always throughout this book, we encourage you to consider the different arguments expressed and then go out to your placement and talk to (and listen to) service users, carers, other students, and professionals. Once you have done this you will be in a better position to decide for yourself how you are going to work as a mental health nurse within this legislation.

Government welcomes passing of Mental Health Bill as vital to community care

Health Minister Ivan Lewis and mental health tsar Professor Louis Appleby both welcomed the final stages of the parliamentary passage of the Mental Health Bill as a vital step towards modern community services.

The Bill, which completed its passage through Parliament on 4 July, will allow psychiatrists to require patients to take treatment following discharge from hospital if they are a risk to themselves or others. It will also strengthen patients' rights by providing advocacy support for anyone who is detained, and create new roles for experienced non-medical professionals.

Health Minister Ivan Lewis said:

'The Mental Health Bill makes mental health law fit for purpose in the twenty-first century. We will consult publicly in the autumn on the Code of Practice and on regulations to underpin the legislation, and a comprehensive implementation programme is in place. As Minister with responsibility for Mental Health, I look forward to implementing these changes within the wider framework of investing in and improving mental health services. We will look to do this in partnership with the many stakeholders in mental health services, and with service users and their representatives.'

Professor Louis Appleby says:

'I am delighted the Mental Health Bill has been passed with all the main government proposals intact, and that we were able to reach agreement with the MPs and peers who expressed concerns about aspects of the Bill.

'These new measures will enable some people with serious mental health problems to be treated in the community under supervision, so that their condition can be properly monitored and steps taken to prevent relapse. This is good for the patients, their families and for the public generally. The Bill will also make it easier for patients with personality disorder to get the treatment they need.'

Department of Health 2007

Mental Health Bill remains a missed opportunity for humane and progressive legislation, says Alliance Office

The Government has missed an historic opportunity to achieve a modern and humane new Mental Health Act, but has made important concessions to protect patients and their families from abuse and neglect, the Mental Health Alliance said today.

As the Mental Health Bill nears completion, Andy Bell, chair of the 77-member Alliance, said: 'The tireless commitment of people who use mental health services and their supporters has achieved real improvements to this controversial Bill.

'We now have a Bill that for the first time gives people a right to an advocate when they are detained and that protects children from being put on adult wards inappropriately. We also have new safeguards over the use of electro-convulsive therapy, for people detained under the Mental Capacity Act, and for the renewal of detention. These are hard won improvements that are a credit to the persistence of activists from across the country.

'But our members will be disappointed today that the Government has rejected changes to many other aspects of the Bill. It has failed to heed the evidence about the risks of significant over-use of community treatment orders and the excessive powers the Bill gives to clinicians. And it treats people with mental health problems as second class citizens by allowing treatment to be imposed on those who are able to make rational decisions for themselves.

'We are now at a crossroads. We call on the Government to start listening to the people who are affected by the Act when it writes the new regulations and to ensure that sufficient resources are made available to mental health services to implement the changes fairly.

'We also call on ministers to take seriously the warnings made by the Commission for Racial Equality about the impact of the Bill on black communities and to take action before it is too late to put this right.'

Mental Health Alliance 2007

The Mental Health Act, England and Wales

In this part of the chapter we give a brief overview of some parts of the Mental Health Act that we think students should be aware of. However, this book is not a legal textbook; you should also refer to the actual legislation and its associated guidelines (some links to this can be found later in the chapter). Firstly, it is useful to consider the structure of the Act as this will help you to understand the way that people refer to it.

You will hear people talking about 'sections' of the Mental Health Act, as well as people 'being sectioned'. These expressions are commonly used but their true meaning is often unclear. For example Section '5(4)' of the Mental Health Act (nurses' holding power) can be found in Part 2 of the Mental Health Act. All *parts* of the Act are split into *sections*. These sections have subsections; therefore '5(4)', which deals with informal holding of patients by nurses, means Part 2 of the Act, Section 5 of Part 2, and Subsection 4 of Section 5. Similarly a patient who has been sectioned for treatment has actually been detained under Part 2, Section 3.

Student activity 2

Part of your work may include personally implementing Section 5, Subsection 4 of the Mental Health Act. This holding power means that you can hold a person for up to six hours or until a doctor attends, whichever is soonest. As you will have seen earlier this is only applicable to mental health service users who are already admitted to mental health inpatient services. There are four reasons why we would implement this section. They are:

1) The person has a mental disorder.

2) The person is a danger to themselves or others.

3) The person is actively seeking to leave the premises and not return.

4) There is no doctor currently available to assess the situation.

It is useful to take some time out now and consider how you will feel when/if you have to implement this section on a person as a qualified mental health nurse. How do you feel about having such power over another person?

How does this work fit in with your own personal and mental health nursing philosophy?

Do you feel that you could do this comfortably and maintain a therapeutic relationship at the same time? We would like to encourage you to discuss this with your clinical assessor, fellow students and your university lecturers. For further reading on some of the ethical considerations raised here, we would recommend Barker and Davidson (1998).

The Mental Health Act provides protection for the mentally ill person and society against actions that may be deemed irrational. The Act achieves this by defining mental disorder and the detailed rules under which doctors make recommendations for compulsory admission. The Act defines mental disorder as follows: 'Mental disorder means any disorder or disability of the mind'; clearly this is a very vague definition! The Act goes on to exclude learning disability as a mental disorder unless the person displays 'abnormally aggressive or seriously irresponsible conduct'. Section 3(2) sets out the criteria for compulsory detention for treatment:

1) The patient is suffering from the specified forms of disorder.

2) Appropriate treatment must be available.

3) Not only must it be necessary for the health or safety of the patient or the protection of others that they receive treatment but it must be shown that treatment cannot be provided unless the patient is compulsorily detained in hospital.

(Remember, all three of these grounds must be met in order for a person to be detained.)

The application for detention must be made by an approved mental health professional or the patient's nearest relative. Two doctors must make written recommendations in support of the application, one of whom must be approved by the Secretary of State for Health for these purposes (under Section 12).

In Box 3.2, we have briefly summarized the sections of the Mental Health Act that we feel are most important for you to know about; again, we would also suggest that you refer to the links at the end of the chapter for more complete guidance.

Offences

The offences covered by Part 9 of the Mental Health Act (see Box 3.1) are not offences perpetrated by those suffering from mental health problems but rather by those caring for them. They include ill treatment, assisting a patient to abscond or avoid recapture, and the creation or possession of a false document. The penalty for these offences is up to six months imprisonment if convicted in a Magistrates Court or two years if convicted in the Crown Court.

Student activity 3

Take some time out to consider and reflect on the following. As a mental health nurse, one of your possible responsibilities under the remit of the Mental Health Act 2007 is explaining the rights patients have whilst held under the Act. If you are based in an inpatient unit, ask your assessor for a copy of the patients' rights leaflet. There is a range available to cover all inpatient sections. Also discuss with them what they do when explaining patients' rights. It is always useful to think about the following:

- *When – what time of day is the most likely to be best for this person?*

- **Who** *is the right professional to inform this person of their rights and should the person's family, carer, or independent advocate be present?*

- **How** *are you going to tell the person their rights? Are you just going to give them the leaflet? How will you check that they have understood their rights?*

- **Where** *will you inform the person of their rights – in a quiet, undisturbed environment where they are free to ask you questions? Or in a busy area of the unit where their confidentiality is likely to be breached?*

- *As mental health nurses we also have a responsibility to record whether the mental health service user has understood their rights –* **how will you check on this?**

We thought the following personal reflection by Victoria Clarke, a mental health nurse, might help you consider ways to approach this important activity.

" On one occasion I was required to inform a mental health service user of their rights under Section 3 of the Mental Health Act. I told them how long the section lasted for, what treatment they would be required to take under the section, and when they could appeal to a Mental Health Review Tribunal. I really thought that I had done quite a good job but now I needed to check whether the service user had understood the content of what I had been saying. He appeared to; he had maintained good eye contact with me and even nodded on occasion. So I passed him the leaflet and asked him to take some time to digest the information I had given him and ask any questions. Unfortunately at this point he tore up the leaflet and ate it. Clearly I had not conveyed the information as well as I'd hoped and I recorded this in the service user's notes. I think this is a good example of how nurses can mistakenly think that they are

Part 1. Application of the Act (including definition of mental disorder)
Part 2. Compulsory Admission to Hospital and Guardianship
Part 3. Patients Concerned in Criminal Proceedings or under sentence
Part 4. Consent to Treatment
Part 5. Mental Health Review Tribunals
Part 6. Removal and Return of Patients Within the UK, etc.
Part 7. Management of Property and Affairs of Patients
Part 8. Miscellaneous Functions of Local Authorities and the Secretary of State
Part 9. Offences
Part 10. Miscellaneous and Supplementary

Box 3.1 The structure of the Mental Health Act

Section of the Mental Health Act	Brief description
Section 2	This provides for a person to be detained for up to 28 days in hospital for assessment (or for assessment followed by medical treatment). It requires two medical recommendations. An application for admission for assessment must be made by an approved social worker/mental health professional or the person's nearest relative. Active treatment is allowed under Section 2 usually after an initial assessment period.
Section 3	Allows a person to be detained in hospital for treatment, initially for up to six months, which may then be renewed for a further six months and after this for a year at a time. An application can be made by the person's approved social worker or their nearest relative; this application must be supported by two medical practitioners.
Section 4	This allows emergency admission to hospital for up to 72 hours and it is based upon one medical recommendation. This Section is supposed to be used in a real emergency where it would be dangerous to delay while awaiting another medical practitioner.
Section 5	This refers to 'holding power' in which a voluntary inpatient can be prevented from leaving hospital. Section 5(2) Allows for a registered medical practitioner to authorize detention for up to 72 hours. Section 5(4) Allows a mental health nurse to detain a patient for up to 6 hours. The number of hours a patient is detained under this section must be subtracted from the 72 hours above. For example where a nurse has detained a person under Section 5(4) for 3 hours, a subsequent Section 5(2) would only last for 69 hours.
Section 17	This section defines the conditions under which leave may be granted to a detained patient. Only the Responsible Clinician (RC) may grant leave. All conditions affecting that leave must be recorded. The RC may not recall a patient once their liability to be detained has expired. (You may notice that in the film of 'Joyce' in Chapter 5 she can be heard asking about this: www.oxfordtextbooks.co.uk/orc/clarke and choose the video link for Chapter Five.)
SCT, CTO	Supervised Community Treatment (SCT) and Community Treatment Order (CTO). If the Responsible Clinician and the approved mental health professional agree that a person should be discharged onto SCT they must make a CTO, which is the authority for the SCT to begin.
Section 37 (37/41)	Section 37 concerns a court's decision that a person should be detained in a mental health facility. This section only applies where the offence committed is normally punishable by imprisonment. Where the offence is very serious an additional restriction order (41) is put in place, which prevents the granting of leave or discharge by anyone other than the Secretary of State.
Section 58 (form 39)	Section 58 deals with treatment that requires consent or a second opinion. For example persons detained under Section 3 must after three months be assessed by a second opinion-approved doctor who will decide whether treatment may continue. If continued treatment is agreed, a form 39 (certificate to treat) will be issued.
Section 117	This makes it the duty of authorities to make arrangements for people who have been detained under Sections 3, 37, 47 and 48 to receive continuing support and care.
Section 132	Under this section a legal obligation is placed on the hospital managers and their employees to ensure that a person understands the conditions of and length of any detention and their rights to appeal. This information must be given verbally and in writing and understanding by the person must be established (see Student activity 3).
Section 136	This allows a police officer to remove someone from a public place and to take them to a place of safety. The intention is that they should be examined by a doctor and an approved social worker/mental health professional with a view to detention.

Box 3.2 Commonly referred to sections of the Mental Health Act

communicating vital information effectively when this is not the case.

Victoria Clarke

2007 Updated Mental Health Act, England and Wales

The following is a partial list of amendments to the 1983 Mental Health Act that will be relevant to student mental health nurses; again, it is not intended to be an exhaustive list of these changes.

- There is now a single definition of the term 'mental disorder' ('Mental disorder means any disorder or disability of the mind', see p. 52) – dependence on alcohol and drugs is not considered to be a mental disorder.
- The 'treatability' clause – this stated that detention under the Mental Health Act must improve a person's condition or at least prevent deterioration, but it has now been removed. It has been replaced by the phrase 'appropriate treatment must be available'. This is a contentious issue as 'appropriate treatment' will have to be tested in the courts for definition. Is detention alone an appropriate treatment?
- 'Responsible Medical Officer' has been replaced by 'Responsible Clinician' (RC). This could mean that in the future, other mental health professionals may become RCs. This is significant because historically this important role has always been held by a consultant psychiatrist.
- 'Approved social worker' has been replaced by 'approved mental health professional'.
- 'Nearest relative' can now be someone over the age of 18, whether or not of the same sex, who has lived with the patient for over five years.

Student activity 4
Part of our work as mental health nurses requires us to assist mental health service users to appeal against the section they are being held under, as well as to represent the service's concerns to Mental Health Review Tribunals (MHRTs) – these bodies have the right to discharge patients from certain sections of the Act if they feel the person has sufficiently recovered to no longer warrant compulsory detention within a mental health unit.

It would be useful at this point to discuss some of these issues with your assessor and colleagues in practice. You may also find the portable documents on the following site useful; the forms used for MHRTs are also included.

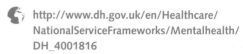 http://www.dh.gov.uk/en/Healthcare/ NationalServiceFrameworks/Mentalhealth/ DH_4001816

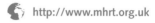 http://www.mhrt.org.uk

The Mental Capacity Act 2005, England and Wales

This Act was intended to provide guidance to anyone working with adults aged 16 or over who may lack the capacity to make decisions for themselves. The aims of this Act were to:

- Support and protect those who cannot make their own decisions.
- Make it clear who can make those decisions.
- Make it clear when and how they can make those decisions.
- Allow people to plan ahead for when they may lose capacity.

Previously there was no clear guidance on whether a person could be considered to be incapable of making their own decisions. Arguably this lack of guidance meant that people were routinely having important decisions made for them. The law was changed so that professionals now have to assume that a person *is* capable of making decisions unless it can be proven that they are not.

One of the most important cases leading up to the development and implementation of the Mental Capacity Act was *HL* vs *United Kingdom* – the 'Bournewood case'. This was a case of a 49-year-old man with autism, HL, who became distressed while travelling by bus to a day hospital. He was taken from the day hospital to a psychiatric hospital, his carers (with whom he lived) were not allowed to see him, and he was not allowed to leave. If he attempted to leave or became distressed, he was medicated. He was not detained under the Mental Health Act, as the hospital felt that it was in his best interests to remain there.

Legal proceedings were brought against the hospital to determine whether HL had been detained and deprived of his liberty. The High Court found that he

1. A presumption of capacity – every adult has the right to make their own decisions and must be assumed to have capacity to do so unless it is proved otherwise.

2. The right for individuals to be supported to make their own decisions – people must be given all appropriate help before anyone concludes that they cannot make their own decisions.

3. That individuals must retain the right to make what might be seen as eccentric or unwise decisions.

4. Best interests – anything done for or on behalf of people without capacity must be in their best interests.

5. Least restrictive intervention – anything done for or on behalf of people without capacity should be the least restrictive of their basic rights and freedoms.

Box 3.3 Mental Capacity Act 2005: Five key principles

The following is an example of the Capacity Act being tested in the courts. This case centres on whether a person whose capacity is impaired by a mental health problem can make important decisions regarding their health and care.

In this case C was a patient in Broadmoor Hospital. A 68-year-old man, he was convicted in 1962 of stabbing his girlfriend and sentenced to seven years' imprisonment. While serving his sentence he was diagnosed with paranoid schizophrenia and transferred to Broadmoor. C suffered from leg ulcers that had become gangrenous. His surgeon considered that he would die without amputation from below the knee immediately. The surgeon also assessed his chance of survival with conservative treatment at less than 15 per cent. C refused to consider amputation, stating that he would rather die with two feet than live with one.

The surgeon carried out the conservative treatment, which averted the threat of imminent death, but was concerned that the gangrene could develop again. He was unprepared to give guarantees that he would not amputate in the future, despite C's repeated refusals.

The court were completely satisfied that although his general capacity was impaired by schizophrenia, C had *understood and retained the relevant information and had arrived at a clear choice*. C was granted an injunction preventing the hospital amputating his foot now or in the future without his express written consent.

This case highlights the fact that all decisions of capacity are case sensitive. Just because C made poor decisions in other areas of his life did not mean he lacked capacity to make any decisions. The defining factor for the court was his ability to understand and retain the information and make an informed choice.

If you wish to know more about this case and others, it is cited in Jones (2007).

Box 3.4 The case of C (Refusal of Medical Treatment), High Court 1994

had not been deprived of his liberty, saying that it was in his best interests to remain in hospital. The Court of Appeal disagreed, saying that he had been detained and that this would only have been legal under the Mental Health Act 1983. The European Court of Human Rights agreed with the Appeal Court that he was unlawfully detained and that his right to liberty under the European Convention on Human Rights (article 5, the right to freedom) had been breached. This case highlighted the need for all people who lack capacity to be properly assessed and only deprived of their liberty in accordance with the law.

The Mental Capacity Act provides a test intended to assess capacity to take a decision at a particular time; note that the definition of incapability refers to that particular decision at that particular time, and that a person is not being generally labelled as 'incapable'. Anyone doing anything on behalf of a person has to consult a checklist of factors to ensure that they are acting in the person's 'best interests', and if the person has previously written statements about their wishes then these must be taken into account.

It is now possible for an individual to appoint someone to act on their behalf in the event of them becoming incapable of making their own decisions in the future. This is called the lasting power of attorney (LPA) and it also allows this person to make health and welfare decisions.

Experiencing mental health legislation – a carer's story

So far we have considered mental health legislation from a legal and professional perspective. The following contribution is intended to give a carer's point of view.

👤 Carer's story: Capacity

My son had a diagnosis of schizophrenia and had returned home to live with us. I knew nothing about schizophrenia, only what I had read in the media – a potential for violence.

It was 2 a.m. when my son woke me; he was really paranoid and delusional. This was my first experience of psychosis. At first I just sat with him hoping that he would calm down. The longer I sat with him and tried to console him the worse he got, he started to frighten me by what he was saying and how he kept banging the table shouting 'no, no', over and over.

By this time I felt he needed medical help, so I phoned the out-of-hours GP. The GP refused to come once I had informed him of my son's diagnosis; this only endorsed the fear I was feeling. If the GP wouldn't come then he must be afraid! He gave me the number for the out-of-hours mental health services; I contacted them expecting someone to come here. Instead I was told to phone the police!

Why should I phone the police? He was ill and in need of medical help, not a criminal. It took 15 hours from my first phone call before I felt I had no choice but to phone the police; it was the only way he was going to get the help he needed. By this time I was quite traumatized; there were about six people who came to my house, which included two police officers. I had to sit in a separate room; no one explained to me what was happening. It would have been nice if someone sat with me while my son was being assessed, someone who would have given me some sort of support and explained to me the process of a section.

When my son was taken away, he was begging and pleading with me not to let them take him. Feelings of helplessness came over me; guilt that I had let my son down by phoning the police and guilty that as a mother, I couldn't help sort out my son's difficulties this time. I later discovered what the banging and shouting was all about; he was hearing voices telling him to attack me!

Once he had been placed on a section I started to ask questions, something that anyone would want to know when it involves someone you care about. Suddenly everything is confidential – my son was not well enough to give his consent. This feels like an iron curtain of silence has been put up; it no longer has anything to do with you. You feel pushed out and excluded, you start getting the feeling that you have done something wrong and there is nothing that you can do about it. It does not feel as if you have any rights at all and that you are used in law only to suit the state when it comes down to putting people under section.

You can be given a leaflet of the rights of the nearest relative; even with this you do not understand what most of it means, nobody sits down and explains it to you. Only that your relative seems to be a property of the state and not part of your family any more. When a family member calls for help they are seeking medical help; having their relative placed under section does not enter their head. I am now aware that a relative can apply for a sectioning; to date I have met and spoken with hundreds of carers and never heard of any carer exercising this right.

When someone ends up needing to be sectioned, there are usually warning signs weeks if not months before a crisis occurs. Family members can see this coming, and often contact services numerous times for help or intervention. The fear of knowing this is coming and being told that their relative has to ask for the help, when they know their relative cannot see that they need help, is the most distressing experience you could imagine. The more stressed the carer becomes, the more this can impact upon their relative and the worse things become. Common sense should prevail here; avoiding a crisis can save a lot of heartache and trauma. Even if you can't force the service user to accept help, intervention and support for the carer could make a lot of difference.

I now work with families and one particular comment I received from a carer who is a senior member of staff at a general hospital said it all. 'I have received mental health awareness training and carer awareness training. Even with all of this training, I could never have imagined how traumatic an experience it was for the carer, until I had experienced it myself.

Pam Pinder

Pam's website 'Carers, Experts by experience' can be found at

http://www.pamshouse.pwp.blueyonder.co.uk/

● **Discussion point**

After a long shift you are very tired and heading home to relax. As you are going along you see a service user you know to be detained and without agreed leave walking along the road. What action do you take? If you decide to go on your way and do nothing, where does this leave you, ethically, legally, and professionally?

Please note that attempting to re-hospitalize the person on your own is not an option as this could place both yourself and that person at risk.

International mental health law

We have asked a range of mental health practitioners and educators from across the world to give their comments about the mental health law as it applies in their own countries. First, we consider Scottish law.

Scotland: a principles-based approach to law

Margaret Conlon is a mental health nurse educator at Napier University in Edinburgh and Hilary Patrick is a human rights lawyer and external lecturer, also at Napier University.

Scotland's mental health and incapacity law and practice is quite distinct from that of the rest of the UK. The Mental Health (Care and Treatment) (Scotland) Act 2003 and the Adults with Incapacity Act (2000) embrace the principles and practice of contemporary mental health nursing in Scotland. Driving these principles is the emergence of an increasingly strong influence of the service user and carer movement. The combination of the legislation alongside the inherent involvement of service users has directly infused into mental health nursing practices and mental health services generally. Thus, there is a gradual shifting in the balance of ideology from a dominant medical orientation to a more progressive, person-centred, and service user-led orientation.

The principles of both of these key pieces of legislation have been further reinforced by *Rights, relationships and recovery – the national review of mental health nursing in Scotland* (Scottish Executive 2006) and the *National Framework for preregistration mental health nursing programmes in Scotland* (NHS Scotland 2008). These documents further progress the core principles of recovery-focused and values-based practice.

A recovery-orientated culture challenges mental health nurses in Scotland to foster nurturing environments within which hope and optimism permeate and service users and carers are recognized as experts of their experience. Scottish Recovery Network (SRN) works to achieve one of the key aims of the National Programme for Mental Health and Wellbeing (Scottish Government 2006) in promoting and supporting recovery from mental health problems. SRN is aligned to Nurse Education Scotland in embedding recovery-based practice in all aspects of mental health services. Recovery-based practice defines the experience of the service user as being key to service culture and mental health care. The incorporation of the tidal model (Barker 2005) in acute and rehabilitation care settings is an example of embedding models of care that resonate with the principles set out in the *10 Essential Shared Capabilities* as well as in legislative policy.

The Mental Health (Care and Treatment) (Scotland) Act 2003 reflects the importance of values-based practice. One of the Act's unique features is to spell out its underlying ethical basis. The Act contains a set of principles, including *benefit, least restrictive alternative, participation* (ensuring service users' involvement in their care), and *respect for carers*. These principles support the development of values-based practice in nursing. The independent Mental Welfare Commission has a legal responsibility to promote and monitor the implementation of these principles, as well as to safeguard the rights and welfare of individuals experiencing a mental illness.

The principle of *participation* leads to significant improvements in service user representation, including:

1) Enabling people to nominate a 'named person' to act as their psychiatric next of kin (s250).

2) The right to independent advocacy (s259).

3) Statutory recognition to advance statements in psychiatry (s275, s276).

Recognition of the importance of autonomy has led to a capacity-based approach to compulsion. Compulsory measures can be used only when mental disorder has 'significantly impaired' a service user's ability to take their own decisions about treatment.

The Act's most controversial feature is the compulsory treatment order, which can authorize detention in hospital or community-based compulsion. Such orders can be justified under the principle of least restrictive alternative, but there remains concern about their use.

Despite this, the Act has been widely welcomed, including internationally. Its principled approach builds on good practice. It attempts to balance protection of vulnerable people with respect for human rights and autonomy. As such it can support, rather than act in opposition to, values-based nursing practice.

Mental health law in Northern Ireland

Anne McKenny and Maureen McMillan are both registered nurses in mental health working as advanced nurses/ specialist practitioners in Belfast Health and Social Services Trust in Northern Ireland.

The mainstay of mental health legislation in Northern Ireland is known as the Mental Health (Northern Ireland) Order 1986. The Order, as it is known, bears a close resemblance to the Mental Health Act 1983 (England and Wales) and Scotland's previous Mental Health Act of 1984. Despite these similarities, the Order has unique distinctions that separate it from other UK mental health legislation. It also differs substantially from the Republic of Ireland's Mental Treatment Act 1945. In this short review it is impossible to acknowledge all the different aspects of the Order but we will attempt to focus on the most pertinent of these.

The Order's definition of 'mental illness' would seem to be the first in UK legislation; it defines mental illness as meaning:

> A state of mind which affects a person's thinking, perceiving, emotion or judgement to the extent that he requires care or medical treatment in his own interests or the interest of other persons.

There is debate about the usefulness of this definition, as it adds little guidance in the decision-making process that occurs when the Order's power to detain is considered.

As a separate category, psychopathic disorder is not recognized within the Order. It does not allow for the detention and treatment of those diagnosed with a psychopathic disorder. Individuals may, of course, be detained and treated under the Order's provision when this disorder coexists with mental illness or severe mental impairment. Fenton *et al.* (1995) recommended that the Order be amended in line with the Mental Health Act 1983 but to date this has not happened.

To be detained under the Order, patients have to be suffering from mental illness or severe mental impairment, and the failure to detain or to discharge would have to 'create a substantial likelihood of serious physical harm'. In making a decision to detain it is necessary that one or more of the following points are evident:

- That the patient has inflicted, or threatened or attempted to inflict, serious physical harm on him/herself; or

- That the patient's judgement is so affected that he/she is, or would soon be, unable to protect him/herself against serious physical harm and that reasonable provision for his/her protection is not available in the community; or

• That the patient has behaved such that other persons were placed in reasonable fear of serious physical harm to themselves.

There is provision for a period of assessment in hospital for up to 14 days, followed if necessary by a detention for treatment, which initially lasts for six months. A medical recommendation (usually by the patient's GP) is completed alongside an application completed by a nearest relative or approved social worker. The common parlance for this is that people are 'formally detained' rather than 'sectioned'.

Patients detained under this provision must be assessed immediately after admission and, if the admitting doctor is not a consultant, this must happen within the initial 48 hours after admission. If further detention occurs, a consultant must see the patient again within the first and second seven-day periods. Thereafter other intervals of consultation must be specified.

Within the Order, Article 10 stipulates that detention for assessment need not be disclosed under certain circumstances, such as declaration to employers. There are no routine managers' hearings and the Mental Health Tribunal hears all appeals against detention.

Unlike other UK mental health legislation, Northern Ireland refers to a combined Health and Social Services, so multidisciplinary working has always been a mainstay of its health and social care provision. Perhaps this is why the Care Programme Approach has never been adopted with the Order. There is no legal duty to provide coordinated aftercare to any detained patient, though 'enhanced' contingency planning for detained patients is seen as best practice and used widely.

Presently, Northern Ireland has provision for the transfer of detained patients between other UK countries. No reciprocal legislation applies between Northern Ireland and the Republic of Ireland.

Mental health legislation across Australia

Mental health law in Australia is somewhat similar to that of the UK. Stewart Gill, working as a mental health nurse in Western Australia, has provided us with an overview of their mental health law as follows.

The Australian Constitution of 1901 established a federal system of government. Under this system, powers are distributed between a national government (the Commonwealth) and the six states and two territories. Each state or territory has its own localized mental health legislation.

State/Territory definitions (from their Mental Health Acts)
New South Wales

Current legislation: Mental Health Act 2007
Primary category: Mental illness
Definition of primary category: Mental illness means a condition that seriously impairs, either temporarily or permanently, the mental functioning of a person and is characterized by the presence in the person of any one or more of the following symptoms: delusions, hallucinations, serious disorder of thought form, severe disturbance of mood, sustained or repeated irrational behaviour indicating the presence of any one or more of the symptoms referred to. A person is mentally ill if the person is suffering from mental illness and owing to that illness there are reasonable grounds for believing that care, treatment, or control of the person is necessary: for the person's own protection from serious harm, or for the protection of others from serious harm. In considering whether a person is a mentally ill person, the continuing condition of the person, including any likely deterioration in the person's condition and the likely effects of any such deterioration, are to be taken into account.

Victoria

Current legislation: Mental Health Act 1986
Primary category: Mental illness
Definition of primary category: A medical condition characterized by a significant disturbance of thought, mood, perception, or memory.

Queensland

Current legislation: Mental Health Act 2000 – subordinate legislation, Mental Health Regulation 2002
Primary category: Mental illness
Definition of primary category: A condition characterized by a clinically significant disturbance of thought, mood, perception, or memory.

South Australia

Current legislation: Mental Health Act 1993 – draft copy of 2007 Bill has now been released for public consultation

Primary category: Mental illness

Definition of primary category: Any illness or disorder of the mind.

Western Australia

Current legislation: Mental Health Act 1996

Primary category: Mental illness

Definition of primary category: If the person suffers from a disturbance of thought, mood, volition, perception, orientation, or memory that impairs judgement or behaviour to a significant extent.

Tasmania

Current legislation: Mental Health Act 1996

Primary category: Mental illness

Definition of primary category: Resulting in a serious distortion of perception or thought, serious impairment or disturbance of the capacity for rational thought, serious mood disorder, involuntary behaviour, or serious impairment of the capacity to control behaviour.

Australian Capital Territory

Current legislation: Mental Health (Treatment and Care) Act 1994

Primary category: Mental dysfunction

Definition of primary category: A disturbance or defect, to a substantially disabling degree, of perceptual interpretation, comprehension, reasoning, learning, judgement, memory, motivation, or emotion.

Northern Territory

Current legislation: Mental Health and Related Services Act 1998

Primary category: Mental illness

Definition of primary category: A condition that seriously impairs mental functioning in one or more areas of thought, mood, volition, or perception and characterized by the presence of at least one of the following symptoms: delusions, hallucinations, serious disorders of the stream of thought, serious disorders of thought form, serious disturbances of mood, or by sustained or repeated irrational behaviour that may be taken to indicate the presence of at least one of the symptoms referred to.

The admission processes under all the Mental Health Acts is closest to the UK system and different from the US and European systems.

Closer examination of mental health legislation in Western Australia

In Western Australia (WA), the Mental Health Act 1996 requires a referral by medical practitioners or authorized mental health practitioners for assessment by a psychiatrist and allows a psychiatrist to make an order for involuntary status, either in the community (Community Treatment Order) or in an authorized hospital. Upon admission to involuntary status, an involuntary patient has access to the Mental Health Review Board, a board consisting of psychiatrists, legal practitioners, and those who are neither psychiatrists nor legal practitioners. The Review Board was established under the Act to review involuntary patients on a periodic (mandatory) basis or upon request. Mandatory reviews are required to occur as soon as practicable and before eight weeks have elapsed since an involuntary order was made. However, a review may be requested at any time and can occur within a short time after request.

The procedure of review is more flexible here than in the US, for example, and illustrates the similarity to the UK, as the Act requires the Board to act according to equity, good conscience, and the substantial merits of the case without regard to technicalities and legal forms. (In general terms, boards or tribunals are created precisely because they provide quicker, more informal, and less 'legalistic' proceedings.)

In WA, the Board is required to consider matters beyond the legislative requirements for involuntary status. It is to have regard primarily to the psychiatric condition of the person concerned and is to consider the medical and psychiatric history and the social circumstances of the person. In WA, there is no mandated legal representation, though as a matter of practice, all patients are advised of their right to legal representation and about the agency (the Mental Health Law Centre). It is still concerning, however, that even with full notification to patients of the availability of legal advice/representation, the percentage of involuntary patients reviewed without representation remains above 80 per cent.

The majority of involuntary patients (approximately 65 per cent) are taken off that status by their psychiatrist within the first 28 days of the order.

Of the patients reviewed by the Board, the rate of discharge of involuntary orders in Western Australia has declined since the Act commenced. In the first months following the introduction of the Act, the rate of discharge was 10 per cent. It has since steadily decreased and is now about 3–4 per cent.

Closer examination of mental health legislation in Victoria

As Stewart has indicated, mental health law in Australia varies from state to state. This example of the legislation in Victoria is provided by David Jones, a mental health nurse who works there.

Victoria in Australia has a similar Mental Health Act to that of the UK, with similar guidelines. The criteria for assessment and admission as an involuntary patient are basically the same, with the exception that it must be the least restrictive for the patient.

As Part 3, Division 2-8(e) of the 1986 Mental Health Act (MHA) states:

> The person cannot receive adequate treatment for the mental illness in a manner less restrictive of that person's freedom of decision and action.

This is a basic tenet that runs throughout the whole of the Act and is the standard in all circumstances. This does not preclude restrictive treatment, as need may demand this, but that it should be restrictive for the shortest time possible.

Within Victoria, to be placed on an involuntary section of the Mental Health Act a request must be made by an adult over the age of 18. A doctor conversant with the Mental Health Act then assesses the individual (for example a psychiatric registrar in an Emergency Department or working in the community). If they agree then a section of the 1986 MHA is commenced; this section lasts for 24 hours, at which point care may be provided in the following settings:

1) An appropriate care facility.

2) The community.

At any point within the 24 hours a psychiatrist should assess the patient and following that assessment determine the care to be provided.
The pathways are:

1) Becoming an involuntary patient in hospital (Section 12).

2) Becoming a voluntary (informal) patient within an inpatient unit.

3) Going to a Community Treatment Order (CTO) in the community.

4) No further follow-up is provided.

Section 12 is open ended, unlike in the UK where treatment sections tend to run for periods of up to six months, and are extendable. The consultant decides on the length of the section, taking into account the least restrictive principle. Independent of the treating team there is a review of the patient's care after eight weeks by the Mental Health Review Board as standard.

The Mental Health Review Board, much like the Mental Health Review Tribunal in the UK, is an independent body set up to review care and detention. The format is the same as in the UK – three members: a lay person, a psychiatrist, and a barrister.

One of the longer-standing tenets of the 1986 MHA is the Community Treatment Order (CTO), which has been implemented in the UK. Here it is one of the most used elements of the Act, insofar as the patient can be treated in their own home within the least restrictive environment available.

However, even though it is seen by professionals as less restrictive, patients still view it as an intrusion in their lives. It is up to the case manager who oversees the individual service plan (ISP) to be as inclusive of the patient's wants and needs as possible, as well as ensuring that care is within the dictates of the plan of treatment (i.e. medication regime, contact with services, and appointments). The idea of inclusion within the process is central to the patient's well-being, and although they can initially be resistive, a majority of patients see benefits in having a case manager to advocate for them.

There remain a proportion of patients who disengage from the service provided or become unwell within the community, and the ability to enforce treatment is then invoked. Either the case manager or the community team, supported by the police, can bring the individual to a community clinic or hospital for review. The psychiatrist then sees the client to assess what the best outcome is. This may be immediate treatment (increase or revision of medications), admission, closer contact (home treatment), or no change in the plan.

The system is not without its problems, and ethical concerns for case managers include coercion within a therapeutic relationship and dealing with clients' distress and potential aggression as a result of forced treatment. If a client is determined to avoid care they can travel to other states, as each state has its own Mental Health Act. There is a level of local agreement between states; however, this is assessed on an individual case-by-case basis. Each state's Mental Health Act is available online.

New Zealand mental health law overview

Robert and Francesca Tummey, who were until recently working as mental health nurses in Auckland, New Zealand, have provided an overview of the law for mental health nurses.

Mental Health (Compulsory Assessment and Treatment) Act 1992 (April 2000)

The New Zealand Mental Health Act (1992) (NZMHA) sets out the circumstances in which assessment and treatment can happen without an individual's consent. The degree of disorder must be such that it:

1) Poses a serious danger to the health or safety of that person or others, and

2) Seriously diminishes the capacity of that person to take care of himself or herself (including consideration of physical health).

New Zealand is bicultural, through integration of *Pākehā* (white European) and indigenous Māori people. Respect of cultural and personal rights is given high importance. Section 5(a) states 'there should be proper respect for the patient's cultural and ethnic identity…' A cultural assessment is a key component of the assessment process. Section 5(b) requires 'proper recognition for the person's family, community, tribe and family group.' Cultural advisors, elders, and interpreters (Section 6) should be consulted.

Duly authorized officers (DAOs) are the front-line operators of the Act and are appointed by Directors of Area Mental Health Services (DAMHS) responsible for the NZMHA in their area. The DAO is a competent, appropriately trained mental health professional whose role is an extension of their clinical duties. They must carry a current DAO identification card at all times.

Application (Section 8) can be made by any concerned individual aged over 18 who has seen the proposed patient in the last three days. Explanation of their relationship to the proposed patient and why they think the person has a mental disorder is necessary. A completed medical certificate is also required from a medical doctor who has seen the proposed patient in the last three days and believes them to have a mental disorder. Application is received by the DAMHS or by the DAO on behalf of the DAMHS.

Once an application is made the individual becomes a 'proposed patient' and the DAO will make the necessary arrangements for assessment. Police assistance can be requested (Section 41) to take the proposed patient to a nominated place for examination. An expert doctor as approved by the DAMHS must carry out the assessment (Section 9). Proposal for assessment must be in writing and issued in the presence of the proposed patient's support or family member. The proposed patient must attend the assessment and cannot refuse.

The expert doctor will issue a certificate for treatment for five days (Section 11) if assessment concludes that the patient is mentally disordered at that time. Patients have the right to ask a judge to review this decision if they do not agree.

Treatment can happen in hospital or a stated place in the community. Before the five day period ends the patient will be assessed to see if they must continue with compulsory treatment. If so, a certificate is issued for a further 14 days (Section 13). The patient is given a written copy of their rights and their rights are monitored by the Review Tribunal and District Inspectors. If deemed necessary, the medical team can apply to a judge to extend the treatment to a Community Treatment Order (Section 29) or Inpatient Treatment Order (Section 30) for six months.

Law and human beings

Having reviewed some of the mental health law that will be relevant to you in your practice, we wanted to remind you of the human cost that mental health law can sometimes impose. The extract on p. 62 is written from a carer's perspective by a blogger who calls herself 'Mr Man's Wife.'

👤 Carer's Story: Sectioned

It was a Sunday morning. I awoke earlier than usual, not having slept very well after being woken during the night by Mr Man repeatedly banging his head on the pillow in an attempt to get the voices to stop. He had been discharged from hospital five months earlier, but the medication he was taking seemed to have less and less effect on his symptoms as time went on. It had been decided some time ago that Mr Man would be admitted into hospital to start treatment of Clozaril (clozapine), but he was still on the waiting list for 'the Clozaril bed'.

Despite a growing history of self-harm, suicide attempts, and psychosis, Mr Man still had no care plan in place, no CPN, and no care coordinator. When I realized how bad the voices were getting, I didn't know what else to do except call the usual 'out-of-hours' doctor's surgery. I explained that Mr Man was waiting to be admitted for treatment with Clozaril, but that in the meantime his condition was deteriorating quite badly. The doctor agreed that I should bring him in to be seen.

The problem was that although Mr Man had previously agreed to go into hospital to start his treatment of Clozaril, whilst waiting to be admitted his symptoms had deteriorated to the point that now he was confused as to whether he was really ill or not. Mr Man refused to get up. To begin with I thought this was merely part of the ongoing problem I had with getting Mr Man to do anything, because of the negative symptoms of his schizophrenia. I called the surgery to explain. I was sure that the doctor wouldn't understand and would think I was wasting his time, but he suggested I try again. Mr Man still wouldn't get up, but this time it became clear to me that it was because he didn't want to be seen by a doctor, rather than just not wanting to get up. This worried me even more because I knew from experience that once Mr Man had lost the insight that he was ill, his delusions would take hold and there would be no reasoning with him. I called the surgery again to cancel the appointment. I felt so helpless. The doctor must have discerned the anxiety in my voice and he threw me a line.

'Are you saying he is refusing to be seen by a doctor?'

Something in the tone of his voice told me what he was thinking.

'Yes,' I replied.

'Are you concerned that he could be a danger to himself?' he asked.

'Yes,' I replied, and I went on to explain that that was why I was so worried; because the voices were worsening and they often tell him to harm himself.

I was so relieved and so grateful when he said he would arrange a home visit for Mr Man to be assessed. Mr Man was a bit sulky with me about that, but once the doctor arrived he agreed to go downstairs to be seen by him. After discussing his symptoms with him, the doctor asked Mr Man if he would go into hospital voluntarily, but he refused. The doctor asked me if I agreed that Mr Man needed to go into hospital, and I did, so arrangements were made for a psychiatrist and a social worker to attend.

Mr Man's mother visited us that day, which had been prearranged earlier in the week. She was obviously confused by the presence of strangers in our home, so I took her into the kitchen and explained what was happening. She was overcome with emotion at the thought of her son being taken into hospital against his will, but for me – as someone who had needed to hide knives and blades, and constantly reassure Mr Man that he doesn't have to slice himself open when the voices tell him to, and that no harm will come to him or me for not doing it – having him 'sectioned' seemed far less traumatic than the thought of his condition deteriorating further.

The whole process was very drawn out with much waiting around, firstly for the appropriate people to attend and then for an ambulance to take Mr Man to the hospital. From the time I called the surgery to the time Mr Man was finally admitted took about 12 hours. During that time Mr Man was anxious but quiet. He didn't argue, and he didn't struggle. He was resolute that he didn't want to go to hospital, but he seemed to have resigned himself to the fact that he would have to. There was no drama, and apart from that edgy feeling of expectation when you're waiting for something to happen, the day was quite boring. I was relieved when the day was over and Mr Man was safely on the ward, although leaving him on the ward was never easy for me.

Mr Man's Wife

http://the-wife-of-a-schizophrenic.blogspot.com/

Reproduced with kind permission of Mr Man's wife.

Summary

In this chapter you have been introduced to mental health law. We have sought to provide you with an overview of mental health law in England and Wales and this is the law that we refer to throughout the rest of the book. Alongside this we have included reviews of mental health law in Scotland, Northern Ireland, Australia, and New Zealand, and for any mental health nursing students working in these countries it may be useful to compare the main issues presented. Common factors in mental health law appear to be an increased effort to provide the least restrictive environment for care delivery and seeking to maintain mental health service users' rights. However, as our carers' contributions demonstrate, this is not always achieved.

In the rest of the book you will be introduced to clinical scenarios, with actors portraying events based on mental health service users' experiences. Some of the scenarios refer to elements of the Mental Health Act and this will be English and Welsh law only. As a student nurse it is likely that you will need to return to this chapter as you progress through this book to remind yourself of aspects of mental health law. We have also placed additional resources and learning materials in the online resource:

www.oxfordtextbooks.co.uk/orc/clarke

and choose the online resources for this chapter. We hope you find this a useful resource that you return to many times.

References and other sources

References

Barker P (2005). **The tidal model: A guide for mental health professionals**. Brunner-Routledge, Hove.

Barker P and Davidson B, eds (1998). **Psychiatric nursing: Ethical strife**. Arnold, London.

Coppock V and Hopton J (2000). **Critical perspectives on mental health**. Routledge, London.

Department of Health (1994). **The Butterworth report**. DH, London.

Department of Health (2007). **Government welcomes passing of Mental Health Bill as vital to community care**. DH, London [online] <http://nds.coi.gov.uk/environment/mediaDetail.asp?MediaDetailsID=2081 40&NewsAreaID=2&ClientID=46&LocaleID=2> accessed 13/05/2008.

Fenton G, Deane E, Herron S, et al. (1995). **The Brian Doherty inquiry**. Western Health and Social Services Board, Derry.

Jones R (2007). **Mental Health Act manual**, 10th edition. Sweet and Maxwell, London.

Mental Health Alliance (2007). **Mental Health Bill remains a missed opportunity for humane and progressive legislation, says Alliance**. [MIND online press release, July] <http://www.mind.org.uk/News+policy+campaigns/Press/MHA030707.htm> accessed 13/05/2008.

National Institute for Mental Health in England/ Sainsbury Centre for Mental Health Joint Workforce Support Unit/National Health Service University (2004). **The 10 essential shared capabilities for mental health**. Department of Health, London.

NHS Scotland (2008). **The National Framework for pre-registration mental health nursing in Scotland**. NHS Education for Scotland, Edinburgh.

Nolan P (1998). **A history of mental health nursing**. Stanley Thornes, Cheltenham.

Rogers A and Pilgrim D (2001). **Mental health policy in Britain: a critical introduction**. Macmillan, London.

Scottish Executive (2006). **Rights, relationships and recovery: The report of the National Review of Mental Health Nursing in Scotland**. Scottish Executive, Edinburgh.

○ Useful web links

Pam Pinder's website: 'Carers, experts by experience'
http://www.pamshouse.pwp.blueyonder.co.uk/

England and Wales
Department of Health (Mental Health Act)
http://www.dh.gov.uk/en/Healthcare/
NationalServiceFrameworks/Mentalhealth/
DH_063423

Mental Capacity Act – Summary
http://www.dca.gov.uk/menincap/bill-summary.
htm#keyprinciples

Mental Health Alliance
http://www.mentalhealthalliance.org.uk/aboutus/
index.html

Office of the Public Guardian
http://www.publicguardian.gov.uk/index.htm

Scotland

National Programme for Mental Health and Wellbeing
http://www.wellscotland.info/index.html

Scottish Recovery Network
http://www.scottishrecovery.net/content/

The Tidal Model
http://www.tidal-model.com

The Mental Welfare Commission
http://www.mwcscot.org.uk/home/home

Australia

Website of the Western Australia Mental Health Law Centre
http://www.mhlcwa.org.au/

Website of the Victorian State Government Mental Health Services
http://www.health.vic.gov.au/mentalhealth

Website of the Western Australia Mental Health Review Board
http://www.mhrbwa.org.au/

New Zealand

New Zealand mental health information
http://www.likeminds.org.nz/

New Zealand Ministry of Health, Guidelines for the Role and Function of Duly Authorised Officers under the Mental Health Act (Compulsory Assessment and Treatment) Act 1992 (April 2000)
http://www.moh.govt.nz/mha.html

Treaty of Waitangi (Bicultural founding document)
http://www.nzhistory.net.nz/category/tid/133

Useful resources: Northern Ireland

Department of Health and Social Services (1986). *The Mental Health (Northern Ireland) Order 1986: A Guide.* DHSS, Belfast.

Department of Health and Social Services (1992). *Mental Health (Northern Ireland) Order 1986: Code of practice.* HMSO, Belfast.

Department of Health and Social Services (1996) *The discharge from hospital (or prison) and the continuing care in the community of mentally disordered people who are thought could represent a future risk to themselves or others.* DHSS, Belfast.

○ Further reading

Australian Government (1986). *The Mental Health Act, Victoria*. Reprint No. 7.

Bowen P (2008). *Blackstone's Guide to the Mental Health Act 2007*. Oxford University Press, Oxford.

Brown W and Kandirikirira N (2007). *Recovering mental health in Scotland. Report on narrative investigation of mental health recovery in Scotland*. Scottish Recovery Network, Glasgow.

Fennel P (2007). *Mental health: The new law*. Jordan's Publishing, Bristol.

Jones R (2008). *Mental Capacity Act manual*. Sweet and Maxwell, London.

Chapter 4
Community mental health nursing care of a person with complex needs

Victoria Clarke and Andrew Walsh

Learning outcomes

This chapter will assist you to:

- Demonstrate understanding of how a recovery approach might be used in practice with a person such as Anthony.
- Demonstrate awareness of the evidence base for the care given to a person with complex needs.
- Understand how care is planned and priorities set for a person such as Anthony.
- Consider the importance of good links with service users and their carers.
- Examine an example of holistic care planning taking into account relevant risk factors.
- Recognize the role of mental health nurses in improving a person's physical health care.
- Identify the effects that social exclusion may have upon a person and consider the role of the mental health nurse in helping to promote inclusion.

Introduction

In this chapter we will consider the care of a person living in the community with complex needs. In the past, the majority of people who suffered from severe and enduring mental health problems would almost certainly have spent their lives living in institutionalized care. Today, the majority of people with such problems live in the community, and the issue of how well (or not) they are supported is a critical one for those working as part of a community mental health team.

In this chapter we introduce 'Anthony', a service user who has a long history of mental health problems. Anthony lives alone, and apart from his brother David, he has little contact with other people. Anthony has been referred to mental health services following a long period in which he has been having a **depot injection** from the nurse at his GP's surgery. He has a complex range of problems including harassment from local youths, possible physical ill health, and housing problems, as well as a deterioration in his mental health state.

Institutions and community care

In the UK, the move from hospital-based care towards a more community-oriented model is a relatively recent one. Many of the care practices and attitudes you may encounter today have their roots in an institutionalized model.

From the 1840s onwards a system of 'lunatic asylums' was developed, the intention being that these should provide a humane and morally disciplined environment for those identified as needing care for mental health problems. They were often linked to county asylums and workhouses and became associated in the public view with both poverty and 'madness'. For ordinary people at this time of great industrial and social change, working conditions were harsh and the asylum policy was intended to provide a degree of social control (Rogers and Pilgrim 2001). A popular ditty of the time illustrates some of the prevailing attitudes:

> Outside the lunatic asylum, I was there and I was breaking stones,
> When up popped a lunatic and said to me 'Good morning Mr Jones,
> How much a week do you get for doing that?'
> 'Sixteen shillings' I cried,
> 'That's not enough to keep a wife and six kids,
> Step inside you silly fella, step inside'.
> (Anon)

As interest in psychiatry evolved, there were developments in both theory and practice, and some changes occurred through new knowledge and ways of thinking about neurology, psychology, and psychoanalysis. Many major shifts and breakthroughs came about via conflict and trauma; the world wars led to significant examinations of mental problems, like 'shell shock' and neuroses, and the work of people like Bion and Foulkes on groups and therapeutic communities emerged following World War I (Harrison and Clarke 1992). When mental hospitals became the responsibility of the National Health Service (NHS Act 1946, incorporated 1948) there was a desire to see change. Inpatient populations were still growing but by 1960, with the work of people like Goffman (1987), 'asylums' and institutional care were being challenged and increasingly perceived as damaging and unhelpful. Government policy of the time started to refer to moving care into the community, but it wasn't until Margaret Thatcher's government of the 1980s implemented NHS reforms and community care policies that mental health services really felt an impact.

From the middle of the 1980s the closure of large psychiatric hospitals began with the replacement of service provision shifting to a system of community-based care. This was partly because it was thought that this would be a cheaper system, but also because prevailing government philosophy held that mental health patients would become 'consumers' of this care, and market forces would hopefully drive change for the better (Nolan 1992).

Community care policy was thrown into crisis by a series of tragic incidents, culminating in the death in 1992 of the musician Jonathon Zito following an attack by a mental health service user called Christopher Clunis. The subsequent inquiry (HMSO 1994) highlighted failures in community mental health care, including poor communication and missed opportunities to properly care for Mr Clunis. A significant factor was lack of resources; staff were doing their best to cope within an overstretched and badly designed system.

Student activity 1

Read the extracts in the box below and consider what image of mental health care or service users reports such as these give?
When you read newspaper articles about people with mental illness, pay particular attention to the language they use and compare it to the style of writing used by charities and academics, such as in the excerpts below.

There is an ongoing debate surrounding the rights of people who have mental health problems. In England and Wales the *National Service Framework for mental health* (Department of Health 1999) states that:

> Any service user who contacts their primary health care team with a common mental health problem should:
> - have their mental health needs identified and assessed
> - be offered effective treatments, including referral to specialist services for further assessment, treatment and care if they require it.

'FEARS are growing over the number of murders by mentally ill offenders. It comes as new research reveals that "stranger killings", often by mentally unstable people, have quadrupled in the last 30 years.'
Perry (2004) writing in the *Sunday Express*.

'Homicides involving psychotics remain constant despite heightened fears about the effects of cuts in the number of NHS beds and a series of chilling murders…'
Timmins (1996) writing in *The Independent*.

'The vast majority of violent crime and homicides are committed by people who do not have mental health problems. In fact, 95 per cent of homicides are committed by people who have not been diagnosed with a mental health problem.

Contrary to popular belief, the incidence of homicide by people diagnosed with mental health problems has stayed at a fairly constant level since the 1990s at between 50 and 60 a year.'

MIND (2006)

'The *Confidential enquiry into homicides and suicides*' shows that serious mental disorders are rare, and affect only four out of every 1000 adults. Serious violence is even more rare – there are between 600 and 700 homicides each year, but few of them are carried out by people with mental health problems.

The enquiry, which took place over a period of 33 months, identified only 39 homicides in England by people in contact with specialist mental health services in the previous year (between five and six per cent of all homicides).'

Royal College of Psychiatrists (1996)
From http://www.mind.org.uk.

In 2004, the *British Medical Journal* published a study that concluded:

'Stranger homicides have increased in the recent years, but the increase is not the result of homicides by mentally ill people and therefore the "care in the community" policy. Stranger homicides are more likely to be related to alcohol or drug misuse by young men.'

BMJ (2004) **328**, 734-37 (27 March)

Standard Three adds that they should be able to make round the clock contact with 'local services necessary to meet their needs and receive adequate care.'

Furthermore, Standard Six states that people caring for a mental health service user should have an assessment of their own physical and mental health needs as well as their own written care plan (Department of Health 1999).

It has been suggested that while service users are now much more likely to be involved in service planning (Commission for Health Improvement 2003) there remains a culture of coercive treatment. Furthermore, this treatment is likely to be oriented towards a medical model, despite suggestions that people often see their problems differently

(Sainsbury Centre for Mental Health 2005). Others have highlighted the effects of social exclusion and discrimination in denying access to opportunities that most people would consider to be a right (Repper and Perkins 2003). A study of service user experiences with clear relevance to Anthony's situation (Read and Baker 1996) found that as well as suffering high levels of abuse, 26 per cent of those surveyed had actually moved home to escape harassment. You may wish to reflect upon how community mental health service users are treated; for example, to what extent do they and the team agree about both the cause of their difficulties and any proposed strategies to help? Also, do service users you meet feel that they are working in partnership with services or are services imposed upon them?

Clinical scenario: Anthony

In this chapter you will meet Anthony and his brother David following Anthony's referral to mental health services. You will find it useful to read the scenario first and then access the brief films that show both Anthony and his brother talking about the situation.

Anthony's story

Anthony is a 45-year-old man who lives alone in a rented flat in an inner city area. He was diagnosed

as suffering from schizophrenia when he was a young man and has had many previous admissions to psychiatric hospitals. He has been receiving a depot injection from the practice nurse at his GP's surgery for several years and has remained relatively stable throughout this time. He does not mix well with other people and at times lets himself become a little neglected. Anthony often appears to be hearing voices although he denies this; on occasions he hints to the practice nurse that the Internet is trying to control him.

Anthony has never worked and spends his time either alone in his flat or in the local library where he goes and spends most of his mornings, although recently he has been complaining that blurred vision is making it difficult to read the newspapers there. Anthony is quite overweight, smokes very heavily, and eats a diet that consists mostly of junk food; he often complains of feeling hungry and gets very thirsty, despite drinking nearly three litres of Coca-Cola and several pints of water on most days.

Because of the medication he has been taking over the past 20 years, Anthony has developed tardive dyskinesia and this makes him pull odd facial expressions. He also has a degree of akasthisia and he is often restless. Anthony often feels tired and listless, which he blames on his medication, although recently his sleep has been disturbed by the need to pass water several times a night as well as more frequently during the day.

Anthony's most important source of support has been his brother, David, who although not living nearby tries to keep a bit of an eye on him and offers extra help when he needs it. He has a school friend who has kept in touch with him and who visits occasionally but apart from this he has no other social contacts.

For several months Anthony has been having problems with local youths who have spotted him in the street and begun tormenting him by calling after him and throwing things; they have now started hammering on his door and running away. Anthony has been quite upset at this treatment and his brother has noticed that he has been becoming more anxious, withdrawn, and suspicious of other people.

One day, David is contacted by Anthony's landlord to say that other tenants of the block of flats have been complaining because he has been shouting and banging till late at night in his flat; also that people are concerned about his unkempt appearance and the fact he has been throwing rubbish out of his flat window. The landlord hints that he may try and force Anthony to move out of his flat if things don't settle down soon. Anthony's friend has also said that he showed him a toy gun that Anthony was intending to use to threaten the people who were tormenting him.

Anthony told his brother that he didn't think life was worth living any more, and David, understandably upset by this, went to Anthony's GP's surgery and told her about all of this; it was at this point that a referral for assessment was made to the local community mental health team.

You can see film of Anthony and his brother at:

http://www.oxfordtextbooks.co.uk/orc/clarke

and choose the video link.

'Typical medication'

As you can see from the scenario, Anthony has been receiving an injection from the practice nurse at the GP's surgery. A 'depot' is an intramuscular injection, the effects of which usually last between two and four weeks, the advantage of this being that people don't have to remember to take lots of tablets (see Box 4.1). Unfortunately, this kind of medication has a range of unpleasant side effects and long-term problems (see Box 4.2). Did you notice any of these features when you looked at the film of Anthony?

> Student activity 2
> *Before you read through Anthony's bio-psycho-social assessment, you may want to review the material in Chapter 2 on assessment.*

Drug	UK trade name
Flupentixol decanoate (flupenthixol decanoate)	Depixol
Fluphenazine decanoate	Modecate
Haloperidol decanoate	Haldol decanoate
Pipotiazine palmitate (pipothiazine palmitate)	Piportil Depot
Zuclopenthixol decanoate	Clopixol
Risperidone	Risperdal
Depot injections typically used in people identified as suffering from schizophrenia.	

Box 4.1 Typical medication

Tardive dyskinesia

Dry mouth

Blurred vision

Flushing

Urinary retention

Constipation

Ejaculatory inhibition

Impotence

Dizziness

Unsteadiness

Muscle spasms and stiffness – may include torticollis (spasms in head and neck) or oculogyric crisis (where a person's eyes roll up painfully).

'Parkinson's'-type symptoms – i.e. limb rigidity, tremor, expressionless face, and shuffling gait.

Akasthisia – restlessness, agitated movements, person often feels uneasy and anxious.

Box 4.2 Some typical side effects/long-term problems

👥 Assessment by CPN

We are going to show you a typical assessment profile for Anthony; this is based on conversation with Anthony as well as information provided by his brother David and a letter received from the practice nurse at the GP's surgery (see Figure 4.1).

> **Student activity 3**
> As you read through the practice nurse's letter and Anthony's assessment profile, consider the following questions:
>
> - Do you agree with the content?
> - Is there anything else you think should be considered?
> - What sort of additional observations would you make?
> - Are there any questions that you would ask of Anthony, David, and/or the practice nurse?

Please note that the authors would encourage you to adopt a critical and analytical approach to all of this; we don't expect that you will agree with everything we have written and we know that other CPNs will have different ways of approaching this. Your task as a student nurse is to think about what makes sense to you and consider why. Now, bearing the above in mind, read through the assessment profiles as you watch the interviews with Anthony and David on the website.

Psychological

Thinking

Patterns of thought: Anthony is demonstrating some negative and disjointed thinking. His thoughts seem to be distressing to him. He seems to be wary and suspicious.

Beliefs: Anthony has said he is misunderstood by his neighbours but wants to protect them. It is, though, important to stress that Anthony may be expressing delusional ideas about both his neighbours and the Internet.

Self-concept: Anthony demonstrates a mixture of both positive and negative notions of self. On the positive side he is motivated and engaged with the news, the Internet, and DIY; negatively, he is lonely and isolated.

Self-esteem: Anthony's self-esteem appears to be quite low. He has stated that 'life is not worth living any more.'

Self-awareness: Anthony lacks awareness of appropriate activities. For example, he has taken to carrying a toy gun with him and appears unaware of the dangers this presents. Anthony also pays less attention than necessary to his personal hygiene and appearance at times.

Dear Mental Health Team,

RE: Mr Anthony Harris

Anthony has been a patient of this surgery for the last 5 years and I have been seeing him to administer his injection (Depixol 200mg every 2 weeks).

He has a long history of Psychiatric care and treatment having been admitted to Bilberry Moor Hall Hospital 4 times since the age of 16 where he was diagnosed as suffering from Paranoid schizophrenia.

In recent years he has appeared to be fairly well on each occasion that he was seen, although he does sometimes look like he may be hearing voices and has hinted to me that he may be worried about the internet in some way.

We have been telephoned by his half-brother (David) who has become concerned about his brother's welfare. On visiting Anthony he does seem to have deteriorated somewhat, he is unkempt (more so than is usual), agitated and his flat is in a state of disarray.

He appears to be obsessed with the internet and has delusional ideas about local people who he feels are persecuting him. Apparently, the neighbours have actually complained to the landlord about his recent behaviour in which he has been shouting and banging in the flat and threw rubbish from the window into the shared courtyard.

It might be worthwhile you having a word with Anthony's brother who is complaining that there has been insufficient help and support given to his brother.
Once again, most grateful for your assistance,

Pat Raven RGN,
Practice Nurse.

Figure 4.1 Referral letter

Personal autonomy and capacity: Anthony has told his friend that he has taken to carrying a toy gun, intending to threaten people who he feels are threatening him. This may suggest that Anthony's capacity to respond appropriately in dangerous situations is compromised.

Feeling

Anthony's mood seems to indicate feelings of hopelessness, sadness, isolation, rejection, and loneliness. He can also be suspicious. He may appear quick-tempered and irritable at times.

Sensory perception

Touch, smell: Nothing unusual in these areas.

Taste: Anthony has indicated an increased thirst.

Vision: Anthony is currently experiencing blurred vision.

Hearing: There is evidence that Anthony may be hearing hallucinatory voices as reported by his practice nurse.

Reality

Anthony's awareness of time, place, and person appears to be appropriate.

Behaviours

Content of speech: Anthony's speech is focused on his felt problems; he mainly speaks about his problems with his physical symptoms and being bothered by local youths. He has stated that 'life is not worth living any more.'

Pace of speech: Anthony's speech is quite rapid at times and is sometimes difficult to understand.

Tone of speech: A little monotonous at times.

Volume of speech: Anthony's speech can be loud, particularly when he is talking about very important issues for him.

Flow of speech: Speech is sometimes disjointed, jumping between subject areas.

Proximity: Anthony remained seated during the interview.

Facial expression: Sometimes 'strange and bizarre' (grimaces at times).

Eye contact/movement: Anthony appears to engage with people well. He has good eye contact that is non-confrontational. When distressed he seems to avoid eye contact and when angry appears to stare.

Movements: Anthony exhibits some restlessness. There is evidence of tremor in both hands.

Social

Social and familial networks

Mother committed suicide when he was young. Anthony's half-brother David believes he was resented and blamed by his stepmother and says that he had a difficult early life. Anthony has occasional contact with an old school friend and his half-sister. Although David does not live locally he has regular contact with Anthony and is 'most important' to him. Anthony feels lonely and misunderstood by his neighbours but wants to 'protect them'.

Employment and engagement in meaningful activities

Anthony visits the library most mornings; he enjoys DIY at home in his flat. He has never held a full-time job.

Finance

It appears that Anthony is in receipt of Disability Living Allowance, which enables him to purchase food, drink, and cigarettes for his personal use and to cover his monthly rent (although it is important to confirm this).

Housing

Anthony lives in a rented flat within the inner city. He shares the outside courtyard space with his neighbours. The flat contains only the most basic amenities and is otherwise sparsely furnished. Anthony's landlord is currently threatening to evict him because of his behaviour; other tenants have been complaining about his shouting and banging till late at night.

Interests

Anthony's identified interests are the Internet and DIY. He demonstrates an interest in the news and frequently uses the local library to read newspapers.

Physical

Current and past physical problems

Anthony states that he is often thirsty, is passing urine a great deal (more than usual), has a disturbed sleep pattern, and has blurred vision.

Current treatment for physical health conditions

He is not receiving any treatment for his physical health conditions currently.

Lifestyle issues relating to physical well-being

There are several lifestyle issues for Anthony at present. Anthony's diet consists predominantly of junk or fast foods; he drinks large amounts of (full sugar) fizzy drinks. Anthony also smokes at least 20 cigarettes per day. He does not take exercise although he frequently walks to his local library. At times, when his mental health deteriorates, Anthony neglects his personal hygiene.

Physical activity

Uses public transport and walks daily to the local public library (distance of journey unknown).

Pharmacist's view

Does the dose of flupentixol decanoate (Depixol) need to be increased? He has 200 mg every two weeks, but the dose could be increased to 300 mg – the usual maximum dose. (Some patients require up to 400 mg a week.)

Anthony has tardive dyskinesia, as shown by his facial movements. The severity should be carefully assessed, as it is potentially irreversible. The association between this side effect and antipsychotic drug use means that the lowest possible dose should be used. Tetrabenazine tablets could be given to treat the tardive dyskinesia.

The **antimuscarinic** drugs procyclidine, orphenadrine, and trihexyphenidyl (Benzhexol) do not improve tardive dyskinesia and may make it worse. They may be used to treat other drug-induced **extrapyramidal symptoms** such as tremor, akathisia, and dystonia (abnormal face and body movements). Anthony has signs of tremor in both hands.

If the screen for diabetes shows that he has the disease, would it be better to change to risperidone injection, which is less likely to exacerbate or cause diabetes? Though Anthony may not want to have a different type of injection.

A useful reference that includes the BNF (British National Formulary) and other information on drugs and evidence-based reviews is:

http://www.library.nhs.uk.

Service user's view

Anthony

What Anthony says about himself describes very well what the experience of mental distress is like: he is very conscious of the loneliness and isolation, about people seeing him as strange, and about how the neighbours and local children react to him. He feels very deeply that people don't understand him, no one understands what it is like to be him, and is clearly distressed by that thought.

It would be too easy to dismiss what he is saying as nonsense, arising from paranoia and the symptoms of whatever diagnosis he has been given (if any). But perhaps he is giving clues as to what might help to alleviate his distress. What can be validated about what he says? Research does suggest that the use of mobile phones may in time cause damage to the brain; it is not illogical for Anthony to 'wonder' (he does not allege) whether the use of the Internet can be harmful.

Anthony does not appear to know that there may be service user groups in his area where he could go to talk to people who are experiencing similar problems.

David

What David says about his brother is a very good illustration of how important it is for practitioners to take the carer perspective into account and to value it. He has thought quite constructively about what his brother's problems might have stemmed from and is himself quite distressed at not being able to access help promptly and effectively for Anthony. He can see quite clearly how things will deteriorate if Anthony is not given help.

He is also distressed about the behaviour of the local children and at not being able to do anything about his brother being stigmatized for being different.

Marion Clark, service user

Sexual health

Anthony has no current partner – no issues were addressed in this area at this time.

Smoking

Anthony is described as a 'heavy' smoker.

Use of prescribed and non-prescribed drugs

Attends for his fortnightly depot injection of Depixol 200 mg. No current knowledge of illicit drug or alcohol use.

Side effects of current or previous medication

Anthony demonstrates some restlessness in his movements as well as tremor; at times his facial expressions can be 'strange'.

Significant histories of family illness

Mother committed suicide when Anthony was a young boy – history and background to this currently unknown.

Current nutritional status

While Anthony appears overweight, his diet indicates that his nutritional status is poor.

Spiritual

Religious and/or spiritual needs and beliefs

Currently unknown

Risk

Risk of Self-harm

Anthony is currently stating that he feels 'life is not worth living anymore.'

Risk of self-neglect

When Anthony's mental state deteriorates, as it has currently, he neglects his hygiene and appearance.

Abuse from others

A gang of local youths are 'harassing' him whenever he goes out and also 'hammering' on his door.

Violence to others

Anthony is now carrying a toy gun; he has told his friend he is intending to threaten the people who are intimidating him.

Current physical, sexual, or emotional abuse

Currently being 'abused' by a local gang of youths, who are physically threatening. Also potentially now by neighbours seeking his eviction.

Past physical, sexual, or emotional abuse

David, Anthony's half-brother, indicates that his stepmother blamed and resented Anthony and he had a difficult early life.

Need for safeguarding children

Unclear status regarding 'gang of local youths.'

Substance misuse

Identify current, recent, and past use of prescribed and non-prescribed drugs

Current prescription Depixol 200 mg fortnightly via intramuscular injection; otherwise no evidence or known past history of substance misuse.

Carers

Identify any carers

Some elements of caring from practice nurse. Closest to his half-brother David, who lives some distance away. Also has occasional contact with half-sister.

Assessment summary

The assessment profile clearly focuses on Anthony's view of his needs and the most important issues for him, but at the same time has to consider any risks from the situation and Anthony's bio-psycho-social state and behaviour. This leads nurses to identify specific priorities for care in negotiation and partnership with Anthony.

Anthony's care plan

Risk

Service User Need/Problem	Goals	Care Plan
1. Possible self-harm. Anthony has said that 'life isn't worth living any more.'	**Short-term goals** Maintain Anthony's safety, contract agreed with Anthony that he will not self-harm but will follow crisis plan. **Long-term goals** Anthony will have renewed sense of hope and purpose in life.	Ascertain intent, plan (if any), previous attempts, and possible methods. Agree a crisis response plan with Anthony (see below). To promote recovery, encourage Anthony to develop support networks and strategies enabling him to anticipate problems and to respond in a more appropriate manner to his difficulties. **Rationale:** *Complies with Standards 1 and 7 of the National Service Framework for Mental Health (Department of Health 1999).*
2. Self-neglect. Anthony's hygiene and appearance worsen as his mental health deteriorates.	**Short-term goals** Anthony will bathe/shower at least every other day. Anthony will change his clothes at least every other day.	Contractually agree to goals with Anthony. CPN to ensure that Anthony has access to wash his clothing and that his bathroom facilities are appropriate to his needs. **Rationale:** *Complies with duty of care requirements, Nursing and Midwifery Council (2004).*
3. Abuse from others – see social care plan.		
4. Risk of violence to others. Anthony has been reported to have started carrying a toy gun with which he intends to threaten the people who are intimidating him.	**Short-term goals** Anthony will cease to carry the toy gun and will dispose of it in an appropriate place. **Long-term goals** Anthony will recognize the inappropriateness of carrying toy weapons and develop alternative approaches to perceived threats.	CPN to explain danger of using a toy gun, which could be seen as a 'real gun' by the people threatening him or by the police. CPN to discuss potentially fatal implications of this. **Rationale:** *Complies with legal requirements, Nursing and Midwifery Council (2004) Code of Professional Conduct, and risk management required by the Department of Health (1991 onwards) in accord with the Care Programme Approach.*

Anthony's crisis response plan

Anthony has stated that he feels 'life is not worth living any more.' The CPN will need to work with Anthony on agreeing what action both parties will take in the event that Anthony feels he is likely to endanger himself in any way.

Personal actions that the CPN could discuss with Anthony

- Relaxation strategies – deep breathing techniques, guided fantasy, muscle tensing/relaxing routine.
- Listening to music.
- Taking a walk, a bath, or a shower.
- Phoning family/friends for support.
- Access possible support from service users/survivors websites.
- Phone CPN's office line and indicate to secretarial support that some contact would be helpful.

A specific time limit needs to be agreed between Anthony and his CPN. For example if Anthony does ring the office the CPN may agree that they will contact him within three hours (See Hostick et al. 1997).

If Anthony does not feel in control after employing these strategies he will need to take the following action:

- Contact CPN on mobile telephone number and ask for support. CPN needs to identify specific contact number that will require an urgent response.
- In the event that the CPN is unavailable, for example out of hours, Anthony will contact crisis intervention/home treatment team – again, CPN needs to identify a specific number to ring for an urgent response.
- In a situation where Anthony feels unable to wait for help to get to him, he should be advised to access his GP, and in an emergency when the GP is closed, his local Accident and Emergency Services.

Social

Service User Need/Problem	Goals	Care Plan
1. To resolve current difficulties with neighbours and landlord.	**Short-term goals** For local neighbourhood officer to assist in conflict resolution. **Long-term goals** For Anthony to feel socially included within his neighbourhood.	CPN to liaise with local neighbourhood office. Organize a meeting with residents. Seek to get a housing officer allocated to Anthony's case. CPN to provide mental health awareness-raising and education at residents' meetings. CPN to attend residents' meetings with Anthony to provide him with support and encourage him to develop friendships with neighbours. CPN to access local service user groups and encourage Anthony to engage with these where appropriate.
2. To reduce risk of harassment and abuse that Anthony is experiencing from a gang of local youths.	**Short-term goals** For Anthony to receive specific assistance from an appointed social worker as a vulnerable adult.	CPN to make urgent referral on Anthony's behalf for a social worker to be appointed to his case.

Service User Need/Problem	Goals	Care Plan
	For local police to monitor situation and make increased 'safe and well' checks.	CPN to work with police community liaison officer to make them aware of the situation and enlist their support in making regular 'safe and well' checks.
	Long-term goals For Anthony to feel safe in his own home.	If prescribed care fails to resolve difficulties, housing officer and social worker may need to collaborate on re-housing Anthony.

The rationale for adopting this approach includes professional, ethical, and policy requirements for the mental health nurse, as well as service user direction in beginning the recovery process. Specific policy drivers include:

- The NMC (2004) and NSF Standard 1 for Mental Health (Department of Health 1999).
- National Institute for Mental Health in England (2004). 'Principle XI – Community involvement as defined by the user of service is central to the recovery process.'
- NHSU (2005). 'Working in Partnership: developing and maintaining constructive working relationships with service users, carers, families, colleagues, lay people and wider community networks. Working positively with any tensions created by conflicts of interest or aspiration that may arise between the partners in care. Challenging inequality: addressing the causes and consequences of stigma, discrimination, social inequality and exclusion on service users, carers and mental health services. Creating, developing or maintaining valued social roles for people in the communities they come from.'
- Department of Health (2006). 'Psycho-social care – Promote mental health and well being, enabling people to recover from debilitating mental health experiences and/or achieve their full potential, supporting them to develop and maintain social networks and relationships.'

See also Piipo J and Aaltonen J (2004). Also, see discussion point below.

● Discussion point: Social inclusion

We debated whether it was appropriate and realistic to include the community mental health nurse in meeting the residents in Anthony's community to raise their awareness of mental health issues. One major concern was the issue of whether this strategy could compromise Anthony's confidentiality. We agreed that any such approach must be carried out with sensitivity to Anthony's rights and wishes at all times. One of the options we considered was that a CPN uninvolved with Anthony's direct care should take on the responsibility for promoting social inclusion and reducing stigma by providing the local community with mental health education; this would avoid any links being made to Anthony's association with mental health services. We also considered whether this type of education should be taken on by community mental health nurses in any circumstances, because of their caseload pressures and requirements from their employing trusts to be involved in the delivery of service user care, not education of local communities.

We also discussed whether this is actually part of the community mental health nurse's role, or whether it should be referred to a social worker as an aspect of social care, not health. Eventually we agreed to disagree. There are clear policy guidelines and very specific drivers that indicate that the Department of Health and a range of government organizations have definite expectations that this aspect of promoting social inclusion for people with mental health problems will happen; however, the debate as to who ultimately has responsibility is one you are likely to come across during your community placements.

Physical needs

Service User Need/Problem	Goals	Care Plan
1. Anthony is concerned that he is often thirsty and passes urine more frequently.	**Short-term goals** Find out cause of unusual thirst, and frequency of passing urine. **Long-term goals** Anthony will re-establish a 'normal' pattern of fluid intake and output, which is appropriate to his health status.	a) Screen for diabetes. b) Measure blood pressure and body mass indicators. c) Begin programme of health promotion: diet, exercise, smoking cessation. d) Ensure prescribed medication is reviewed as soon as possible. CPN to liaise with practice nurse at GP's surgery and ensure she is involved in the screening and health promotion process. See the separate boxes for plans to tackle diabetes, diet, exercise, and smoking. **Rationale:** *Interventions are based on existing ill health diagnostic criteria and the medical model.*
2. Anthony has disturbed sleep.	**Short-term goals** Find out Anthony's current sleep pattern. **Long-term goals** Re-establish Anthony's preferred sleep pattern.	Ask Anthony why he thinks his sleep is disturbed now – has anything changed? What is his normal sleep pattern? Ask Anthony to monitor his sleep pattern. Give advice re: sleep hygiene. **Rationale:** *Interventions are based on existing ill health diagnostic criteria and the medical model.*
3. Anthony has blurred vision.	**Short-term goals** Establish cause of blurred vision. **Long-term goals** Anthony will have clearer vision to a level satisfactory to him.	Ascertain if Anthony's blurred vision is due to: a) diabetes, b) prescribed medication, c) normal ageing.

Service User Need/Problem	Goals	Care Plan
		Encourage Anthony to have an eye test. Encourage him to monitor time spent at the computer, and educate about distance and breaks. **Rationale:** *Interventions are based on existing ill health diagnostic criteria and the medical model. Underpinned by and in accordance with national guidelines and policies.*
4. Anthony experiences tremors, restlessness, and 'strange' expressions at times.	**Short-term goals** Establish cause of Anthony's problems. **Long-term goals** To reduce tremors, restlessness, and strange facial expressions to a level Anthony feels able to manage.	Discuss with Anthony the length of time he has been having these experiences. Assess their frequency, intensity, number of times they occur each day, and their duration. CPN to ask MDT to review medication to either exclude side effects or alter prescription as necessary to alleviate. **Rationale:** *Interventions are based on the medical model, which informs the specific choice of intervention.*

See also: Allen *et al.* (2004), Duffin (2005), and Olsen *et al.* (2005).

Anthony's Health promotion plan – diabetes

Typical NHS screening for diabetes (type 2, or late onset; see www.nhsdirect.nhs.uk/articles/alphaindex.aspx) would include the following battery of tests. You will find explanatory information on each of these tests on the relevant website.

- Abdominal obesity, waist to hip ratio, and body mass index assessments.

www.eatwell.gov.uk/healthydiet/healthyweight/bmicalculator

- Blood pressure measure to exclude or recognize hypertension.

www.netdoctor.co.uk/health_advice/examinations/measuringbloodpressure.htm

- Random blood glucose – finger prick test. If the results indicate that glucose levels are above 7 mmol per litre, this suggests that diabetes may well be present and further tests are required.
- Urine test for glycosuria.

- Lipid profile – blood testing for high LDL and cholesterol levels and low HDL to exclude or diagnose dyslipidaemia.

- Fasting blood glucose analysis.

- Glucose tolerance test.

- Baseline glycosylated haemoglobin (HBA 1C).

www.labtestsonline.org.uk/understanding/analytes/lipid/glance.html

The treatment of type 2 diabetes is largely centred around lifestyle changes, healthy diet, getting appropriate levels of exercise, and losing weight, but some people may require medication to help. This can include oral hypoglycaemic agents such as **glibenclamide**; and certain weight-reducing drugs are occasionally used, such as **orlistat**. The CPN working with Anthony would work with the **primary health care team** in order to establish a thorough and regular screening of Anthony within his GP practice setting.

They would also educate both Anthony and the team about Anthony's antipsychotic medication, as this can potentially cause weight gain, a key indicator in diabetes. At the same time they would raise awareness that some of the symptoms of diabetes, for example in Anthony's case thirst, polyuria, and blurred vision, are relatively common side effects of antipsychotics. Whether the outcome for Anthony is a diagnosis of diabetes or not, the CPN will still need to offer an appropriate programme of health promotion and education to Anthony and monitor the effectiveness of these sessions. According to his assessment and care plan, the CPN would need to offer Anthony specific sessions on the following areas: healthy diet; smoking cessation; getting exercise; and sleep hygiene. We have included some examples of what you could do with Anthony; however, these are not meant to be exhaustive and need to be adapted for individual service users' needs.

Health promotion session 1 – healthy eating

- Stage 1 – Carry out a baseline assessment. Ask Anthony to keep a food and drink diary for one week and establish whether he would like to be weighed throughout the changes to see if this approach is helping him to lose weight.

- Stage 2 – Start with minor and maintainable changes. Encourage Anthony to drink at least six glasses of water a day, drink less fizzy drinks, and add or maintain five portions of fruit and vegetables every day. Ask him to continue with his food and drink diary but also to include how he sleeps, how he feels, and what he's thinking about food.

- Stage 3 – Encourage Anthony to eat at regular times during the day and to always have breakfast, lunch, and dinner. Encourage him to avoid big, heavy meals at the end of the day and not to eat after 7 p.m. If he gets hungry in between mealtimes, advise Anthony to have ready small, healthy snacks such as fresh fruit, seeds, and small portions of unsalted nuts. Discuss with him the constituents of a healthy diet; what should be incorporated into his daily intake.

- Stage 4 – Using Anthony's area of interest, the Internet, to encourage him to access relevant sites to promote self-help and autonomy in relation to a healthy diet. Encourage him to access sites such as:

www.eatwell.gov.uk

www.eatwell.gov.uk/healthydiet

www.eatwell.gov.uk/healthydiet/healthyweight

Encourage him to avoid foods high in saturated fats and fried foods and get him to recognize these foods by reading food labels. Advise him about the meaning of some food labels that are currently in use, such as the traffic light system (mainly green labels indicate go ahead, but always within reason; amber labels suggest some caution should be used when eating these foods; and mainly red labels indicate that these are foods to eat little of and rarely). Also advise him that most food labels will have some green, some amber, and some red sections. Encourage him to access **www.eatwell.gov.uk/foodlabels/trafficlights.**

Health promotion session 2 – getting moving

Before Anthony can be advised about exercising he would need to see his GP and determine appropriate levels of activity. As with any health promotion strategy, the idea is to start with minor and maintainable changes. In certain parts of the UK, GPs are now prescribing exercise for people and this can help to keep costs down. Many local council facilities will offer discounts for people on benefits or prescribed exercise programmes.

It is also useful to associate exercise with pleasurable activities. Anthony likes to go to the library; encouraging him to walk there or to use a library further away over time, which would increase his activity levels, could be a useful strategy. The CPN would need to ask Anthony what he enjoys doing and target those areas.

Starting off with simple and free activities is always useful and walking is an excellent first option. Many parks, in collaboration with the NHS, have measured walking areas to encourage people to get active; finding something local for Anthony is a useful start point. As his confidence grows, seeking to enhance his social networks by joining walking associations could also be a useful approach. As previously observed, Anthony enjoys using the Internet so the CPN could encourage him to access the following websites to help him design his own exercise programme:

www.dh.gov.uk/PolicyAndGuidance/HealthAndSocialCareTopics/HealthyLiving

www.mentalhealth.org.uk/html/content/exercise_depression_booklet_patient.pdf#search=22%exercise%22

http://hcd2.bupa.co.uk/fact_sheets/html/exercise.html

www.weightlossresources.co.uk/exercise/take_5_plan

www.ramblers.org.uk

www.nhs.direct.nhs.uk/articles/alphaindex.aspx

www.florahearts.co.uk

The CPN would be looking for 30 minutes of activity at least five times per week, and would then gradually build this up with Anthony to enhance his general health and fitness.

Health promotion session 3 – smoking cessation

- Stage 1 – Carry out a baseline assessment. Ask Anthony to monitor when and where he smokes and record any triggers to his smoking. Also discuss with Anthony his health awareness and the dangers of smoking; encourage him to identify why it would be appropriate for him to stop. Discuss Anthony's preparedness and motivation to stop smoking. Identify strategies that Anthony would like to employ in stopping smoking. Consider whether he wants to stop, reduce the amount he smokes, use nicotine replacement therapy, or other alternatives such as hypnotherapy.

- Stage 2 – Start with minor and maintainable changes. Encourage Anthony to have his first cigarette later in the day than usual; encourage him to clean his teeth before smoking and to drink a glass of water. Encourage Anthony to use simple relaxation techniques such as slowed breathing instead of smoking. Motivate Anthony to set a target stop date, one that he chooses and feels confident in. For example some people will choose to give up on New Year's Eve to start the New Year smoke free. Try to establish a date of significance with Anthony that he can work towards.

- Stage 3 – Using Anthony's interest in the Internet, encourage him to access relevant sites promoting autonomy and self-help in relation to stopping smoking, such as:

www.ash.org.uk

www.bupa.co.uk/health_information/asp/healthy_living/lifestyle/smoking/

A useful guide for nurses is provided in Percival (2006).

Health promotion session
4 – sleeping pattern

Anthony has stated that he is not sleeping well. There is a need to identify what exactly this means to Anthony. Encourage Anthony to record the following in a diary by his bed: what time he goes to bed; if he is awake for long periods in the night; and if his sleep is disturbed. Anthony has also complained of polyuria, which could be contributing to his perceived poor sleeping patterns.

Once the CPN has established some sort of baseline assessment of Anthony's sleeping pattern, it is essential that they determine what would be appropriate in sleep terms for Anthony. Simple changes like establishing a routine, going to bed and getting up at the same time each day, can help. Strategies employed could include sleep hygiene mechanisms such as removing televisions, stereo equipment, phones, and computers from the bedroom so as to reduce distractions; all of these would be useful in Anthony's case. Limit caffeine drinks and nicotine intake before bed. Encourage Anthony to avoid heavy meals or exercise late in the evening. Also get Anthony to consider a winding down period before bed when he carries out relaxation and might have a warm bath. Some people recommend wearing warm socks to bed as this convinces the body that you are ready to sleep sooner because your feet are cosy – a cautionary note: it doesn't work for everyone. Several of the recommendations for exercise, diet, and smoking cessation should also assist Anthony in re-establishing appropriate sleeping patterns.

Student activity 4

http://www.oxfordtextbooks.co.uk/orc/clarke

and choose the video link.

Review the online video interview with Anthony; the priorities set are risk, social, and physical needs.
Would you agree with these priorities?
How would you try to help Anthony with his needs?

Care planning

Having done the assessment and identified the priorities of care, mental health nurses now need to try and develop a care plan in partnership with the client (note that this issue is explored further in Chapter 2). You should consider the care plans suggested for Anthony, bearing in mind that these are *suggestions* – ideally we hope that you will adopt a critical/analytical approach to these, using them as a starting point for your own plans.

You will see that in places, the content of the care plans overlap; in these circumstances there is no need to duplicate planning. Also, we have not stuck rigidly to the same format in each case where this is not necessary; for instance, we couldn't identify long-term goals in each case. Care plans are meant to be practical guides to *help* the process of nursing care and shouldn't be treated as a bureaucratic exercise.

You will be busy enough preparing plans without making more work for yourself by doing the same thing twice!

Implementation

Implementing Anthony's care requires specific mental health nursing skills. Your assessor from practice will be expecting you to demonstrate certain standards as recommended by the Nursing and Midwifery Council (NMC), but as you will be working with people like Anthony in a community setting you must also demonstrate *safe*, *effective*, and *efficient* capabilities in meeting these standards. This part of the chapter considers four of the NMC standards in relation to both Anthony and the work you are likely to be doing in a community mental health team setting and offers some examples of the necessary skills and example documentation.

NMC Standard D

" Engage in, develop and disengage from therapeutic relationships through the use of appropriate communication and interpersonal skills. "

Important mental health nursing skills that you need to demonstrate include the core conditions as recommended by Rogers (1951): empathy, warmth, genuineness, and **unconditional positive regard**. You also need to demonstrate listening and attending skills (Egan 2002). Your facial expression should show warmth and concern and you should smile where appropriate to the circumstances. Good use of eye contact helps to show that you are listening but it is important that this isn't too intense as staring makes people feel uncomfortable. Your gestures need to be calm and relaxed and you need to avoid making the service user feel that their personal space is being invaded. Although what you say is important, it is also necessary to consider *how* you say it; for instance, consider the effect that your pace, pitch, and tone of speech can have on an interaction. Calm and clear is effective and you should vary this as determined by the service user's needs.

Student activity 5

Basic communication skills are identified in Chapter 2 on p. 29–33; review the section on basic aspects of engagement. Consider the following questions and make a note of your ideas:

- *How will you encourage Anthony to trust you?*
- *How will you demonstrate to Anthony that you are genuinely interested in him?*

NMC Standard E

" Create and utilize opportunities to promote the health and well-being of patients, clients and groups. "

Student activity 6

Review the material provided on Anthony in relation to smoking cessation, healthy eating, and exercising. Pick an example from your clinical placement and work on a health promotion package for that service user. You can use this material as supporting evidence for your clinical assessor and in your portfolio; make sure that if you do so, you ensure service user confidentiality.

NMC Standard F

" Undertake and document a comprehensive, systematic and accurate nursing assessment of the physical, psychological, social and spiritual needs of patients, clients and communities. "

NMC Standard G

" Formulate and document a plan of nursing care, where possible, in partnership with patients, clients, their carers and family and friends, within a framework of informed consent. "

Student activity 7

Review the assessment and care plans provided on Anthony as this will be useful preparation for practice. It might be useful to practice both your assessment and care planning skills with your clinical assessor and in partnership with a service user. Again, this work is appropriate supporting evidence for your clinical assessor and your portfolio; ensure that service user confidentiality is maintained.

Practice

You would need to show both Anthony and your mentor that you are honest, reliable, and can behave professionally; for example being punctual is important, as lateness may be seen as trivializing people's concerns.

You should also consider your general approach, for example, do people feel that they can speak to you? How might you show you are listening and showing concern? Learning to reflect on your practice (see the following section) is essential if you are to fully develop your skills as a mental health nurse.

What your clinical assessor may expect from you when working in the community

Consider the following while working with the community mental health team.

Preparation

Before visiting any service user(s), be prepared:

- Be self-aware; consider what message you are sending in terms of your general appearance and approach.
- As a student you need to read through any existing information about the service user(s).

Consider:

- Why are we visiting this service user?
- Are any interventions required?
- Ask your assessor what is expected of you during the visit.
- Are there any approaches that this service user dislikes/prefers?
- Is there any risk that you need to be aware of? (Your placement area should have a 'lone worker' policy in place and you should make yourself aware of this.)
- Are there any intended outcomes from this visit?

Once there:

- Always adopt a courteous, formal approach; ask permission to enter the service user's home (have your identity card ready), don't sit until asked, and make sure you know what they prefer to be called.

- Sometimes CPNs are required to carry emergency mobile phones for urgent calls. If this is the case, ensure that the service user is aware of this potential disruption before commencing any interventions; otherwise ensure that all mobile phones are switched off.
- Many CPNs make notes as the visit progresses, although some find this distracting – you might be advised to discuss this with the CPN you are working with. These can help to show that you are taking seriously what is being said; however, do be careful to ensure that the service user is aware of what you are doing and be prepared to share these notes.
- Carry out appropriate activity and ensure that this is within a time frame to suit the service user. Always work with respect and in partnership, and before finishing summarize the visit and anything that has been agreed together.
- Remember that any care plans should be mutually agreed and shared between the service user and CPN.
- Finally, set a date and time for your next appointment if this is appropriate.

After visiting:

- Record the details of the visit in the service user records and discuss intervention/action with your assessor.
- Feedback the relevant information to the appropriate multi-professional team members. This may be verbally or in written form, for example a letter to the service user's GP.

Two practising CPNs suggested a list of Dos and Don'ts (Box 4.3, p. 88).

Evaluation

In this part of the chapter you are encouraged to reflect upon and analyse your clinical practice in relation to service user satisfaction and its effectiveness. We will also provide some consideration of what your personal tutor and university lecturers will expect from you once your clinical placement is completed.

> ◣ **Student activity 8**
> *Reflection*
> *After completing a community visit with your assessor, carry out the following activity. Analyse what you did*

with the service user, employing a simple SWOT analysis approach (see Box 4.4).

Analysing clinical work in this way helps you to become a reflective practitioner (see especially Schön 1987). This means that you always consider what you've done and why and whether you could have done things differently. The following activity encourages reflection, placing the service user as advisor and expert, while showing your desire to work in partnership.

MORECAMBE BAY HOSPITALS NHS TRUST

Dos
Be prepared
Plan what you will do
Ensure your personal safety
Consider 'risk'
Promote independence
Discuss time-limited nature of relationship
Maintain existing support networks
Ask questions of the CPN – show interest
Research/study around the problems you encounter

Don'ts
Clock watch
Fidget
Look bored or disinterested
Overstay your welcome
Promote dependency
Worry about admitting you don't know something

Box 4.3 Dos and Don'ts

Strengths

- What did you do well with this service user?

- What were you particularly happy with in your work with this service user?

Weaknesses

- Where did you feel that you could have improved in your work with this service user?

- Was there anything lacking in your approach?

Opportunities

- What do you need to know to do things better?

- Is there any research or reading that you could do to improve your knowledge and approach to assist this service user?

Threats

- Was there anything you wished you had done differently?

- Did you feel out of control?

- Did you feel uncertain of what to do at any time?

Box 4.4 SWOT analysis

Student activity 9
Service user feedback
Try asking the following questions of the service user:

- *Do you feel that I have understood what you've told us?*

- *I would like us to work together in trying to deal with your problems. Is there anything I can do to make you feel we are partners in this?*

- *As a student nurse, what do you think I could do to improve?*

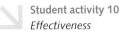

Student activity 10
Effectiveness
Having previously documented an assessment and formulated a care plan, from this analyse each of the care plan segments for their effectiveness. Consider whether the element of care is:

* *Prescribed in accordance with national policies and guidelines.*

* *Utilizing a specific theoretical model to inform the approach, for example psycho-social interventions.*

* *Based on existing mental health diagnostic criteria.*

* *Underpinned by specific published research suggesting that this is the best approach.*

Discussion points

Risk

You will have noticed, both from reading this book and from reflection on your clinical experience, that risk and risk management are important aspects of mental health nursing. In this chapter we have introduced you to specific issues around risk in the context of caring for Anthony. It is worth reiterating that as a minimum when you think about risk in a nursing context, you should consider the following basic components in Figure 4.2.

In analysing the care prescribed for Anthony we should consider the implications of the mental health nurse's action or inaction. The harm Anthony is experiencing from a gang of youths has led to his readiness to carry an imitation gun. This presents us with a serious dilemma. On one hand, we may live in areas of increasing violence and crime where self-defence is seen as acceptable within that context. Asking Anthony to destroy his imitation gun may leave him feeling increasingly vulnerable and unable to defend himself against a perceived violent threat. In any future conflict with this gang, if Anthony is hurt or seriously injured or worse, could we, in part, be responsible for this outcome?

On the other hand, the likely escalation of any potentially violent encounter, the possibility of police involvement (including armed response teams) and the need to uphold the law of the land would lead the mental health nurse to agree to the action prescribed on Anthony's care plan.

However, we are presented with additional dilemmas. If Anthony refuses to destroy the imitation gun, whom do we inform? Do we have a responsibility to inform the police, considering Anthony is not planning to commit violence but rather to defend himself if necessary? As mental health nurses, we need to develop alternative response strategies with Anthony. We could encourage him to adopt a range of personal safety measures to enhance his feelings of safety, for example carrying a mobile phone, or travelling at different times and by different routes to avoid contact. However, to some extent it does sound as if this 'gang' may well be targeting Anthony; his encounters with them seem to be increasing and the level of threat he perceives also seems to be worsening.

Social exclusion

> Social exclusion happens when people or places suffer from a series of problems such as unemployment, poor skills, low incomes, poor housing, high poor health and family breakdown.
>
> Social Exclusion Unit, Office of the Deputy Prime Minister 2004.

If you briefly pause to consider the above definition in terms of Anthony's situation, it is easy to see how he might be considered to be experiencing social isolation. Faulkner and Biddle (2002) remind us that as long ago as 1796, the founders of the York Retreat considered physical well-being as essential to the care of

To Self

From others → **Harm** ← To others (Including staff)

Neglect

Figure 4.2 Basic components of risk

people with mental health problems, but we might reasonably ask how much consideration is given to this matter in modern mental health care. It should be noted that mental health services have been criticized for not paying sufficient attention to the physical care needs of our clients (Muir-Cochrane 2006).

In the UK, the Black report attempted to draw attention to the powerful evidence for links between ill health and poverty (Townsend *et al.* 1988, see also Wilkinson 1996). At the time of its initial publication it would be fair to say that this report was received unenthusiastically (Morris 1995) but in recent years the issue of health inequalities has at least been achieving a higher policy profile. In an attempt to address this problem, the UK Government established the Social Exclusion Unit (Office of the Deputy Prime Minister 2004) with the intention of trying to consider policy solutions across different government departments.

In terms of mental health, the *National Service Framework for mental health* (Department of Health 1999) highlights figures that suggest that people living with mental health problems also have high rates of physical morbidity, and that people with schizophrenia, for example, may have mortality levels 1.6 times that of the general population (Harris and Barraclough 1998).

More recently, the Chief Nursing Officer's review of mental health nursing (Department of Health 2006) identified one of the ten essential shared capabilities for mental health nurses as being the ability to 'Promote physical health and well-being for people with mental health problems'. Obviously we should consider these factors when meeting with a client such as Anthony (see 'physical needs' section of the care plan, p. 81).

Evaluating the service

If you are undertaking final year clinical experiences you will probably be involved in a range of strategies that the team/service use to evaluate their provision. It would be useful for you to familiarize yourself with clinical governance strategies, including audit and service user surveys. It is appropriate for you to discuss with your assessor any ideas you may have to improve the service and/or experience for other students. Most clinical assessors will expect senior students to demonstrate a move towards independence and autonomy and evidence of thinking as a qualified nurse; similarly your personal tutor and university lecturers expect you to demonstrate a proactive approach to learning at this stage.

Evaluating yourself

Preparing your portfolio for review

Universities recognize the need for all students to be lifelong learners and maintaining a portfolio of learning is a strategy frequently employed. The NMC recommends that all nurses keep a portfolio of evidence of their ongoing professional development and learning.

> **Student activity 11** – Portfolio review
> *Consider the following questions as you read through and check your portfolio.*
> *What should be in your portfolio?*
> *Where should it be in your portfolio?*
> *How should it be presented in your portfolio?*
> *Have I included all of the correct materials?*
> *Have I provided sufficient evidence to support my claims of learning?*

Summary

This chapter has introduced you to some of the important issues in mental health nursing practice; it builds on ideas introduced in the first chapters, such as the recovery approach and engagement skills. You have had an opportunity to explore typically encountered mental health nursing approaches to the care of people such as Anthony and his brother. It is intended that this chapter will help you to understand the complexity of a person's needs and the likelihood of multiple issues arising in people with mental health problems. It clearly demonstrates the need for mental health nurses to use a bio-psycho-social perspective

when working in partnership to help people. You have also been introduced to the changing environment of mental health nursing and the move to community mental health care.

The necessity of considering a person's physical health has been stressed, as well as the importance of holistic health promotion.

This is the first of our clinical chapters in which you are introduced to the films of our 'service users'; these are intended to give you an idea of how people really express their problems. Obviously these cannot replace real life experience and we would recommend that if you really want to understand people then you must take every opportunity to spend time with mental health service users. The materials in this chapter provide you with the opportunity to begin reflecting on and applying this learning in your clinical practice. It is essential that you broaden and deepen your knowledge and to aid you in this we have identified some further appropriate reading.

You may also find it helpful to work through our short online scenario, intended to help you to consider and actively work through issues raised by Anthony's case.

@ http://www.oxfordtextbooks.co.uk/orc/clarke

and choose the online resources for this chapter.

References and other sources

References

Allen D, Harvey S and Smith S (2004). Enduring mental illness and physical health care. **Practice Nursing, 15**(7), 356-60.

Commission for Health Improvement (2003). **What CHI found in mental health trusts.** Commission for Health Improvement, London.

Department of Health (1999). **National Service Framework for mental health: Modern standards and service models.** DH, London.

Department of Health (2006). **Best practice competencies and capabilities for pre registration mental health nurses in England: The Chief Nursing Officer's review of mental health nursing.** DH, London.

Duffin C (2005). Physical health needs of patients with mental illness are overlooked. **Nursing Standard, 19**(43), 10.

Egan G (2002). **The skilled helper: a problem management and opportunity-development approach to helping.** Brooks/Cole, Pacific Grove, CA.

Faulkner G and Biddle S (2002). Mental health nursing and the promotion of physical activity. **Journal of Psychiatric and Mental Health Nursing, 9**(6), 659.

Goffman E (1987). **Asylums: Essays on the social situation of mental patients and other inmates.** Penguin, Harmondsworth.

Harris EC and Barraclough B (1998). Excess mortality of mental disorder. **British Journal of Psychiatry, 173,** 11-53.

Harrison T and Clarke D (1992). The Northfield Experiments. **British Journal of Psychiatry, 160,** 698-708.

HMSO (1994). **The report of the inquiry into the care and treatment of Christopher Clunis: presented to the Chairman of North East Thames and South East Thames Regional Health Authorities.** HMSO, London.

Hostick T, Newell R, and Ward T (1997). Evaluation of stress prevention and management workshops in the community. **Journal of Clinical Nursing, 6**(2), 139–45.

MIND (2006). **Dangerousness and mental health: The facts.** http://www.mind.org.uk/Information/Factsheets/Dangerousness.htm accessed November 2006.

Morris JN (1995). Pride against prejudice: Lives not worth living. In B Davey et al., eds. **Health and disease: A reader,** pp. 107–110. Open University Press, Buckingham.

Muir-Cochrane E (2006). Medical co-morbidity risk factors and barriers to care for people with schizophrenia. **Journal of Psychiatric and Mental Health Nursing, 13**(4), 447-52.

Nolan P (1992). **A history of mental health nursing.** Stanley Thornes, Cheltenham.

Office of the Deputy Prime Minister (2004). **The Social Exclusion Unit.** Office of the Deputy Prime Minister, London.

Olsen R, Peacock G and Smith S (2005). Practice development. Developing a service to monitor and improve physical health in people with serious mental illness. **Journal of Psychiatric and Mental Health Nursing, 12**(5), 614-19.

Percival J (2006). Innovations in smoking cessation. **Nursing Standard Essential Guide, 20**(47), August.

Perry A (2004). Focus: growing murder toll of the mentally unstable monsters in our midst. **Sunday Express,** 12 September.

Piipo J and Aaltonen J (2004). Mental health: integrated network and family-oriented model for cooperation between mental health patients, adult mental health services and social services. **Journal of Clinical Nursing, 13**(7), 876–85.

Read J and Baker S (1996). **Not just sticks and stones: A survey of the discrimination experienced by people with mental health problems.** MIND, London.

Repper J and Perkins R (2003). **Social inclusion and recovery: A model for mental health practice.** Balliere Tindall, Edinburgh.

Rogers C (1951). **Client-centered therapy: its current practice, implications and theory.** Constable, London.

Rogers A and Pilgrim D (2001). **Mental health policy in Britain: A critical introduction.** Macmillan, London.

Sainsbury Centre for Mental Health (2005). **Beyond the Water Towers: The unfinished revolution in mental health services 1985–2005.** SCMH, London.

Schön D (1987). **Educating the reflective practitioner.** Jossey Bass, San Francisco.

Timmins N (1996). Facts challenge fear of the mentally ill. **The Independent (London),** 15 January.

Townsend P, Davidson N, and Whitehead M (1988). **Inequalities in health: The Black Report and the health divide.** Penguin, London.

Wilkinson R (1996). **Unhealthy societies: The afflictions of inequality.** Routledge, London.

✺ Useful web links

Mental Health Foundation
http://www.mentalhealth.org.uk/

National Library for Health
'Aims to be the best health library and information service in the world.' You will need an ATHENS ID to fully access this, which your librarian will be able to advise you about.
http://www.library.nhs.uk/?autoLogin=0

Rethink website
http://www.rethink.org/how_we_can_help/campaigning_for_change/physical_health/whats_the.html

The Sainsbury Centre for Mental Health
'We work to improve the quality of life for people with mental health problems by influencing policy and practice in mental health and related services.'
http://www.scmh.org.uk/80256FBD004F6342/vWeb/wpKHAL6S2HVE

❷ Sources of help and advice

Be-frienders Worldwide
http://www.befrienders.org

MIND
http://www.mind.org.uk

Samaritans
http://www.samaritans.org.uk

◔ Further reading

Barker P, ed (2003). **Psychiatric and mental health nursing: The craft of caring.** Hodder Arnold, London.

Department of Health (2001). **Making it happen: A guide to delivering mental health promotion.** DH, London.

McDonald G and O'Hara K (1998). **Ten elements of mental health, its promotion and demotion: Implications for practice.** Society of Health Education and Health Promotion Specialists, UK.

Norman I and Ryrie I (2004). **The art and science of mental health nursing: a textbook of principles and practice.** Open University Press, Maidenhead.

Sainsbury Centre for Mental Health (2006). **Prevalence, how common are mental health problems?** http://website.scmh.org.uk/80256FBD004F6342/vWeb/wpKHAL6GUENF accessed August 2006.

Chapter 5
The nursing care of an adult in crisis with mental health problems

Simon Steeves and Chris Smith

Learning outcomes

This chapter will assist you to:

- Examine 'crisis' and what that means for a service user.
- Demonstrate knowledge of the signs and symptoms of bipolar affective disorder.
- Demonstrate awareness of the evidence base for the care given to a person with this diagnosis.
- Understand and apply risk assessments.
- Understand the process of planning care.
- Consider legal and ethical components of care, including empowerment versus safety.
- Begin to understand some of the models used in mental health nursing.
- Demonstrate knowledge of the available help for people, including pharmacology, talking therapies, and who can deliver this care.

Introduction

In this chapter we will look at the issues arising from an acute crisis in two people's lives. Two differing crises with separate needs and outcomes but similarities in risk assessment and planning of care will be discussed. First you will meet Joyce, a mature family woman who has a history of mental health crises. You will also meet Andrew, a young man who is very troubled by his current circumstances, which have led to a significant mental health crisis.

Dictionary.com defines crisis in many ways, and there are two useful definitions here:

- A stage in a sequence of events at which the trend for all future events, especially for better or for worse, is determined; turning point
- The point in the course of a serious disease at which a decisive change occurs, leading either to recovery or death

So we will examine the nature of a crisis, what must be done about it, and what we need to do in the future to either prevent recurrence or minimize its impact. We will pay special attention to the risks included in both definitions to ensure our outcomes are for better not worse and lead to recovery not death. In mental health nursing there is, historically, difficulty in accepting death, whereas in all other branches of nursing it is accepted that a percentage of clients will die. For example in oncology, surgery, and neonatal care it is accepted that death may occur, but in our branch of nursing it causes angst, blame, and fear. In light of this we will discuss risk assessment and planning in some depth.

Clinical scenario: Joyce

Joyce is a 57-year-old woman, now divorced, with three children who are all now grown up and leading their own careers. The eldest is a highly respected solicitor. Joyce has a long history of bipolar affective disorder. She has, when in low mood, attempted suicide on several occasions. Some have been very serious attempts, one requiring the administration of acetycysteine (**Parvalex**) to redress her symptoms. For the last 18 months she has been living in Cedar Lodge, a rehab and recovery unit, following her most recent relapse. Her progress appeared to be successful until about six or seven weeks ago. She had formed a relationship with a younger man, Mark, whom many of the staff distrusted. Recently she had exhibited changes in behaviour. Most noticeably she had begun to disappear for long periods of time, possibly drinking more than normal and drawing out unusually large sums of money. Her mood appeared to be becoming elated and she was apparently more chaotic. For example she would request repeat prescriptions for her **lithium** well before they were due, citing problems like she'd lost her tablets, someone must have taken them, or they were not correctly dispensed. Reports were coming in from neighbours in the locality that she had been pestering them. Staff also reported that her absences were lengthening.

She finally absconded from the unit and the staff were unable to locate her. Missing persons procedures were implemented but local police appeared to give them low priority as it was assumed she had run off with her boyfriend and the unit could not identify evidence for high risk. Due to overwhelming demand for beds, Joyce's place had had to be reallocated so there was no possibility of her returning to Cedar Lodge. Three days later she was found in an extremely disturbed state (apparently following a row with her boyfriend) and arrested under Section 136 of the Mental Health Act 2007. She was seen in cells for a Mental Health Act assessment and detained under Section 3, and was admitted to a local acute admission ward.

Student activity 1

View the 'Joyce – admission' video and try to identify anything you think is significant in the first interview.

http://www.oxfordtextbooks.co.uk/orc/clarke

and choose the video link.
Complete the multiple choice quiz that you will find online.

http://www.oxfordtextbooks.co.uk/orc/clarke

and choose the online resources for this chapter.
You may also wish to refer to the section on the nursing process in Chapter 2.

👤 Joyce's admission – a service user's viewpoint

I would like to know what it was that made Joyce so angry, annoyed, and provocative, and indeed she challenges the interviewer about how he would feel in the circumstances.

The interviewer seems caught between on the one hand making sure his predetermined set of questions is answered, which makes him appear unwilling to engage with Joyce as a person and how she is viewing the world at that particular point, and on the other hand trying to develop some sort of conversation.

But of course he does have a 'duty of care', which in turn needs to be examined to ensure that it is not being used as an excuse to deny service users the attention they need or to cover up inadequate services.

Joyce is asked how she is feeling, but is she asked about how *she* understands her situation? She has tried to give her views at some time – 'you lot don't believe anything I say' – but it is not clear that a real discussion with Joyce has ever taken place. Does this come from the view that what mental health service users say and do is bizarre, meaningless, and incomprehensible, whereas in fact the person may well be articulating quite well how s/he understands the situation?

Marion Clark, service user

✏ Lithium: a pharmacist's perspective

While on the ward, the lithium treatment would be assessed and it would be a good opportunity to check the plasma lithium level. The dose of lithium may need to be increased when the hypomanic episode is over, to prevent future relapse. If the level is low, compliance should be examined before increasing the dose. In the film, Joyce was complaining of feeling cold, which could be a symptom of lithium toxicity. Other symptoms are blurred vision, paraesthesia, ataxia, tremor, cognitive impairment, muscle weakness, hyperextension of limbs, mild »

» drowsiness and lethargy, anorexia, vomiting, and diarrhoea.

Admission to the ward itself may have a beneficial effect if the environment is calming and uncrowded. If the sleep/wake cycle is greatly disturbed the routine on the ward can help re-establish this to a more normal pattern. Haloperidol has a sedative effect, which can be useful, but it has a risk of movement disorders, particularly at higher doses. Atypical antipsychotics may also be used. Risperidone and olanzapine are available as tablets that melt in the mouth. If symptoms are severe, an injectable form of medication may be given. The different forms of injection offer flexibility with treatment. Haloperidol is available as both short-acting and long-acting injections, Olanzapine is available as a short-acting injection, and risperidone is available only as a depot or long-acting injection. There are issues around giving an injectable drug if the patient does not agree and would need to be restrained in order for it to be administered. Consider whether the Mental Health Act offers any assistance in this situation.

For guidance on the management of bipolar disorder go to **http://www.nice.org.uk/CG038** (July 2006).

Assessment

Today, mental health nurses are much less likely to focus on assessment based on medical diagnosis, tending now towards a more person-centred approach (Barker 2003). This approach considers not only people's problems in living but also their strengths. Here it is stressed that it is important when assessing to consider the impact on the individual. The use of diagnosis to inform assessment and care is impractical. We know of people who suffer the same illness but who react to it in totally differing ways. The use of signs (what the nurse observes) and symptoms (what the person tells us) is useful as a guide but will not give us the whole picture about an individual and their perception of their crisis. It is also important that the assessor makes no assumptions or judgements. For example, let us consider pain. Different people react to pain in differing ways depending on their own circumstances, situation, and abilities. People used to poverty and starvation will accept far more suffering before it impacts on their lives than people used to being well fed. Boxers will accept much harder blows and more pain than the average person. So you can see that your own personal judgement about the impact of hunger or a blow to the head is related to you and cannot be assumed to have the same impact on another person. Therefore the use of the diagnosis that Joyce has bipolar affective disorder will not give us the whole picture about the nature of her crisis or its impact on her.

Having seen the video of the first assessment, you will already have begun the process of assessing Joyce. It is important though that the assessment process is supported by knowledge. As previously stated, we must avoid jumping to conclusions. For example when Joyce swears loudly at the nurse, is this symptomatic of disinhibition or just the result of Joyce being angry at her situation (see Box 5.1)?

What more do we need to know to confirm what we think is happening? There are several questions in the quiz that may have shed light on the answer to that question. Joyce is demonstrating 'clang association'; this is defined in Merriam Webster's *Medical dictionary* (Webster 2003) as 'word association (as in a psychological test) based on a sound rather than a

---

Disinhibition is a condition that manifests itself in several mental health problems. Most of us have our behaviours inhibited, or you might say controlled, by many factors. What our parents or society have taught us, our religion or personal beliefs, and our culture or social norms will affect our behaviour. We have belief systems imprinted on us as young people and can be conditioned to behave in certain ways by our society. We all know of some behaviours that are not deemed acceptable by our society or peers. In some mental health problems this imprinting and conditioning is overridden and the person's behaviour can become extreme and high risk.

Box 5.1   Disinhibition

meaning.' This is evident when Joyce states that she is 'fine and you'll be fined if you don't let me go.' This symptom is common in those people suffering from hypomania, one of the poles in bipolar affective disorder. Her mood is also quite volatile and she can go from anger to sadness very quickly. She is also demonstrating extreme vulnerability caused by her disinhibition. She was arrested following approaches she made to men (complete strangers) asking for help in creating her 'special baby' and flirts with the assessing nurse, referring to her lack of underwear. Her dishevelled state can also be indicative of her mental state, although this is not always true. We need to know what her usual appearance is like to make any kind of judgement. So what do we know from our interview?

Assessment form

Assessment date:	5 Dec 2007	**Assessment time:**	11:00 hrs
Assessment location:	Ward Four	**Assessor(s):**	WM Simon Steeves

Presenting problem including person's perceptions of their problems

- Joyce does not accept she is unwell
- Joyce has a long history of bipolar affective disorder
- She is complaining of feeling physically unwell including dizziness and diarrhoea
- She reports that she is sleeping only a few hours each night – feels exhausted
- Joyce states that she was unjustly detained as she was not doing anything to warrant this
- She appears to be preoccupied with ideas of creating a 'special baby'
- Joyce states that she had a falling out with her current partner
- During the assessment Joyce appeared angry and agitated; she was noted to be emotionally labile and at times disinhibited

History

- Joyce is 57 years of age
- She has a long history of bipolar affective disorder
- Until recently Joyce was living in a local care hostel
- Joyce left the hostel some days ago without informing anyone of her plans
- Joyce was found a few days later in a very agitated state in the city centre. The police report that she was approaching men in the street asking them if they would father her child. They arrested her under Section 136 of the Mental Health Act 2007
- Joyce appears to have separated from her current partner
- Joyce has taken overdoses in the past, which on at least one occasion was life threatening
- Joyce is now homeless

Summary of past treatment and response

- Joyce has previously been treated with antipsychotic drugs, mainly haloperidol. She finds this makes her very drowsy and has in the past become quickly depressed
- Joyce has a history of non-compliance with medication
- Joyce has required supervision when recovering from a psychotic episode as she will quickly relapse

Previous mental health history

- As previously stated, Joyce has been diagnosed with bipolar affective disorder and has previously suffered both hypomanic and depressive episodes

Alcohol and substance misuse

- Tends to drink more heavily when becoming unwell
- No known history of illicit drug use

Forensic history/contact with criminal justice system

- Although frequently arrested, has always been treated under the Mental Health Act; never charged with any offence

Family history

- Joyce is reluctant to discuss her family
- Joyce has three children, none of whom has had any contact with mental health services except about their mother

Personal history

- Joyce is now homeless
- She has a boyfriend whom the family do not like and will not meet
- Joyce is in denial about her illness and has never accepted either the diagnosis or the prescribed care
- She has had residential placements in the past but reports that she dislikes the restrictions on her life
- Joyce is divorced from the father of her three children. He has no contact

Present circumstances

Carers/significant others/appropriate adults:
- Eldest daughter, a solicitor who manages Joyce's funds
- Mark, her boyfriend

Family/significant relationships:
- Joyce has three children but their relationship is strained

Social network:
- Joyce has little or no social network

Employment/Education:
- School career was average but no higher education
- No employment history as she chose to be housewife and mother

Leisure:

- Joyce is interested in art and will paint and sculpt
- No other hobbies or interests

Housing:

- Joyce was in a hostel until recently
- Joyce is now homeless

Finances:

- Joyce's financial affairs are very poor. Her eldest daughter is trying to sort them out

Activities of daily living:

- Joyce's self-care is poor at the moment
- Joyce is refusing to do anything just now and becomes angry when asked to do things
- Joyce's diet and fluid intake is poor

Childcare responsibilities and child protection issues:

- N/A

Physical health history

Smoking, blood pressure, obesity

- Joyce is overweight
- Joyce is reporting dizziness and diarrhoea but refuses physical examination

Diversity issues

- Joyce is from a white British background
- When stable, she is articulate and able to talk about her experiences clearly

Spirituality issues

- Joyce does not state any religious beliefs but alludes to spiritual events in her life

Mental status examination

- Joyce appeared emotionally labile during the assessment
- She complained of being unlawfully detained and alluded to her going to have a 'special baby', but would not elaborate
- Joyce was at times sexually disinhibited during the interview
- Joyce exhibited signs of hypomania, garrulousness, clang association, and possibly delusional thinking
- Joyce's presentation is chaotic and her personal appearance dishevelled

Physical status examination

BMI

- Refused any physical examination.

Information from other sources

* Report from home manager

Risk and safety issues

* Joyce has a history of self-harm
* Joyce is sexually disinhibited, putting her at risk
* Joyce is to be nursed on level 2 observations

Physical, psychological, social, and spiritual formulation

* Joyce appears to have suffered a relapse in her illness
* Joyce is currently unable to make decisions about her life
* Joyce has little or no social network

ICD 10 diagnosis:　　　　Hypomania

Care Programme Approach (CPA) Indicators

* Enhanced CPA to be used as Joyce will continue to be at risk even during recovery

Outcome of assessment

Including views/preferences of the service user and carer, treatment options discussed, what was decided and by whom

* Joyce will require medication to reduce the severity of her symptoms
* Joyce has been detained under Section 3 of the MHA 2007
* Joyce has refused to be informed of her rights under the Mental Health Act 2007
* Short-term care plan in place to be reviewed daily
* Observation level two to be reviewed hourly

Assessor

Name: S Steeves　　　　　　　　　　**Designation:**　　W M
Signature:　　　　　　　　　　　　　**Date:**　　　　5 December 2007

Assessment summary

There are three main areas to summarize about this assessment. Firstly, we must stick to the facts we know and not make assumptions. You will note the use of phrases like 'Joyce appears to' or 'Joyce states that'. These phrases are used to give the broadest possible information but not to prejudice anyone who may read it. Secondly, the assessment includes mental state assessment and risk assessment. These two assessments always go hand in hand and are discussed in more detail elsewhere in the chapter. Finally, under the heading of 'outcome of assessment', note the review times. Joyce's level of observation must be continuously reviewed to make these as least restrictive as possible and move more quickly to Joyce being able to take control over her own situation.

Care planning

The care plans that we must consider fall into four main categories:

- Short-term goals/plans.
- Long-term goals/plans.
- Risk management plans.
- Contingency plans.

In any of these aspects of planning we need to consider the acronym SMART. It stands for:
Specific,
Measurable,
Achievable,
Relevant, and
Time-related
(adapted by Steeves, 2007).

Specific

When writing a plan, the action to be taken and the goal to be met must be specific. For example instead of writing 'The person can have leave from the ward', the care plan should state the exact conditions of that leave. The care plan could say that the person may leave the ward at a certain time for a specified length of time. It could also say where the person may or may not go and who they may go with. In the case of a detained patient, Section 17 of the Mental Health Act 2007 will apply and these conditions and the detail of the planned leave are a legal obligation to be carried out by the Responsible Medical Officer/ Clinician, often the ward consultant (see Box 5.2).

Measurable

The goal or plan must be measurable for us to gauge the progress of our care. This is easy in a physical illness like diabetes as the treatment regime's effects can be measured using a blood sugar monitor. One way in which we can measure mood is to ask the person to place themselves on a scale from one to ten, where one is extremely sad and ten is happy. Other measures could be the length of time a person can sit at rest or how many hours sleep they get a night.

Achievable

The goal or plan you set must be achievable. If a person is admitted with advanced dementia it is not reasonable plan for them to return to independent living. It may be reasonable to plan for them to go into supported accommodation. Planning for a severely thought-disordered person to manage their own medication is similarly unachievable in the short term, so although that independence may be our long-term goal, our short-term goal would be to help the person to order their thoughts.

Relevant

There are some interpreters of the SMART goals who will say that the 'R' stands for 'realistic'. Although this makes sense, realistic and achievable are somewhat the same in my opinion. I prefer 'relevant', as it is necessary to consider culture, religion, gender, mental

Joyce was detained under Section 3 of the Mental Health Act 2007. The criteria for this are:

- The person must be suffering from an illness of a nature or degree that warrants detention.
- There must be no alternative treatment to detention.
- Appropriate treatment must be available (Mental Health Act 2007).

All three of these criteria must be met.

What evidence do you find in Joyce's first interview that supports this detention?

Joyce was arrested under Section 136 of the Mental Health Act 2007.

This states:

'A police officer may remove a person from a public place, or a place normally accessible to the public, to a place of safety because they believe the person to be suffering from mental illness and presenting a risk to safety of self or others.'

Joyce has asked what Section 17 is. Section 17 is the legal agreement for leave from the hospital for a detained patient. It was highlighted by the case of Mark Zito, who was killed by Christopher Clunis, and must contain in writing the length of leave, the date of leave, the purpose of leave, and any conditions or restrictions upon that leave.

Box 5.2   Mental Health Act law

capacity, and intellectual capacity. For example if we expect a person with poor English and a borderline learning disability to understand and agree with their care plan, we must use terms and language that they are comfortable with.

Time-related

Your plan must also be time-related. Using a time limit allows us to evaluate our care plans, giving limits to when we would have expected them to have been effective. However, be generous with time as some things take longer than others. For example if you tell a person that the antidepressant tablets they are starting should work in four weeks and they do not, they will in all probability stop taking them. Antidepressant medication can take up to six weeks to work in some cases. It is vitally important that all care plans include review dates so that progress is monitored. That way, what is working for the client can be continued and what is not working can be changed.

Short-term goals/plans

For Joyce our short-term goals are threefold. Firstly, we need to maintain her safety and ensure she comes to no harm. As already discussed, we have detained Joyce for her own safety. Secondly, we need to ensure that planning for her future is well under way. This can only be done with Joyce's assent and concordance; therefore the third component of our short-term plans is simply to lessen the severity of her condition so that we may begin to work with her. What we want to achieve is the reduction of the severity of her symptoms. At present she is very chaotic and any therapeutic process will be impeded by this. We want to establish the therapeutic relationship, which

will improve the likelihood of success for our long-term goals (see Box 5.3). The treatment most usual in symptom reduction is pharmacology. The most common drug used in this case is haloperidol. Our goal is to introduce this drug at 5 mg three times a day initially. This must be reviewed on a daily basis as the risk of causing Joyce to swing into depression is great. Ideally we will adjust the dose downwards as Joyce's symptoms lessen. This treatment should be discontinued before Joyce's mood becomes euthymic (see Figure 5.1).

Note: There is no time line as all mood swings are individual to the person.

> **Student activity 2**
> *View the video of Joyce and her boyfriend Mark meeting with Simon. Make notes on anything you find significant. Do you think the short-term goals have been met?*
>
> http://www.oxfordtextbooks.co.uk/orc/clarke
>
> *and choose the video link.*
> *After watching the film you will also find it helpful to undertake Online quiz 2.*
>
> http://www.oxfordtextbooks.co.uk/orc/clarke
>
> *and choose the online resources for Chapter 5.*
> *Now before proceeding, try writing an updated care plan for Joyce (you may wish to use the blank care plan template provided online).*

Long-term goals/plans

Long-term goals and plans for any person must include several aspects. The first thing that must be discussed is compliance versus concordance. Put simply, compliance is doing something because of the perceived threat of what will happen if you do not.

Problem	Action	Person responsible	Review date
Joyce is exhibiting hypomanic symptoms, causing her distress and putting her at risk	To start antipsychotic medication	Ward doctor	Daily
Joyce has no accommodation	Allow Joyce time to discuss her hopes for her future	Named nurse	Next ward round

Box 5.3   Short-term care plan

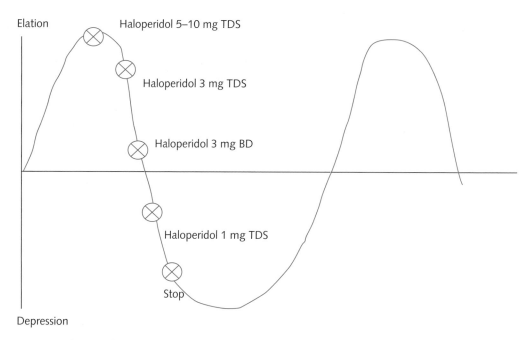

Figure 5.1 The use of haloperidol in symptom reduction

For example a person may accept regular injections of **depot** medication because, if they do not, they will be re-sectioned and taken back into hospital.

Concordance, on the other hand, is the person understanding the care plan and agreeing with it. It implies that the practitioner and the person work together and produce a contract. Concordance will obviously increase the success of any plan made and decrease the chance of relapse.

It is also important to remember our SMART goals. This idea still applies even to longer-term goals. We must make all our goals fit this framework, as without this we may confuse the person we wish to

help and unwittingly set goals that will never be successful. I remember a consultant psychiatrist telling someone who had lost their licence for drink driving to hire a chauffeur. This person was in a low-paid salesman's job!

The outcomes of our plans must also fit in with the individual's life. There are influences around us that dictate limits on our behaviours. For example when planning the discharge of someone, we have to take into account the needs, wishes, and abilities of the carer. The person may not be discharged to their own home but to their parent's house. This means that the plans may have to take into account the

Concordance and compliance: Pharmacist's view

Compliance indicates that a patient is taking the correct medication at the correct time and in the right way, and refers to the end result. Concordance describes a process (discussion between prescriber and patient) and a final agreement. Concordance can improve compliance due to increased understanding, but some compliance problems can remain, for example if a patient simply forgets to take medication. In the process of concordance, the patient is given an explanation of the reasons for wanting to use the chosen medicines and the benefits of treatment, as well as any possible adverse effects. There would be discussion around these topics and an agreement or compromise is reached whereby the patient agrees to follow a plan. Not all patients may want to be involved in concordance, as some would rather be told what to take. All the health professionals involved in the patient's care must understand the reasons behind treatment decisions for concordance to be meaningful and in order to be able to answer any questions the patient may have.

feelings, morals, and practices of the parents as well as the person being treated.

Finally, we must consider the risks to the people we are caring for.

Risk assessment

There are three main points to consider in risk assessment. Firstly, risk assessment is a continuum. The assessment you make now is only valid for that split second unless you factor in what might change. Someone who seems quite stable and safe when talking to you in a room might walk out the door and receive some news that changes everything. So, when doing risk assessments, never be afraid to discuss what may affect the way a person feels at present.

Secondly, do not underestimate the complexity of risk assessments. When at school I was taught to risk assess crossing a road. Look left, look right, look left again, and if nothing is coming, cross the road. This risk assessment misses several factors. How wide is the road and how long will it take me to cross? How is my health, will this make the crossing longer? How fast is the traffic? How high is the kerb, will I slip and fall? What's the weather like, is it icy, will I fall over in the middle of the road? Okay, you get the point. In risk assessment we must cover all eventualities.

Finally, consider is it necessary to cross this road at all, or if it is, is there a crossing/underpass/bridge nearby?

Conceptual models in psychiatry

Conceptual models in psychiatry are best described as the differing philosophies that underpin the way in which practitioners work. They vary in their fundamental beliefs about how people's lives may come into mental health crisis and how the problems should be treated. Each model represents an evidence-based, logical set of ideas that enable the practitioner to try to understand the nature of the crisis or problem. The model used will also inform the actions taken, as planned interventions, and allow the practitioner to predict outcomes for the client.

Tyrer and Steinberg (2006) describe four conceptual models (see also Chapter 1), which are:

- The disease model (also referred to as the biomedical model).
- The psychodynamic model.

● Discussion point

Can a person who is diagnosed with a mental health problem but is now asymptomatic and in complete remission, although still taking treatment, still be said to be suffering from that illness?

The report into The Edith Morgan Unit led by Blom-Cooper (1995) discusses this at some length and concludes that if relapse is the likely outcome of the cessation of treatment then that person may be found to be still 'suffering from that illness'. The Legal and Ethical Special Interest Group of the Mental Health Act Commission cited in Jones (2003) emphasized that there should be good proof that a person is not well purely because the medication has not left their system, and good evidence that they still have significant mental health problems.

● Discussion point

Advocates of a certain model may at times come into conflict with other models. It may be argued that practitioners must be proficient in several models in order to address complex problems. For example Joyce needs to be in control so medication (disease model) may be used, before we can assist her to understand her thought processes in order to control the effects of her condition (cognitive-behavioural model). Conversely it can be argued that practitioners should be proficient in their chosen model, and not as the old saying has it 'Jack of all trades and master of none'.

- The cognitive-behavioural model.
- The social model.

All these models will be described and discussed, but it is also necessary to include one further model:

- The humanistic model.

The disease model

The disease model assumes that mental illness is caused by physical and chemical changes, primarily in the brain. Therefore the main and sometimes only treatment is to reverse these changes by correcting the chemical imbalance or to remove or repair the physical cause. Its priority is to relieve symptoms and restore **homeostasis**. This model places the sufferer in the role of being 'sick' and requiring the assistance of a medical practitioner to make them well again. Although this model is not popular, one might argue, it is an important model in caring for people. As seen already, Joyce would have difficulty in utilizing any of the other models until the severity of her symptoms was reduced. There are also client groups who rely on this model. Some people, for example, want to go to see their GP and be told what is wrong with them and what will make them well. The reassurance is positive for them. People who are parents and have had a sick child may also have found this approach reassuring.

The psychodynamic model

This model, which has its philosophy historically grounded in the work of Freud and Jung (Gross 2005), assumes that mental illness is caused by unconscious forces in a person's **psyche**. It assumes that some of our feelings, emotions, or thoughts are unconsciously affecting our well-being. We protect our idea of self by using unconscious defence mechanisms that may impact on our behaviour. An example of this may be found in someone who has suffered abuse at the hands of someone far more powerful than them. Because they cannot express their anger at that person (perhaps it's their employer), they internalize that anger and when upset by someone of their own status or lower display excessive anger. So the main aims of treatment in this model are to make the person aware of the motives behind their behaviour, and to identify conflicts, fixations, and complexes using this knowledge to differentiate between coping strategies that work and those that perpetuate the problem.

The cognitive-behavioural model

This model assumes that mental illness is caused by abnormal, internal cognitions or thoughts that dictate behaviours and learned responses. The person has learned unsuccessful strategies that lead them to think about themselves in a negative light and also to be thought about by others as being odd and abnormal. Abnormal learning can be corrected using 'relearning' techniques. Therapists using cognitive-behavioural therapy may help people by changing 'unhelpful' thoughts into 'helpful' thoughts. For example when we pass someone we know in the street and they do not recognize us, an unhelpful thought may be 'They do not like me', or 'I have made them angry'. The therapist may try to reframe this thought into 'They seem distracted, I hope they are alright'. The different thoughts will dictate very different reactions. The first may make us defensive or upset, while the second will make us consider how we may help that person. So treatment will try to control the antecedents, behaviour, and consequences in order to facilitate relearning and retrain the individual to use more appropriate and successful intra and interpersonal strategies.

The social model

There is sufficient evidence to show that good mental health can be supported by social factors. These include things like:

- Housing/shelter.
- Finances.
- Social network.
- Occupation.
- Loving relationships.

This model assumes that lack of any of these factors can cause the person to suffer mental health problems. Therefore the main focus of therapy will be to redress the lack of any of these factors in the person's life. This model does not regard the person as 'ill' but as disadvantaged. It proposes that given quality in these areas, the individual would not require medical help. It dismisses the idea that the person is behaving in an abnormal way because of 'madness' but rather as a reaction to the lack of support in their lives.

The humanistic model

This model assumes that the individual client is the one who should say what is wrong, find ways of improving things, and determine the conclusion of therapy. Some of the most important people in this model were Carl Rogers and Abraham Maslow (Gross 2005). Rogers saw people as basically healthy and good and striving to do the best they can. This model was also referred to by Rogers as the **person-centred** approach (1951). In therapy, the practitioner will strive to be non-directive. The client knows what is best for them and will come up with the answers if this approach is used. This model uses three very important priorities:

- **Congruence** – genuineness or honesty with the person.
- **Empathy** – to see the person's life through their eyes and understand them.
- **Respect** – unconditional positive regard towards the person.

> **Student activity 3**
> *Having read the section on conceptual models, view the video of Joyce talking to the community mental health nurse (CMHN). What model do you consider the CMHN is using?*

📼 http://www.oxfordtextbooks.co.uk/orc/clarke

and choose the video link.
After watching the film, you will also find it helpful to undertake Online quiz 3.

ⓦ http://www.oxfordtextbooks.co.uk/orc/clarke

and choose the online resources for Chapter 5.

Contingency planning/ relapse prevention

This will be considered in greater depth in the following chapter, but it is important to stress having watched the last video that Joyce asked several 'What if' questions without receiving any answers or support. In any care plan it is important to consider the 'What if'. It is reassuring to know that if things start to go wrong you have a plan. If Joyce had been given names, strategies, and contact numbers she would have been much more secure.

Care planning only ends when the person has no further need of our services. From first contact and short-term goals (immediate needs), to the long-term goals (what will keep the person in control), to the plans for 'What if' is a cycle that only ends if we are successful and no longer required.

> **Student activity 4**
> *Evaluating care*
> So far, you have seen the journey Joyce has made from admission through to her preparation for discharge. Bear in mind what you have heard Joyce say on the videos, as well as what was written by the service user. Now consider how effective you think her care has been and what changes you would have made, if any?

Clinical scenario: Andrew

We will now go on to consider the assessment, planning, implementation, and evaluation of the care of a 19-year-old man (Andrew) by a CMHN following referral by the family doctor. This consideration will place special emphasis on risk assessment as a distinctly separate and yet intrinsic element of the care given to Andrew, in light of the nature of his referral to service.

It will debate the nature of risk, both generally and in the context of deliberate self-harm (DSH) and suicide. It will illustrate the relevance of evidence-based practice to the assessment and care processes. It will consider complex and diverse issues that arise from Andrew's scenario, and how these dynamics influence the work of the CMHN following a risk-led referral.

Meeting Andrew

The previous day, Andrew's mother had returned home to discover Andrew constructing a noose from the garage rafters. He was emotionally distraught

and unable (or unwilling) to rationalize his alarming actions. His mother had never witnessed this kind of behaviour from him and panicked; the family doctor was duly notified and a home visit rapidly ensued. After considerable persuasion, Andrew eventually spoke with the doctor and made a key disclosure. This involved an impending, temporary move out of the family home and into a hotel, as a requirement of a vocational course he was engaged in. He would have to live-in for four weeks. As this deadline approached, Andrew had become increasingly concerned, depressed, and anxious. The doctor prescribed a short-term course of anxiolytic medication and arranged a CMHN home visit for the next morning.

Andrew is the youngest of three boys and has no contact with his father and little contact with his brothers. His father cut himself off from the family since leaving them when Andrew was aged 14. His brothers are now married with their own families and live abroad.

Andrew's support network is limited to just his mother, who has not entered into a new relationship since the breakdown of the family unit and who, increasingly, resorts to alcohol – primarily to overcome an insomnia problem. She has been taking antidepressant medication for many years. Outside of Andrew, who she has always regarded as her 'baby', her only real interests are her pet cats, crosswords, and needlework. She has been well provided for by her divorce settlement and lives in a detached house in a prosperous area. Andrew has mild learning difficulties for which he used to attend a special school, on a private basis, prior to commencing the vocational course in catering.

He does have interests outside of his ambition to become a chef, such as football, but lacks the physical skills necessary to do this competitively (a matter of some regret for him). The progression from special school to college of further education has rendered him more isolated and he misses the company of his schoolmates and contemporaries. He does not find it easy to make new friends and is particularly shy in the company of girls.

Student activity 5

Having read the information above, which gives you the context of the situation, have a look at the video link of Andrew.

http://www.oxfordtextbooks.co.uk/orc/clarke

and choose the video link.
As you watch the film it would be appropriate for you to consider the following questions:
What do you notice about Andrew's presentation – make brief notes.
Does your observation lead you to any thoughts or feelings?

If you are finding it difficult to focus on specific issues, initially you may want to think about:

- Non-verbal communication, including eye contact, posture, gestures.
- Verbal communication – did what Andrew said about himself suggest to you that he had good self-esteem and self-worth?

You may want to reflect on what you have written and perhaps discuss these issues with your clinical mentor or student nurse colleagues.

Andrew – a service user perspective

Just because Andrew was found making a noose does not necessarily mean he will or even wants to actually go ahead and commit suicide!

He may be literally at the end of his tether but is actually engaging in a much safer exercise. Sometimes knowing there is even the possibility of a permanent way out is all that is needed for a person to try to cope with life.

Andrew, aware only of self-help, could not ask for outside help within his very claustrophobic relationship with his mother. He, after all, thinks he is the one to take on all the responsibility. He had no one to turn to; his only hope the **possibility** of a way.

His face lights up when he talks about college – **is this for show or for real?** He has low self-esteem,

» but with the right help and encouragement he may gain confidence as he takes up the opportunity to gain new skills and a sense of achievement.

Remove stressful environmental factors; add hope and empowerment and he would find it easier to cope.

His first sentence is an altruistic one. Although he does not verbalize it, it's he who needs support, as he winces at the enormity of his responsibility. His only companion is his mother. He feels very isolated as a carer. Who is caring for Andrew?

With only his Playstation for company and no male role models, he misses his brothers, not to mention his father. Male family members were essential points of reference for Andrew, providing camaraderie, banter, and emotional succour, but now he has only his mother. The roles are reversed; he has become the 'parent', she the child. They are both still enduring the grieving process. Andrew is also grieving for his former life of family stability.

Playstation games offer escapism but isolation is the price. His needs for affiliation are not being met; he has no friends for moral support and fun, no chance of exploring his sexuality – only shopping with his mother! (Shopping – another addiction for *her*?)

He feels he does not fit in and the stress of college, of four weeks away (worried about the socializing side and leaving his mother?), and 'all the *normal* boys at college'.

He wishes he could be like them, like his brothers; feeling he is not good enough. We have to question if indeed catering was his choice or his mother's. He feels he may be the only son who lets her down. All this responsibility, the fear of failing – (his mother?), and his father's absence puts enormous stress on Andrew.

With such social and emotional isolation, is it any wonder he has a negative self-image?

Alongside this fear is the fear of letting his very real emotions be revealed; he tries to put on a brave face and swallows down his emotions, possibly worrying about worrying his mother and letting her down.

She seems a very controlling factor, but then we get a glimpse of his long-lost autonomy and independence when he becomes angry with her.

Tracey Holley, survivor

👥 Assessment

Prioritizing assessment based on risk

As facts unfold and interpretations are made, it will become apparent that a mid- to long-term strategy is required in order to assist Andrew. The exact 'shape' of this strategy cannot usually be immediately deduced and requires further time with Andrew and greater information gathering. The CMHN must swiftly address issues of Andrew's safety as their initial action in the assessment phase, using an apparent attempted suicide as the 'starting point'.

Assessment (1): Risk and risk assessment

The assessment of risk is acknowledged as not being an exact science (Kemshall and Pritchard 1997).

Definitions of it are diverse and tend to be either vague or over-simplified, for example: 'An attribute/ habit [such as smoking] or exposure to some environmental hazard that leads the individual to a greater likelihood of developing an illness. The relationship is one of probability and as such can be distinguished from a causal agent' (Popular Dictionary of Nursing 1996); 'To be exposed to the chance of injury or loss' (Collins Dictionary 2007).

The term 'risk' often has a negative connotation; however, others suggest that our core beliefs overlook the positivity contained within the definition (Smith 1998). In this perception of it, risk is considered a dynamic process that changes according to circumstances and need. This may be considered in context with Andrew's impending live-in; there had been no previous risk behaviour from him, so what then are the catalysts for this change and what meanings do they have for him? How does he regulate difficult emotions? Does he possess problem-solving skills? If not, then would he be less at risk if he learned some?

All these (and other) considerations may contribute to the evolving plan of care for Andrew. Research suggests there are three psychological deficits associated with increased risk:

- Poor problem-solving skills (Schotte and Clum 1987).

- Hopelessness about the future (Beck *et al.* 1989).

- Inability to regulate difficult emotions (Macleod *et al.* 1992).

Student activity 6 – Discussion point

What do you understand by the term creative risk taking? You may want to consider Buchanan-Barker and Barker's work around this subject (Buchanan-Barker and Barker 2005). Do you consider that this is relevant in Andrew's case? There is a potential debate over the serious nature of Andrew's suicide attempt. Consider your likely responses. Would you want to ensure Andrew's safety above his independence and autonomy?

The risk assessment process has been defined as 'A gathering of information and analysis of the potential outcomes of identified behaviours. Identifying specific risk factors of relevance to an individual, and the context in which they may occur. This process requires linking historical information to current circumstances – to anticipate possible future change' (Morgan 2000: 2).

Risk assessment tools

These vary in design and purpose but are an essential component of assessment. Following any suicidal behaviour, particularly of a violent nature (such as hanging), here are just some of the things the CMHN must assess:

- Severity of episode and methodology.

- Evidence of planning.

- Nature of discovery.

- Access to means.

- Triggering factors.

- Continuing suicidal ideation – directly expressed or inferred.

- Previous suicide attempts and/or self-harm.

Good risk assessment should be free of ambiguity and not be entirely based upon anecdotal evidence (Smith 1998). Some might assign a numeric value to the assessed risk, on the basis that the perception of it will

not be solely inferred from subjective criteria, e.g. unspecific statements such as 'I just wanted it all to stop' are not clear statements of suicidal intent. Risk indicators may take many forms and the number of assessable criteria could be large. You will note from discussion with Andrew in the video clips that he did not speak of suicide in even the vaguest of terms.

Student activity 7

Revisit the video and consider any indications from Andrew's verbal and non-verbal communication that may suggest he is considering suicide.

http://www.oxfordtextbooks.co.uk/orc/clarke

and choose the video link.

Andrew's verbal behaviour on the matter of suicide, along with the non-verbal content, seems only mildly guarded and defensive – almost embarrassed. He does not feel that his mother had any right to raise the matter with an outside party. He does not express hopelessness and conveys some sense of positivity for the future, e.g. he speaks of his ambition to become a chef. See Tables 5.1 and 5.2 for examples of how numeric criteria could be applied to assess risk in Andrew's case. We will assume that Andrew has scored 2–4 (low to moderate perceived level of risk) and that the suggested action forms the basis of the care planning process.

Assessment (2): Mental capacity

Some feel that mental capacity should be assessed and recorded on every contact with the client. This is especially pertinent where that contact has implications for: decision-making (in the client's best interest); treatment proposal (including further referral or informal admission); or planned intervention involving the CMHN. It should be remembered that a person's mental capacity is not fixed and can fluctuate for a number of reasons such as intoxication, trauma, illness, etc. It should also be remembered that the client *does not have* to prove they have mental capacity; it is the CMHN's task to prove that they do not. Furthermore, the presence of intoxication, illness, (physical or mental), or trauma should not be taken to mean that the client therefore lacks capacity. Of key importance is the intention of the Mental Capacity Act (2005) to replace 'common law', which had no

Table 5.1 Risk indicators

Criteria	Risk value	Total
Wrote suicide note	2	2
Bought rope	2	4
Isolated location	2	6
Does not regret actions	2	8
Still wants to die	2	10
Expressed hopelessness	2	12

Table 5.2 Perceived level of risk

Numerical interpretation	Perceived level of risk	Suggested action
Total = 0–2	No/low risk	No further referral. Capacity and psychosocial assessment. Establish therapeutic rapport. Evaluate risk fortnightly.
Total = 2–4	Low to moderate	Evaluate weekly. Increase visits. Notify GP.
Total = 4–6	Moderate to high	Evaluate ×2 weekly. Crisis response strategy. Notify GP.
Total = 6–8	High	Evaluate ×3 weekly. Consider RMO referral. Notify GP. Evaluate crisis response strategy.
Total = 8 or more	Imminent/very high	Consider home treatment/crisis team referral. Consider informal admission or MHA assessment if necessary. Notify GP.

legal statute, no evidence base in practice, and therefore was not definable.

The basic rules of capacity:

- Is the client able to understand information?
- Do they retain the information?
- Do they believe it?
- Are they able to weigh up this information in context with appropriate decision- making relevant to their best interest?
- Do they understand the risks, side effects, or potential undesired outcome of the proposed intervention(s)?
- Have they communicated their decision in some identifiable form?

Considering Andrew's 'slight' learning difficulties, which render him with a degree of cognitive impairment, are these having some impact on his mental capacity and, if so, how is this demonstrable? Does the perceived level of risk change once we are able to contextualize his actions in relation to their meaning(s) to him? If the perceived risk is changed by such considerations, what interpretations may be inferred from his actions?

Do these actions have underlying functionality, say, to communicate distress or to emphasize the existence of a problem/crisis? Could they more accurately be described as self-harm (as opposed to suicidal)? Before discussing further assessment we will consider the phenomena of deliberate self-harm (DSH) and its link with suicide.

Deliberate self-harm

DSH has been suggested as a broad term describing many acts that result in 'personal harm' (MIND, 2007). These encompass various behaviours such as lacerating, burning, and self-poisoning – as *direct* manifestations – but also include failing to attend to emotional and/or physical needs (including eating distress and addictive behaviour). You may consider examples of lifestyle, possibly even your own, in order to deduce the various ways in which people may, consciously or otherwise, cause personal harm: smoking, drinking, poor diet, lack of exercise, etc. In young people, it has been suggested that pressures come from various sources (such as families, peer groups, school) that engender complicated issues within the young person, e.g. living up to expectations, underachieving, conforming. In this model, difficult emotions arise (such as hopelessness, despair, frustration, low self-esteem) and self-harm may provide a medium for the ventilation of these. Viewed this way, self-harm could be perceived as a coping strategy.

The likelihood of repeated acts of self-harm may therefore be high and this is problematic insomuch as there is a strong statistical link (more than 30 per cent) between repeated self-harming behaviours and the incidence of suicide. This information may be found in Standard Seven of the *National Service Framework for mental health* (Department of Health 1999).

This incidence includes the intentional taking of one's life and the risk of death by recklessness. In addressing the issue of suicide prevention, by way of targets for mental health, the *National Service Framework* (Department of Health 1999) suggests a reduction in the suicide rate – in England and Wales – of one fifth by 2010. No true figure for the annual suicide rate is known (usually because of the lack of 'evidence' that death was intended, resulting in an open coroner's verdict); however, it hovers around 5000 per annum (Meltzer *et al.* 2002). Clearly, contextualizing Andrew's actions is a vital element of the CMHN's work. The assumption of risk – purely in terms of suicide (as opposed to self-harm) – is erroneous (Babiker and Arnold 1997).

> **Student activity 8**
>
> Visit http://www.dh.gov.uk, access the National Service Framework for mental health (Department of Health 1999), and look at Standard Six: Caring about Carers. Having read briefly what this standard requires, review the film of Andrew's mother, Mrs J. Do you think that we need to be offering a specific service on the basis of Standard Six to Mrs J? What criteria, taken from Standard Six, have you based your decision on? You will also be referred to this Standard again in Chapter 6 and throughout your practice, so you do need to become familiar with it and with all of the standards of the National Service Framework.

Assessment (3): Psychosocial assessment

This form of assessment is considered best practice in the assessment of self-harm (National Institute for Clinical Excellence, second draft, Department of Health 2004) as it addresses issues of risk and need. It also posits that such actions may be placed in a social context, by way of consideration of a wide number of criteria: living arrangements, work, debt, personal relationships, recent/significant life events, psychiatric history, previous episodes (of self-harm/attempted suicide), drug and alcohol use, psychological factors. When all is considered, the formulation should include issues of long-term vulnerability (difficult relationships with parents, overprotective parenting styles); short-term vulnerability (lack of social support, work/health-related problems); and precipitating factors (Situational/stress triggers, relationship difficulties) (Department of Health 2004).

In summary then, Andrew's assessment highlights a possibility of further self-harm/suicide risk, and possibly impaired cognitive ability with implications for his mental capacity. Also highlighted in the psychosocial element of the assessment are his long- and short-term vulnerabilities and precipitating factors.

Care Planning

Care planning (1): Andrew and his mother

Considering Andrew's personal circumstances, within the framework(s) of assessment outlined previously, the CMHN must now make interpretations based on the information gained in the assessment stage of the care process. The relationship between Andrew and his mother is a significant component of this; although they enjoy a close relationship, it is reasonable to state that some distance exists between them in spite of their closeness.

Both Andrew and his mother would seem to be isolated since the breakdown of her marriage and, while having protective feelings towards her, Andrew also appears to have other, more awkward feelings, e.g. anxiety about her well-being. This is brought into sharp focus in his statements about how she will manage when he is away. Another example is suggested in his statements about events of the previous day, in which Andrew is clearly resentful of his mother for mentioning his attempted self-harm. This theme (of the distance between them) is also reflected in the little time they spend together, beyond Andrew assisting with cooking or shopping duties. Andrew spends long periods of time in his room watching videos and playing computer games. He seems to have no coping strategy (for the impending move) that is adequate to dispel his anxiety over her, or the demands that the required 'live-in' place upon him.

His resultant actions (the episode with the noose) may be viewed as a form of problem externalization and, if this is true, it may suggest that his actions carry underlying functionality; however, the CMHN would be wrong to suppose that the greater part of his anxiety is more attributable to one particular element of his dilemma than the other.

He may have concerns about his mother's coping strategy, as this relates to her consumption of alcohol; he most certainly appears to have low self-esteem and no peer group support from which he may draw healthy self-esteem. This is certainly a matter to be addressed in the evolving plan of care; the rationale for this is the manner and frequency in which his low self-esteem arises at the assessment stage. Andrew makes various statements that reflect this, e.g. when speaking of his college mates: 'People don't want to speak to me very much', and then 'I'm a misfit'. When speaking of his brothers: '...I'm not as good as they are'. His mother, when speaking of Andrew and his aspirations to be a chef, states '... it's easier to do certain things yourself if you want them done quickly'. Equally, she believes that Andrew 'has all he needs at home', which might seem to imply that she does not agree with the need for him to live-in for a month or believe in his ability to achieve his ambition. All of this provides *subjective* evidence for the low self-esteem issue; the *objective* evidence is, to some extent, provided by his mother but is bolstered by the CMHN's interpretation of the situation, and by empirical study of the matter.

Acknowledged consequences of low self-esteem include stress, loneliness, depression, relationship difficulties, impaired academic performance, and under-achievement (The Counselling and Mental Health Centre 1999).

Care planning (2): Stress

The same empirical study suggests the existence of the second issue to be addressed in the plan of care for Andrew: stress. In terms of definition the word *stress* is rather like the term *risk* insomuch as no single or universal definition of it exists (Cox 1978, Gross 2005). Also like risk, it is truly a subject that is more easily understood through as wide a knowledge base as possible. Essentially, and for all the lack of 'commonality' (inherent in the subject), one could more easily ask 'How is it manifest and what result does it have on an individual?' That it is potentially harmful is widely agreed upon. This is measurable in terms of disruption to all aspects of a person's health, i.e. mental, physical, emotional, spiritual, etc.; it can cause significant relationship difficulties and, generally, impairs quality of life. Perhaps the primary aim of the assessing CMHN should be to focus upon the manifestation of stress in Andrew in relation to his safety and well-being.

An essential principle, or aim, of good care, this line of thought is strongly derived from cause–effect principles. It is also apparent in the engineering model. The analogy with the effect of stress on a human being comes from physics, which indisputably shows that stress (loads) placed upon a material will produce deformity. Further considerations are important:

- The degree of stress required to produce damage is not the same in any two individuals. People's ability to cope with stress is equally variable.

- People, unlike metal, are sentient and have a potentially greater number of ways in which the stress reaction is expressed.

- Is the true nature of stress intrinsic (within the individual), or extrinsic (the result of an environmental or situational stressor)?

Our modern biological understanding of stress is based upon research in the 1950s by Hans Selye (1978) in what he termed the *general adaptation syndrome*. This theory, it has been suggested, can be used to interpret all human responses to stress. Selye's (1978) contention is that, if it is to survive, the human body must adapt to the repeated stress to which it is subjected. His stress model proposed three stages, which are shown in Figure 5.2. Selye (1978) suggested that, in cases of protracted, overwhelming stress, death could occur.

Although simplistic in its linear approach to analytical thinking, we have assessed Andrew as potentially at *risk* (of suicide/self-harm) due to internal factors (low self-esteem, learning disability, poor problem-solving skills) and external factors (demands of his course, concerns over his mother, alienation from peers, social exclusion). This, in turn, has created stress

and frustration resulting in a stress reaction (the episode with the noose) and, therefore, increased risk. The twofold plan of care points toward the aim of effective management of these issues with the goal of reducing both – their success, or lack of it, will be reviewed at the evaluation phase of care.

Andrew's care plan should reflect the monitoring of perceived risk alongside, or as an integral feature of, the overall plan. This overall plan, by now, will also reflect the greater gathering and analysis of data from the assessment phase (see Figure 5.3 and Box 5.4, Andrew's care plan).

Implementing the care plan

The above care plan will have been fully discussed with Andrew and he will be aware of deadlines and dates for significant actions arising from it. The approach to Andrew has so far been **humanistic** (client-centred); however, the whole ethos of care evaluation is to focus upon the effectiveness of the intervention(s) contained within the care plan. If subsequent evaluation shows it to be ineffective, the approach may have to be revised, modified, or changed completely. Consideration must be given to ways in which its effectiveness might be monitored. These could include measurable outcomes,

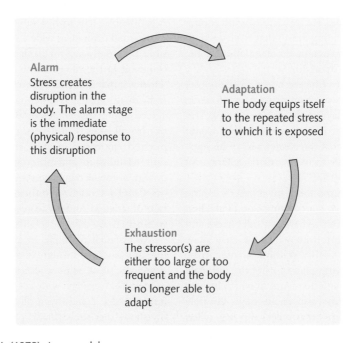

Alarm
Stress creates disruption in the body. The alarm stage is the immediate (physical) response to this disruption

Adaptation
The body equips itself to the repeated stress to which it is exposed

Exhaustion
The stressor(s) are either too large or too frequent and the body is no longer able to adapt

Figure 5.2 Selye's (1978) stress model

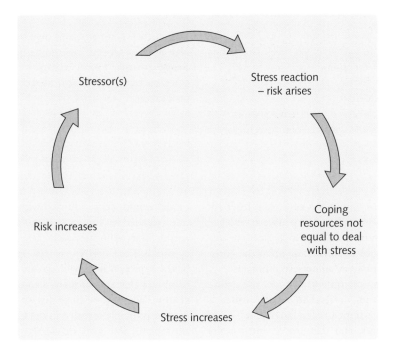

Figure 5.3 Risk/stress cycle

Client: Andrew J
Perceived level of risk: 2–4 (low to moderate)
Risk evaluation: Weekly
CPA level: Standard

Care plan (1) Identified problem: low self-esteem
Andrew has expressed ideas of low self-esteem. He sees himself as a misfit and feels that others don't want to engage him. His problem is exacerbated by long-term issues arising from experience of abandonment and his learning difficulty, reinforcing the view that he is 'not as good as others' (i.e. school peers and siblings). He is shy of girls, has never had a close/sexual relationship and is socially isolated. He shows motivation to learn and is training to be a chef but has no peer group support due to above issues. Negative feelings may be enhanced by impending 'live-in' and the resultant stress this induces.

Care plan (1) Intervention(s) and rationale
Discussed with Andrew increasing his social network and accessing available support from college. He agrees with the principle but the prospect arouses anxiety, which is malleable to support, reassurance, and logical positivism. By increasing his support network, outside of home life, Andrew's social exposure should increase along with the opportunity to learn new skills and receive positive strokes from others. He responds well to a humanistic approach. Have arranged to escort him to local friendship group in two weeks. Have also contacted student support services at college, who have agreed introductory meeting and will also participate in crisis response strategy. Arrange visit involving Andrew and mother to discuss the impending move, logistics, and plan(s) to support. Andrew to continue on anxiolytic medication.

Care plan (1) Goals/aims/outcomes
There is a probable link between Andrew's low self-esteem, stress, and risk behaviour. The strategy is to facilitate his increased ability to cope using short, achievable steps. Ideally, Andrew will be in a position to actualize and identify in himself the ability to overcome obstacles. He may especially gain a sense of self-worth by receiving acknowledgement from his peers. He may then be proactive in building healthy self-esteem. It is possible that the short-term result of confronting these obstacles will be to increase his experience of stress. Maintain contact at current

level until a week before 'live-in'. Will then increase contact to two visits per week plus phone contact and crisis response.

Care plan (1) Evaluation
Evaluation will take place upon every contact with Andrew (visits, phone contacts, and crisis response)

and if there are problems that require the care plan to be amended, this can be done promptly. If things go well, formal care plan review will take place once weekly. Review usefulness of anxiolytic medication.

Box 5.4 Andrew's care plan

accomplishing goals within the care plan, feedback from Andrew and others (mother, people at college), visible improvements in dealing with stress or evidence of better problem solving, or upon the emergence of any anticipated or unforeseen problems.

This is an opportune time to consider the nature and purpose of care, in relation to the issues it addresses. We have assumed that a tangible self-harm or suicide risk exists, and that this is intrinsically linked to the dual problems of low self-esteem and stress. The rationale is that in addressing these two problems, the risk factor will be reduced; however, until we are satisfied that this is the case, this risk must be managed. One model of risk management defines the process as: 'A statement of plans, and an allocation of individual responsibilities, for translating collective decisions into actions; this process should name all the relevant people involved in the treatment and support – including the client and appropriate informal carers' (Morgan, 2000: 2).

This can only be achieved with engagement. The process really has to begin with the principle of rapport building and the establishing of a defined, consistent approach to Andrew. At another level, there is a distinction to be made between the manner in which planned interventions are carried out and the way in which the CMHN behaves towards Andrew the rest of the time (when not performing planned interventions).

For example psycho-educational approaches, such as **cognitive behavioural strategies**, may be better suited to those interventions that seek to foster in the client different thinking/behaviour towards certain problems, such as managing anxiety (see Chapter 8). Heron (1990) suggests that the very behaviour of the CMHN – regardless of whether they are carrying out planned care – *is* an intervention in itself: 'An intervention is any identifiable piece of verbal or non-verbal behaviour, which is part of the practitioner's service to the client' (Heron 1990: 3). This particular

model would seem to fit well with the 'non-planned' care extended to Andrew in that it neither suggests an agenda nor delineates tasks, resulting in an 'open' approach. The CMHN may well opt for an **evidence-based** approach in providing care to Andrew, which combines elements of more than one model of intervention. When we evaluate this we identify the adherence to principle revealed in the CMHN's work. The aims, plans, and goals are clearly stated and rationalized; significant persons are identified; contingency plans are made. This will maximize support and safety for Andrew at a time when his potential exposure to stress-inducing circumstances is reasonably anticipated. This approach involves him fully in the process, states the timing of care plan review, and has some degree of flexibility.

Consideration of Andrew's relationship with his mother

The plan also specifies the need to directly include Andrew's mother in the care process. This is significant in many ways: he has indicated that at least some of his anxiety arises from his concern about her while he is away from home. Additionally, his mother may have her own anxieties about Andrew, and these two elements combined may impact on the situation in some way. Arranging to see them together is a good opportunity to gain insight into these dynamics and to make plans to allay or minimize any stressors – on either party's side.

Student activity 9
Revisit the two videos and consider the relationship between Andrew and his mother.
From looking at both of the videos, do you think that you would be able to draw any conclusions about the nature and dynamics of their relationship?

http://www.oxfordtextbooks.co.uk/orc/clarke

and choose the video link.

As we noticed earlier, Standard Six of the *National Service Framework*: Caring about Carers (Department of Health 1999) suggests that the needs of carers also be assessed; this is focused into three basic elements – information, support, and care. The policy goes on to state that, by *carer*, it means 'an individual who provides regular and substantial care for a person on care programme approach (CPA)' (Department of Health 1995). This suggests that carers, so defined, have an assessment of their own 'caring, physical and mental health needs', along with a written care plan that they retain. It specifies that this is 'implemented in discussion with them'. On one hand you could suggest that Andrew is self-caring and able to perform activities of daily living with little or no care required on his mother's part, beyond taxi-ing him to and from college – the term 'substantial care' is not exactly defined and may prove problematic in terms of Mrs J being formally assessed as a carer. On the other hand, there is a contention that Andrew would not survive independently from his mother and therefore it is her care that maintains him within the community. While she is not financially compromised, it is her independent means that support both of them. This should not deprive her of the entitlement to information or practical support; neither should it imply that her ability and competence to support Andrew are being questioned. If, in the course of the planned meeting, any matters are raised that are actually issues *between* them (or *for* them as individuals), the opportunity to discuss their nature/solution may arise. Examples could include Andrew's anxiety over his mother's drinking or her anxiety over how Andrew will cope away from home. The care plan to support Andrew in a structured way during the live-in period may in itself lessen her anxieties.

Student activity 10

It is necessary for you to consider interviewing both Andrew and his mother together. Andrew is a dependent and lives at home, therefore we are likely to be actively involving his mother as his main carer in monitoring and supporting the care we prescribe and alerting us to changes in his mental health state or increased risks.

What issues would you raise during this interview?

Think about some of the concerns that both parties have raised. How would you attempt to deal honestly and openly with these difficult, sensitive, and challenging issues, which are likely to lead to significant changes within their relationship? These might include Andrew's mother's alcohol use, Andrew's infantilization, Andrew's desire for external relationships, and possible future separation.

You will also need to consider what skills you would employ during this interview. Revisit Chapter Two as a starting point if you need to. Discuss mental health nursing skills with your clinical mentor. Having identified appropriate skills together, ask your mentor to assess your abilities to employ them within a clinical environment during your next interview of a mental health service user and their carer. It is essential that you follow the guidelines identified in Figure 5.4 before you carry out this activity. The acronym 'TOP' is a clever memory aid.

Summary

We hope that in this chapter you will have considered the notion of working with people in crisis. Both Joyce and Andrew are going through times of great stress, which carry high risk for them and those around them. We hope you will have learned not to fear these crises but to manage them effectively, reducing harm to those suffering them and to others. The skills used in this chapter of interviewing, risk assessing, care planning, and evaluating demonstrate techniques used to achieve this. You will have noticed throughout that empowerment of the individual and autonomy given to them in achieving their goals is paramount. It is often said that people with mental health problems do not know what is best for them and cannot make decisions. That may be true, however questionable, but it should be our gold standard that we will strive to empower people and give them control over their lives. There should be institutional acceptance of individuals, however different they may be from our norms, and all practitioners should strive towards partnership working.

The student should now understand the processes involved in caring for people in crisis and some of the skills you have practised can now be transferred to

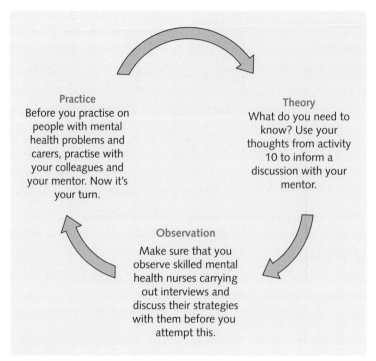

Practice
Before you practise on people with mental health problems and carers, practise with your colleagues and your mentor. Now it's your turn.

Theory
What do you need to know? Use your thoughts from activity 10 to inform a discussion with your mentor.

Observation
Make sure that you observe skilled mental health nurses carrying out interviews and discuss their strategies with them before you attempt this.

Figure 5.4 Guidelines for learning

placement. Don't be afraid to try care planning or interviewing but remember 'TOP' (see Figure 5.4). Nursing is one of the few professions where students get to practise on real people.

In the next chapter you will see this empowerment and autonomy become even more important. In crisis work we affect people's lives for, hopefully, as short a time as possible. In rehabilitation and recovery we may be involved for longer times, even the rest of someone's life. Giving them the lead in controlling their future can be a challenging but rewarding aspect of mental health nursing.

References and other sources

References

Babiker G and Arnold I (1997). **The language of injury: Comprehending self-mutilation**. British Psychological Society Books, Leicester.

Barker P (2003). **Psychiatric and mental health nursing**. Hodder Arnold, London.

Beck AT, Brown G, and Steer RA (1989). Prediction of eventual suicide in psychiatric inpatients by clinical ratings of hopelessness. **Journal of Consulting and Clinical Psychology**, **57**, 309-10.

Blom-Cooper L (1995). **The falling shadow: one patient's mental health care 1978-1993**: Duckworth, London.

Buchanan-Barker P and Barker P (2005). Observation: the original sin of mental health nursing? **Journal of Psychiatric and Mental Health Nursing**, **12**(5), 541-9.

Collins English Dictionary (2007). Harper Collins, Glasgow.

Cox T (1978). **Stress**. Macmillan, London.

Department of Health (1995). **The care programme approach**. HMSO, London.

Department of Health (1999). **National Service Framework for mental health: Modern standards and service models for mental health**. DH, London.

Department of Health (2004). **National Institute for Clinical Excellence, 2nd Draft for Consultation**. DH, London.

Dictionary.com (2008). [online] <http://dictionary.reference.com/> accessed 21/12/2007.

Gross RD (2005). **Psychology: The science of mind and behaviour**, 5th edition. Hodder Arnold, London.

Heron J (1990). **Helping the client: A creative practical guide**. Sage, London.

Jones R (2003). **Mental Health Act Manual**, 8th edition. Sweet & Maxwell, London.

Kemshall and Pritchard (1997). **Good practice in risk assessment and risk management 2: Protection, rights and responsibilities**. Jessica Kingsley Publishers, London.

Macleod A, Williams J, and Linehan M (1992). New developments in the understanding and treatment of suicidal behaviour. **Behavioural Psychotherapy, 20**, 193-218.

Meltzer H, Lader D, Corbin T, Singleton N, Jenkins R, and Brugha T (2002). **Non-fatal suicidal behaviour among adults aged 16 to 74 in Great Britain**. ONS, London.

Mental Capacity Act (2005). DH, London.

Mental Health Act (2007). DH, London.

MIND (2007). **Understanding self-harm**, revised edition. Mind Publications, London.

Morgan S (2000). **Clinical risk management: A clinical tool and practitioner manual**. Sainsbury Centre for Mental Health, London.

Popular Dictionary of Nursing (1996). Paragon Book Service and Magpie Books with the Oxford University Press.

Rogers C (1951). **Client centred therapy: Its current practice, implications and theory**. Constable, London.

Schotte D and Clum G (1987). Problem solving skills in suicidal psychiatric inpatients by clinical ratings of hopelessness. **Journal of Consulting and Clinical Psychology**, 57, 309-10.

Selye H (1978). **The stress of life**. McGraw Hill, New York.

Smith M (1998). **Working with self harm**. Handsell Publishing, Gloucester.

The Counselling and Mental Health Centre (1999). **Better self-esteem**. The University of Texas at Austin.

Tyrer and Steinberg (2005). **Models for mental disorder: conceptual models in psychiatry**, 4th edition. John Wiley, Chichester.

Webster M (2003). **Webster's New World Medical Dictionary**, 2nd edition [electronic resource] http://www.medicinenet.com/script/main/hp.asp from the doctors and experts at MedicineNet.com. Wiley, New York.

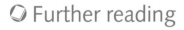 Online Resources Centre

If you have not done so already, you may find it helpful to work through our short online quizzes intended to help you to consider and actively work through issues raised by the cases in this chapter:

 http://www.oxfordtextbooks.co.uk/orc/clarke and choose the online resources for this chapter.

Further reading

Department of Health (2000). **National confidential enquiry into suicide**. DH, London.

Chapter 6
Mental health nursing in a rehabilitation and recovery context

Marjorie Lloyd

Learning outcomes

This chapter will assist you to:

- Understand the principles of rehabilitation and recovery in relation to discharge planning.
- Identify how recovery principles can contribute towards managing risk.
- Develop a therapeutic relationship based upon trust and hope.
- Identify the bio-psycho-social and spiritual needs of a patient being discharged from hospital.

Introduction

In this chapter we return to the story of Anthony and his brother David, who we originally met in Chapter 4, and Joyce, who first appears in Chapter 5. Previously we considered the role of the mental health nurse in working with people experiencing acute mental health crisis. This chapter seeks to consider how as mental health nurses we might go on to work with these people to support their rehabilitation and reintegration into the community. The chapter opens by outlining some key principles of recovery and proceeds to demonstrate how these ideas might be implemented in working with both Anthony and Joyce.

Recovery?

> The way I was feeling my sadness was mine. When I was in hospital staff rarely took time to find out what this was like for me. Not taking the time often fuelled what I was thinking: 'I'm not worth finding out about.'
>
> Nigel Short (2007: 23)

This service user describes how it feels to live with mental illness continuously throughout their lives, not just while they are in hospital. Professional staff may contribute to this feeling if care planning becomes too focused upon symptoms and treatment rather than person-centred care and recovery. In this context, recovery should not be seen as a new concept;

rather it can be traced back at least 200 years to one of the earliest asylums, the Tuke Retreat in Yorkshire.

> For it was a critical appraisal of psychiatric practice that inspired the Tuke at York to establish a clinical philosophy and therapeutic practice based on kindness, compassion, respect and hope of recovery.
>
> Roberts and Wolfson (2004: 37).

Later, during the 1960s, The Vermont Project (an American psychiatric facility) also published research on successful rehabilitative practice that was based upon 'faith, hope and love' (Eldred *et al.* 1962: 45). However, much of the current focus upon recovery practices is based on longitudinal studies in America, particularly Ohio. During a review of mental health services in Ohio, service users were asked to identify what was important to them. This resulted in the *Emerging Best Practices* document that is recommended guidance in the UK today (NIMHE 2004). The guidance defines recovery as follows:

> Recovery is what people experience themselves as they become empowered to manage their lives in a manner that allows them to achieve a meaningful life and a positive sense of belonging in their community as defined by the person in recovery.

It also states that:

> Users of services are able to recover more quickly when their:
>
> - Hope is encouraged, enhanced or maintained
> - Life roles with respect to work and meaningful activities are maintained
> - Spirituality is considered
> - Culture is understood
> - Education needs, as well as those of family and significant others, are identified
> - Socialisation needs are identified
> - They are supported to achieve their goals.
>
> NIMHE (2004: 2)

The care plan must therefore take account of the client's concerns in order to restore the balance towards hope and recovery, which may also include faith in taking risks. *The 10 Essential Shared Capabilities* (Department of Health 2004: 3) state that best practice can be achieved when:

> Promoting safety and positive risk taking [involves] empowering the person to decide the level of risk they are prepared to take with their health and safety. This includes working with the tension between promoting safety and positive risk taking, including assessing and dealing with possible risks for service users, carers, family members and the wider public.

(See also Chapters 2 and 5 for further discussion of this point.)

Student activity 1

Watch the video of Anthony talking about his illness and what it means to him. Make some notes about what you think his needs might be. These will be listed further on in this chapter so you can test your assessment skills.

www.oxfordtextbooks.co.uk/orc/clarke

and choose the video link.

Clinical scenario: Anthony

Anthony's discharge plan: Assessment

When listening to Anthony in the film, there is evidence that he has some insight into his illness that can be developed further in order to help him learn to cope with and recover from a serious mental illness (SMI) such as schizophrenia. *The National Service Framework for mental health* (Department of Health 1999b: 129) defines SMI as follows:

- There must be a mental disorder as designated by a mental health professional (psychiatrist, mental health nurse, clinical psychologist, occupational therapist, or mental health social worker) and **either**
- During the previous six months there must have been a score of 4 (very severe problem) on at least

one, or a score of 3 (moderately severe problem) on at least two, of the Health of the Nation Outcome Scale (HoNOS) items 1–10 (see Box 6.1). (This excludes item 5, 'physical illness or disability problems'.)

or

- There must have been a significant usage of services over the past five years as shown by:
- A total of six months in a psychiatric ward or day hospital, or
- Three admissions to hospital or day hospital, or
- Six months of psychiatric community care involving more than one worker or the perceived need for such care if unavailable or refused.

There are 12 items on the HoNOS, which since its original invention has been developed to address specific areas such as older people with mental health problems, secure settings, children, learning disability services, and acquired brain injury. For more information visit the Royal College of Psychiatrists website: http://www.rcpsych.ac.uk.

Box 6.1 Health of the Nation Outcome Scale (HoNOS)

Stages of the grieving process include:
Denial – refusing to acknowledge that anything has changed, e.g. 'There is nothing wrong with me'.
Anger – an emotional attributional response to acknowledging the change.
Bargaining – an attempt to return to life before the change by setting goals and conditions in an attempt to ward off the change event, e.g. 'If I stop smoking cigarettes the problem will go away'.
Depression – emotionally, the person is getting ready to accept the loss; this may be experienced as feeling powerless to stop the change.
Acceptance – understanding and recognition of the consequences of change.
(Kübler-Ross 1969)

Box 6.2 Stages of the grieving process

NIMHE (2004: 2) suggests that:

" People who are in recovery from mental illness/distress move from a state of dependency to independency. Many factors influence their current level of functioning. Consequently, movement is not linear. "

This is supported by Thornicroft (2006) who suggests that when a person is described as 'lacking in insight', it means that they have very little self-awareness of themselves and their own behaviour. However, he goes on to suggest that there is some evidence that lack of insight is a psychologically protective mechanism against the loss of the life that was known before the development of the illness. The client continues to act as if they had not been ill, as a form of denial against accepting the realization that they are suffering from a mental illness. This is a frequently used coping mechanism when someone does not want to accept some information that will affect them, sometimes quite drastically, and in some cases fatally. Perkins and Repper (2004) suggest that the most well-known work on dealing with loss is that of Kübler Ross (1969), who identified five stages of the grieving process common to people dealing with loss, and in particular the ultimate loss – death (see Box 6.2).

An understanding of the client's perception of their illness thus enables the nurse to work with them towards a recovery approach to managing the changes brought about by the illness. The important factor in helping the client to develop a recovery approach is to progress at the client's own pace, noting when they feel ready to take more responsibility over managing their illness and their lives. The Chief Nursing Officer's (CNO) review of mental health nursing (Department of Health 2006: 4) recommends that:

" Mental health nurses should incorporate the broad principles of the recovery approach into every aspect of their practice. This means working towards aims that are meaningful to service users, being positive about change and promoting social inclusion for mental health service users and carers. "

Pat Deegan (1988: 15, cited in Davidson 2003), emphasizes the need to help clients and their carers accept that change has happened and that the ability to live with mental illness must be developed in response to, not in spite of, the change. Deegan (1988: 15) suggests:

" In accepting what we cannot do or be, we begin to discover who we can be and what we can do. "

The CNO (Department of Health 2006: 18) recommends in her report that:

" ... the key principles and values of the recovery approach will inform mental health nursing in all areas of care and will inform service structures, individual practice and educational preparation. These values will recognize the need to:

- value the aims of service users.
- work in partnership and offer meaningful choices.
- be optimistic about the possibilities of positive change.
- value social inclusion. "

However, Davidson (2003) warns that there may be some significant differences between the recovery approach and rehabilitation services. The latter, as suggested, are provided and controlled by professionals, whereas recovery is a personal experience, which can be achieved without any professional intervention at all. Furthermore, he suggests that some rehabilitative practices can delay recovery, if they impede the development of hope, trust, and responsibility through paternalistic practices. Repper and Perkins (2003) identify the difference as recovery being an individual journey, whereas rehabilitation is the way in which practitioners help begin the journey. They suggest that:

" ... symptom reduction is neither a necessary nor sufficient condition for recovery. "

Let's turn now to Anthony's assessment (see Box 6.3). Not all of the issues in the box can be addressed at one time, so it is necessary to consult with Anthony on how the identified needs can be prioritized. It will be important for Anthony to begin his recovery by focusing upon what is important to him, which may not be what is important to professional staff or his brother (Davidson 2003, Department of Health 2004).

Biological needs

- Managing symptoms and psychotic episodes.
- Managing medication.
- Addressing side effects of medication.
- Addressing physical health needs, e.g. diet, exercise, sleep etc.

Psychological needs

- Coping with illness.
- Developing trusting relationships.
- Managing stress.
- Relapse prevention.
- Early interventions.

Social needs

- Developing wider social network.
- Developing social skills.
- Expanding social roles.

Spiritual needs

- Developing hope of recovery.
- Developing self-awareness of living with serious mental illness.

Box 6.3 Anthony's bio-psycho-social and spiritual assessment

Planning

In the 1970s, it was suggested that stress may play a role in the development of schizophrenia (Spence 2005). The stress/vulnerability diathesis theory (predictability/susceptibility) by Zubin and Spring (1977) led to the development of psycho-social interventions (PSI) as a popular rehabilitation model (Williams 2002, Baguley and Dulson 2004).

At the same time, the theory of high expressed emotions (EEs) in families and carers was being recognized as a significant factor in a person's relapse signature (see also Chapter 8, Box 8.4). The theory identified the negative behaviours demonstrated by relatives and carers showing high expressed emotion as over-involved, over-critical, and/or hostile (Baguley and Dulson 2004). These behaviours were thought to develop in families because of difficulties coping with the changes that SMI can lead to, and research indicates they may contribute to a relapse in people with SMI.

Student activity 2
If you wish, you could watch the video of Anthony's brother David being interviewed and consider whether he shows high EEs. Does the nurse assess this aspect of David's involvement in any way?

🔊 www.oxfordtextbooks.co.uk/orc/clarke

and choose the video link.
While the move into community care developed as medication choices grew in the 1990s, it became increasingly recognized that professionals needed to work in each of the bio-psycho-social areas in order to help people recover from mental illness. Spence (2005) suggests that this new approach was not intended to cure people of all their symptoms, but to help sufferers and their families cope and manage the illness so that it caused as little disruption to their lives as possible (Department of Health 2001a, Repper and Perkins 2003).

A 1994 review of mental health nursing entitled *Working in partnership: A collaborative approach to care* (Department of Health 1994) suggested that community mental health workers were not addressing the needs of people with SMI, but spending much of their time with less severely ill people who became known as the 'worried well'. Mental health nurses were encouraged along with other mental health workers to develop a psycho-social approach to mental health service provision, and psycho-social

intervention (PSI) skills became a requirement of mental health staff and educational curricula. The report was also the first to suggest that nurses in mental health care became community mental health nurses (CMHNs) to represent their health-promoting role, rather than community psychiatric nurses (CPNs). See Figure 6.1 (p. 122) for an amalgamation of the evidence that contributed to the PSI approach.

In the same decade, many reviews found that mental health services both in hospital and in the community had failed to meet the needs of people with serious mental illness. The Care Programme Approach (CPA) was developed and implemented alongside the recommendation of psycho-social interventions being offered to all people suffering from SMI (Department of Health 1999b, Baguley and Dulson 2004). This approach to mental health care was further supported in 2006 when *10 High impact changes for mental health services* (Care Services Improvement Partnership 2006) were developed by the Department of Health to improve the efficiency and the effectiveness of care provided to people with SMI. The guidance outlined in the document made the following recommendations in developing mental health services in hospital and the community:

1) Treat home-based care and support as the norm for the delivery of mental health services – *avoiding hospital admission where possible.*

2) Improve flow of service users and carers across health and social care by improving access to screening and assessment.

3) Manage variation in service user discharge processes – *aiming to improve the discharge process.*

4) Manage variation in access to all mental health services – *to improve consistency in service provision.*

5) Avoid unnecessary contact for service users and provide necessary contact in the right setting – *to improve efficacy of the service.*

6) Increase the reliability of interventions by designing care around what is known to work and that service users and carers inform and influence – *identifying good practice and evidence-based interventions.*

7) Apply a systematic approach to enable the recovery of people with long-term conditions – *supporting people with long-term conditions.*

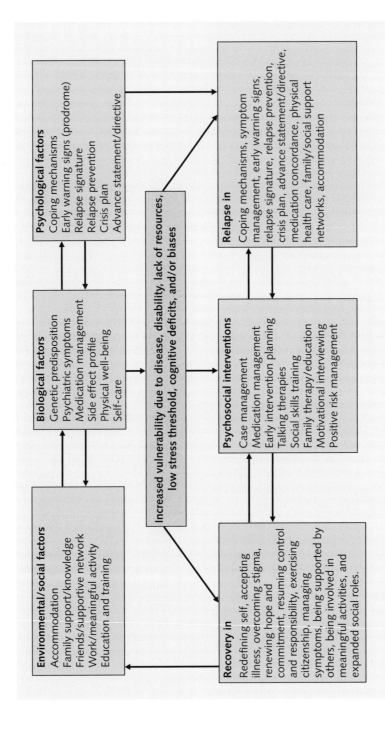

Figure 6.1 A combined psycho-social/recovery approach

8) Improve service user flow by removing queues and reducing waiting time.

9) Optimize service user and carer flow through the service using an integrated care pathway approach – *developing a whole systems approach*.

10) Redesign and extend roles in line with efficient service user and carer pathways to attract and retain an effective workforce.

Implementation

To lessen the likelihood of relapse in a person living with an SMI, effective support systems need to be in place. Anthony will need a great deal of support in his daily life to help him take control of his illness and learn how to manage it. The *10 high impact changes for mental health services* (Care Services Improvement Partnership 2006) provide some guide as how this support can be achieved for Anthony, but it also requires a knowledge of evidence-based interventions and service provision to be fully implemented.

> **Student activity 3**
> *Now watch the video of Anthony and his brother talking to a mental health nurse:*

www.oxfordtextbooks.co.uk/orc/clarke

and choose the video link.
Try to identify a number of areas in which Anthony could be helped and supported to manage his illness and consider how you might address these needs.

The *10 essential shared capabilities* (Department of Health 2004) also recognize that mental health nurses must work in partnership with service users and their carers to promote recovery and provide service user-centred care. Anthony will be leaving hospital and going back home with 'aftercare under supervision', as anyone who is detained on a Section 3 of the Mental Health Act (1983) is entitled to the provision of aftercare (under Section 117 of the Act) by local statutory agencies, e.g. NHS and local authority. In addition to this criterion of the 1983 Act, under the amended Mental Health Act (2007), Anthony fulfils the criteria for treatment in the community under a Community Treatment Order (CTO), because:

A. The patient is suffering from mental disorder of a nature or degree that makes it appropriate for him to receive medical treatment;

B. It is necessary for his health or safety or for the protection of other persons that he should receive such treatment;

C. Subject to his being liable to be recalled as mentioned in paragraph (D) below, such treatment can be provided without his continuing to be detained in a hospital;

D. It is necessary that the responsible clinician should be able to exercise the power under Section 17E(1) to recall the patient to hospital; and

E. Appropriate medical treatment is available for him.(Mental Health Act 2007: 31).

This new section of supervised community treatment (Section 17A–G and 20A–B, Mental Health Act 2007) is intended to reduce the risk of relapse in the community by providing comprehensive care planning for recovery and fast access to treatment. Supervised CTOs were implemented in October 2008 to enable clients to remain in their own homes while receiving care under the Mental Health Act (Department of Health 2007a). An Assertive Outreach Team (see models of case management further on in this chapter), under CPA care coordination, will provide support that has a more intensive approach to implementing Anthony's care plan (Department of Health 1999a, 2001a).

Anthony's care plans

Now read Anthony's care plans (on pp. 126–129) and see where and how his needs might be addressed.

Anthonys' care plan

Biological

Service User Need/Problem	Goals	Care Plan
1. Management of symptoms, psychotic episodes, and medication.	**Short-term goals** Anthony will feel more in control of his illness.	Mental health nurse will provide information and education on managing symptoms with medication.
	Long-term goals Anthony will understand how his illness is affected by medication and symptom control.	**Rationale:** *Promoting recovery – The 10 essential shared capabilities (Department of Health 2004).* *NSF Standard One, Mental Health Promotion (Department of Health 1999b).*
2. Physical health needs, e.g. diet, exercise, sleep.	**Short-term goals** Anthony will be able to identify his physical health needs.	Mental health nurse will liaise with local GP services to provide regular health checks and advice. Anthony will be provided with regular appointments by GP and/or practice nurse to maintain appropriate health standards.
	Long-term goals Anthony to manage his physical health needs with support from local services.	**Rationale:** *10 high impact changes for mental health services (Care Services Improvement Partnership 2006)* *1. Treat home-based care and support as the norm for the delivery of mental health services.* *2. Improve flow of service users and carers across health and social care by improving access to screening and assessment.*

● Discussion point: Biological health needs

There is growing evidence that the physical health needs of mental health service users are neglected by mental health professionals. Unfortunately, if the client's health needs are neglected, they may become physically unwell and concordance with medication can be affected. Simply attending to the client's health needs through some basic observations may prevent complications with medication for the client later. Early interventions around symptom and medication management may also prevent a relapse, which can have devastating effects upon recovery (Department of Health 2001a). Monitoring physical health needs can take place in the GP's surgery or in prearranged medication clinics. It is important to identify where this monitoring role will take place to aid evaluation of the care plan at regular intervals. Basic observations might include:

- Sleep pattern.
- Fluid and dietary intake.
- Blood pressure/vital signs monitoring.
- Weight monitoring.
- Exercise advice.
- Smoking cessation advice.

Psychological/Spiritual

Service User Need/Problem	Goals	Care Plan
1. Coping with illness and managing stress through relapse prevention and developing early warning signs profile.	**Short-term goals** Anthony will be able to identify some aspects of his illness that may contribute to a relapse. **Long-term goals** Anthony will identify and recognize his own relapse signature.	Mental health nurse to discuss with Anthony individual early warning signs and triggers. **Rationale:** *NMC (2004) Standard H – based upon best available evidence, apply knowledge and an appropriate repertoire of skills indicative of safe and effective nursing practice. 10 high impact changes for mental health services (Care Services Improvement Partnership 2006): 6. Increase the reliability of interventions by designing care around what is known to work and that service users and carers inform and influence – identifying good practice and evidence-based interventions.*
2. Developing trusting relationships to help cope with illness.	**Short-term goals** Anthony will become familiar with key people who can help him recover. **Long-term goals** Anthony will be able to identify and contact key people in his support network.	Members of the Assertive Outreach Team to introduce themselves to and work with Anthony on his care plan on an agreed, regular basis. **Rationale:** *Promoting safety and positive risk taking – The 10 essential shared capabilities (Department of Health 2004). NSF Standards 4 and 5, Effective Services for People with Severe Mental Illness (Department of Health 1999b).*
3. Develop self-awareness of living with serious mental illness through hope and recovery.	**Short-term goals** Anthony will become aware of useful skills in helping him cope with his illness. **Long-term goals** Anthony will identify his own unique recovery approach to living with mental illness.	Care coordinator and Anthony will identify and recognize unique recovery approach through support mechanisms identified. **Rationale:** *Promoting recovery – The 10 essential shared capabilities (Department of Health 2004). NSF Standard 1, Mental Health Promotion (Department of Health 1999b).*

● Discussion point: Enabling Anthony's journey to recovery

Anthony will need to be able to trust those people who are involved in his care when he returns home so that he can rely upon them to support his mental health recovery. The success of the care plan will depend upon a collaborative approach to attaining goals in the short and long term (NMC 2004, Department of Health 2004). Empowering Anthony to move forward from achieving the short-term goals to the long-term goals will depend upon time and resources available to Anthony, the care coordinator, and other members of the multidisciplinary team involved in the care plan. *You should never set a client up to fail because resources are not in place to support the care plan*. If needs are unmet, this should be addressed by reporting to your manager using appropriate documentation. However, some actions can be taken that will ensure the development of

respect and trust between Anthony and the team, which will aid the implementation of the care plan. These might include:

- Arranging to meet with Anthony at an agreed time, place, and date.
- Writing down (or even using electronic methods, e.g. text messaging) the arrangements so that Anthony does not forget.
- Always arriving and leaving on time.
- Contacting Anthony to let him know if you are going to be late or absent.
- Arranging to meet again as soon as possible so that Anthony knows when the next meeting is.
- Making sure Anthony has access to transport (if meeting outside his home) and money to get there.

Sociological

Service User Need/Problem	Goals	Care Plan
1. Develop wider social network.	**Short-term goals** Anthony will explore his social network with support from the Assertive Outreach Team. **Long-term goals** Anthony will identify places he can go to receive support outside of the Assertive Outreach Team.	Members of the Assertive Outreach Team to help Anthony identify places in which he can develop a social network, including leisure, meaningful occupation, and/or employment opportunities. **Rationale:** *10 high impact changes for mental health services (Care Services Improvement Partnership 2006):* *5. Avoid unnecessary contact for service users and provide necessary contact in the right setting – to improve efficacy of the service.* *7. Apply a systematic approach to enable the recovery of people with long-term conditions – supporting people with long-term conditions.*
2. Develop social skills and expand social roles.	**Short-term goals** Anthony will practise social skills with members of the Assertive Outreach Team.	Members of the Assertive Outreach Team will role model social skills and provide feedback to Anthony in order to help him develop his social skills, e.g. communication and assertiveness skills.

Service User Need/Problem	Goals	Care Plan
	Long-term goals Anthony will be confident in accessing support outside of the Assertive Outreach Team to meet his needs for recovery.	**Rationale:** *NMC (2004) Standard E – create and utilize opportunities to promote the health and well-being of patients, clients, and groups.* *Providing service user-centred care – The 10 essential shared capabilities (Department of Health 2004).*

Evaluation

Because Anthony has been discharged back to his home in the community within the parameters of the Mental Health Act (2007), there will need to be rigorous evaluation of his rehabilitation and recovery. However, as suggested by Davidson (2003), rehabilitation is provided by professionals whereas recovery comes from the client. Therefore, a careful balance for Health and both rehabilitation service provision and a recovery approach in supporting Anthony in his home should help reduce his mental, social, and physical disability associated with his diagnosis of schizophrenia. When evaluating care provision it is frequently observed that mental health workers refer back to the original assessment in order to observe changes in presentation, frequency, and level of need. However, it is also possible to evaluate care provision from a service level and to use social policy guidance to support the evaluation. For example the National Institute for Health and Clinical Excellence (NICE) have produced guidance on the treatment of schizophrenia and the use of atypical antipsychotic medication.

Student evaluation

Following your evaluation of Anthony's assessment and care plans, discuss your findings with your mentor and/or your tutor.

- What would you do differently and why?
- What would influence your decision about Anthony's care?
- How could mental health social policy and/or law support your decision?

Service user evaluation

Mental health care provision should always include service user and carer evaluation of service delivery. This could take place when the care plan is being reviewed at a multidisciplinary meeting, or it could take place between one mental health worker and Anthony and/or his brother. This would reduce the stress of discussing their needs in a large meeting and it would ensure that the meeting stays focused upon the needs of the client.

Student activity 4

Review the care plans produced for Anthony's care using the 10 high impact changes for mental health services (see p. 123). This will enable you to think about how social policy might look in practice and to generate a few questions of your own.

Student activity 5

Reflect, preferably in writing, upon a multidisciplinary team care planning meeting that you have attended. How did you feel about the process and were the needs of the client discussed and addressed from their viewpoint?

Clinical scenario: Joyce

Joyce's discharge plan: Assessment

> " Recovery is not about 'getting rid' of problems. It is about seeing people beyond their problems – their abilities, interests, possibilities and dreams – and recovering the social roles and relationships that give life value and meaning. "
>
> (Repper and Perkins 2003: ix)

Student activity 6

Watch the films that introduce Joyce into this chapter:

▶ **www.oxfordtextbooks.co.uk/orc/clarke**

and choose the video link.
Make notes of the skills staff use to help Joyce begin her recovery. You may want to refer to your notes later in the chapter.

Joyce has been admitted to hospital following a relapse in her mental health, which has led to her being admitted involuntarily. This decision will have been taken by the multidisciplinary team if they felt that Joyce was at risk of harm to herself or others. We know that this is not Joyce's first contact with the mental health services for the following reasons:

- Joyce already has a diagnosis of bipolar disorder, which means that she has previously been assessed.

- Section 3 of the Mental Health Act is for treatment up to six months and is renewable.

- Section 2 of the Mental Health Act is for assessment up to 28 days and is not renewable.

- Sections 4, 135, 136, 5(4), and 5(2) should only be used in an emergency:
  - To detain someone in hospital for up to 72 hours (Section 4); or
  - To remove them to a place of safety from a public place (136) or from their home (135); or
  - By a registered nurse to detain a voluntary patient for up to six hours or until a doctor arrives (5 (4)) or by a doctor (or approved clinician) for further assessment (5 (2)).

(Callaghan and Waldock 2006, Mental Health Act 2007).

Joyce will also have the right to appeal against her detention to the hospital managers and to a mental health review tribunal, and it is the responsibility of the nurse to inform Joyce of her rights.

Student activity 7

Now watch both films, listen carefully, and read your notes – do you notice the nurse mention her rights under the Mental Health Act to Joyce?

▶ **www.oxfordtextbooks.co.uk/orc/clarke**

and choose the video link.

Identifying and allocating resources

Part of your assessment will include identifying and allocating resources so that Joyce can be provided with adequate care in the community. According to *The National Service Framework for mental health*

Areas identified by Joyce, her carer(s), and the nurses in the scenarios that may represent a risk to Joyce remaining in the community:

1. Vulnerability to *exploitation* – sexually and financially, from herself and others.

2. Loss of *accommodation* – if unable to pay bills due to above and chaotic lifestyle.

3. Relapse in *symptoms* – if not concordant with medication and community follow-up.

4. *Self-care* – at risk of neglect due to symptoms of disorganized thinking and behaviour.

5. Loss of *occupation* – if time management skills are poor or symptoms result in hyperactivity.

Box 6.4 Discharge plan risk assessment

(Department of Health 1999b), Joyce's care falls within the category (NB this is not a medical diagnosis) of severe mental illness (SMI). This is because she has a diagnosis of a mental disorder (bipolar disorder) and a recent admission to hospital under Section 3 of the Mental Health Act 2007. Joyce will have a right to aftercare under Section 117 of the Act (Department of Health 2007a) and records of this may be inspected by an independent mental health advocate.

Following admission to the ward, the multidisciplinary team will be preparing for Joyce's discharge as part of a 'whole system' approach (Onyett 2004, Department of Health 2007b). This will begin with an initial assessment and history taking that will provide the staff with information on how Joyce spends her time, what support networks are available to her, what her strengths and weaknesses are, and what risks might prevent Joyce maintaining her place in the community (Perkins and Repper 2004, Spence 2005). Risks of mental illness are often exaggerated by inaccurate media reporting and so it is important to assess risk calmly and fairly (McCann and McKeown 2002). Once identified, risks are often easy to reduce if not eliminate, but for some risks there may need to be positive risk-taking decisions made to support Joyce when she returns home. *The National Confidential Inquiry into homicide and suicide by people with mental illness* (Department of Health 2001c) recommends regular auditing to improve risk assessment.

Student activity 8
From what you know of Joyce, what risks do you think might present in her discharge plan? Some ideas are provided further on in this chapter but try to identify as many as you can and compare your findings with those ideas.

Some of the risks might also be identified when using the Health of the Nation Outcome Scale (HoNOS – Department of Health 1999b) to identify levels of severity and to evaluate Joyce's care and discharge plan (Wing et al. 2000). James and Mitchel (2004) argue that HoNOS is not an assessment tool but an outcome measurement tool that will provide services with a quick identification of areas of need. This information can then be used as a baseline for further, more in-depth assessment of certain areas such as mood, social skills, mental state examination, etc. (Department of Health 1999b).

Discharge care planning will therefore influence any further admissions to hospital and will help the community teams plan with Joyce for any future crisis or relapse in her symptomatology. Evidence suggests that early intervention will reduce relapse and help the service user maintain some control or power over her illness (Baguley and Dulson 2004, Rayne 2005). This is especially important when national and local policy supports the recovery approach to mental health care (Department of Health 1999b, 2001a, 2004, 2006, 2007, Perkins and Repper 2004, Spence 2005). Based on the information provided in the scenarios, Joyce's care plan should address the issues listed in Box 6.5 that will contribute to Joyce's recovery.

Carer assessment: Mark

The *National Service Framework*'s (Norman and Ryrie 2004, Department of Health 1999b) Standard Six identifies that all carers who provide a substantial amount of care should have their own needs assessed and be provided with their own care plan. In the scenario on p. 99, Joyce's partner Mark, who said he was also her carer, accompanied Joyce but his role was not addressed throughout the interview. Mark was showing signs of frustration in the scenario with which the nurse refused to engage. However, some carers who have experienced this assessment process have suggested that it recognizes their role and provides them with the opportunity to talk about their experiences as a carer (Department of Health 2001b).

Student activity 9
Consider your response to the following alternative scenario for Mark as if you were assessing his needs as a carer – what would his care plan contain?
Mark has known Joyce for the past two years. Mark says he loves Joyce and wants to take care of her. However, sometimes he finds it very frustrating when she takes no notice of him, flirts with other men, and spends all her money on silly things that she does not need. When Joyce behaves like this Mark feels that she cannot be left alone but he needs to go out sometimes for his own stress-relieving activities. Mark enjoys sport and going to the pub once or twice a week with his friends. He has not been able to do either of these things for some time now and he is considering how long he can stay with Joyce while she is like this. Mark thinks that Joyce's medication is affecting their relationship too. He wants to know if it is doing her any harm and how long she will need to take it.

You have met Mark twice now (he also appeared in Chapter 5) and you will come across him again in Chapter 7. Keep in mind what you have seen so far.

Biological

- Side effects of medication.
- Medication concordance.
- Relapse prevention.
- Coping with the illness.
- Recognizing and managing symptoms, which include abnormally elevated, irritable, and expansive mood, pressure of speech, flight of ideas, grandiosity, distractibility, increased goal-directed activity (wants a baby, to buy clothes, etc.), disinhibition (sexually and financially).

Psycho-social

- Fear of becoming ill again.
- Lack of control over her illness.
- Inability to cope with home life.

Sociological

- Loneliness.
- Isolation.
- Loss of relationships.
- Volatile relationships.
- Lack of knowledge about the area in which she lives.

Spiritual

- Lacks confidence in own ability to recover.
- Dependency upon professionals.
- Lacks self-confidence.
- Loss of hope.
- Lacks self-esteem.
- Loss of community/group cohesion.
- Poor relationship skills.

Box 6.5 Joyce's bio-psycho-social and spiritual assessment

Planning: the Care Programme Approach

The Care Programme Approach was originally identified in the NHS and Community Care Act (1990) as the best way to support people with long-term conditions in the community (Spence 2005, Norman and Ryrie 2004). This Act also made it clear that people should be treated at home wherever possible and that a system of multidisciplinary case management should be put in place to support people in their own homes. There is a variety of models of case management that can be implemented and Wilson (2002) describes six models of case management that have been identified in the literature:

- Brokerage case management model – the person is allocated a professional who will access resources on their behalf but rarely provides the interventions themselves.

- Clinical case management model – the professional who carries out the assessment is allocated the client to their caseload and provides the interventions needed.

- Assertive outreach case management model – the person is allocated to a team of professionals who will support the person in their own home and

help them to maintain their place in the community by providing extra support around daily living tasks.

- Crisis intervention and home treatment case management model – this model provides intensive care in the home for short periods of time.

Joyce's care plans

Risk

Rationale:
Department of Health (2001a). The journey to recovery – The Government's vision for mental health care. DH, London.
NMC (2004). Standards of proficiency for preregistration nursing education. Nursing and Midwifery Council, London.

Service User Need/Problem	Goals	Care Plan

1. Vulnerability to exploitation – sexually and financially, from herself and others.	**Short-term goals**
	To avoid Joyce being exploited while she is vulnerable and to reduce frequency of exploitation.
	
	Long-term goals
	To enable Joyce to have more control over her money and her relationships with other people.
		Ascertain risk areas, e.g. where does Joyce keep her money, house keys, etc.? Encourage her to use safe resources, e.g. open a bank account, secure locks on doors.
		    Help Joyce to develop budgeting skills on an everyday basis.
		    Refer to welfare rights officer for financial assessment and support.
		    Help Joyce socialize in a way that is safe from exploitation.
		    Provide information on social support as outlined in **social care plan**.
		    Help Joyce to identify and report signs of exploitation and abuse (see discussion point).
		
		Rationale: *Promoting safety and positive risk taking – The 10 essential shared capabilities (Department of Health (2004).*
		    NSF Standards 4 & 5 – Effective services for people with severe mental illness (Department of Health 1999b).
		    NMC (2004) Standard H – based upon best available evidence, apply knowledge and an appropriate repertoire of skills indicative of safe and effective nursing practice.

Service User Need/Problem	Goals	Care Plan
2. Loss of accommodation if unable to pay bills due to above and chaotic lifestyle.	**Short-term goals** Joyce to manage day-to-day requirements of keeping her home. **Long-term goals** Joyce will secure her accommodation with regular upkeep of maintenance and amenities.	Joyce will be helped to run her home on a day-to-day basis. Joyce will develop a routine of homecare. Provide support in coping with day to day issues as outlined in **psychological care plan**. Refer Joyce to housing officer if appropriate to help her maintain her accommodation. **Rationale:** *NSF Standard 1 – Mental health promotion (Department of Health 1999b).*

3. Relapse in symptoms if not concordant with medication and community follow-up.	**Short-term goals**
	Joyce will follow a systematic approach to managing her symptoms.
	
	Long-term goals
	Joyce will feel comfortable managing her own symptoms with little support.
		Help Joyce renew her prescription each week or as required.
		    Help Joyce to remember to take her tablets at regular intervals using a system that she is comfortable with.
		    Ensure Joyce attends regular outpatient appointments with her psychiatrist to review her medication.
		    Provide medication management support outlined in **biological care plan**.
		
		Rationale: *Promoting recovery – The 10 essential shared capabilities (Department of Health 2004). NSF Standard 1 – Mental health promotion (Department of Health 1999b).*

4. Self-care at risk of neglect due to symptoms of disorganized thinking and behaviour.	**Short-term goals** Joyce will be able to manage her self-care on a daily basis with support. **Long-term goals** Joyce will manage her self-care needs independently of support from others.	Mental health worker to prompt Joyce when required to maintain her self-care, e.g. regular haircut, washing, shopping for food, cooking, laundry, sleep, and relaxation. Mental health worker to encourage Joyce to develop a routine for the above and act as a reminder to reduce chaotic nature of the illness.

Service User Need/Problem	Goals	Care Plan
		Mental health worker to encourage Joyce to explore her coping mechanisms and develop ways of managing her illness as outlined in **psychological care plan**. **Rationale:** *Working in partnership – The 10 essential shared capabilities (Department of Health 2004). NSF Standards 4 & 5 – Effective services for people with severe mental illness (Department of Health 1999b). NMC (2004) Standard E – Create and utilize opportunities to promote the health and well-being of patients, clients, and groups.*
5. Loss of occupation if time management skills are poor or symptoms result in hyperactivity.	**Short-term goals** Joyce will identify activities that are meaningful to her and be supported to pursue unless in conflict with care plan. **Long-term goals** Joyce will develop a network of meaningful activities and support systems to maintain them.	Encourage Joyce to explore opportunities available to her. 　Joyce will be provided with appropriate support and advice in relation to effects upon benefits, etc. 　Support Joyce to attend various activities in order to gain experience and make choices that are relevant to her needs. 　Refer Joyce to occupational therapist to assess and support occupational needs. **Rationale:** *Respecting diversity – The 10 essential shared capabilities (Department of Health 2004).* 　*NMC (2004) Standard M – demonstrate knowledge of effective inter-professional working practices which respect and utilize the contributions of members of the health and social care team.*

● Discussion point: Safeguarding of vulnerable adults

Because of the nature of her illness, Joyce may at times of crisis be vulnerable to exploitation and abuse from people who should be supporting her. However, many incidents of abuse by staff, the public, or her carers may go unreported due to negligence and/or ignorance. Under The Mental Capacity Act 2005, negligence is now a criminal offence that could result in a fine or imprisonment. Negligence can mean that although staff or carers may be aware that someone is taking advantage of Joyce's trust, they may not think it is important enough to report it or may simply not recognize it as an act of abuse. Clinical supervision is an appropriate arena to discuss your concerns and how to report them. However, if you are not sure of how to help Joyce identify abuse, the government document *No Secrets: Guidance on developing and implementing multi-agency policies and procedures to protect vulnerable adults from abuse,* provides the following examples in identifying abuse (Department of Health 2000: 9):

- **Physical** – including kicking, slapping, punching, hitting, misuse of medication, restraint, or inappropriate sanctions.

- **Sexual** – including rape, sexual assault, or acts to which the vulnerable adult has not consented or could not consent or was pressured into consenting.

- **Psychological** – including emotional abuse, threats of harm or abandonment, deprivation of contact, humiliation, blaming, controlling, intimidation, coercion, harassment, verbal abuse, isolation, or withdrawal from services or supportive networks.

- **Financial** or material abuse – including theft, fraud, exploitation, pressure in connection with wills, property, inheritance, or financial transactions, or the misuse or misappropriation of property, possessions, or benefits.

- **Neglect** and acts of omission – including ignoring medical or physical care needs, failure to provide access to appropriate health or social care or educational services, the withholding of the necessities of life such as medication, adequate nutrition, and heating.

- **Discriminatory** abuse – including racist, sexist, that based upon a person's disability, and other forms of harassment, slurs, or similar treatment.

Biological

Service User Need/Problem	Goals	Care Plan
1. Concordance with medication and understanding side effects.	**Short-term goals** Joyce will develop a system for taking her medication regularly with support. **Long-term goals** Joyce will be able to manage her medication with little support.	Mental health nurse to encourage Joyce to develop system for taking medication that will help her to understand the relation of medication to symptom reduction. Mental health nurse to provide information and education on the drugs used, their side effect profile, and the management of side effects experienced by Joyce. Mental health nurse to encourage and support Joyce to attend regular medication reviews with her GP and

Service User Need/Problem	Goals	Care Plan
		her psychiatrist, to improve communication between the two, and to ensure changes in medication are made swiftly.
		Rationale: *Providing service user-centered care – The 10 essential shared capabilities (Department of Health 2004).* *NSF Standards 2 and 3 – primary care and access to services (Department of Health 1999b).* *NMC (2004) Standard B – practice in accordance with an ethical and legal framework, which ensures the primacy of the patient and client interest and well-being and respects confidentiality.*

2. Prevent relapse by developing coping skills.	**Short-term goals**
	Joyce will identify her relapse signature with her care coordinator.
	
	Long-term goals
	Joyce will be able to identify relapse triggers and access appropriate help.
		Care coordinator to encourage Joyce to identify signs that occur prior to a relapse in her mental health, e.g. sleep/eating patterns, patterns of activity, etc.
		    Care coordinator to help Joyce to prepare a **crisis plan** and/or an **advance decision** and share with appropriate agencies (see separate crisis plan).
		    Care coordinator to identify coping skills that have been/are effective in helping Joyce manage her symptoms.
		
		Rationale: *Practising ethically – The 10 essential shared capabilities (Department of Health 2004).*
		NSF Standards 4 & 5 – Effective services for people with severe mental illness (Department of Health 1999b).
		    NMC (2004) Standard E – Create and utilize opportunities to promote the health and well-being of patients, clients, and groups.

Example Crisis Plan for Joyce

1. Previous triggers that have led to a relapse (relapse signature)
Argument with boyfriend
Spending money excessively, i.e. over and above daily living needs and/or in excess of budget
Lack of contact with friends/family
Lack of sleep
Excessive (binge) eating
Excessive alcohol intake (over and above safe limits on a regular basis)
Rapid thoughts or not being able to switch thoughts off

2. Level of importance to Joyce (1 being very important and 10 being of no importance)

Rapid thoughts or not being able to switch thoughts off	2
Argument with boyfriend	1
Lack of contact with friends/family	4
Lack of sleep	2
Excessive (binge) eating	5
Excessive alcohol intake (over and above safe limits on a regular basis)	5
Spending money excessively, i.e. over and above daily living needs and/or in excess of budget	3

3. Coping mechanisms
   1. *Obtain important phone numbers to access support in a crisis (including out-of-hours services)*
      Include the phone numbers here
      Doctor ....
      Practice nurse ....
      Care coordinator ....
      Friend/family ....
      Local voluntary organizations ....
      Crisis telephone lines ....
   2a. *Discuss the following areas (identified in my relapse signature above as important in preventing a relapse – Section 2) with doctor/care coordinator as soon as possible to identify coping strategies:*
      Sleep pattern
      Relationship with boyfriend
      Rapid thoughts/inability to control thoughts
   2b. *Discuss the following areas of my relapse signature above with doctor or care coordinator if they are becoming a frequent problem (specify how long, e.g. over two weeks):*
      Excessive (binge) eating – over a month
      Excessive alcohol intake (over and above safe limits on a regular basis) – over a week
      Spending money excessively, i.e. over and above daily living needs and/or in excess of budget – over a month
      Lack of contact with friends/family – over a month

4. Crisis interventions (and advanced statement, but this could also be a separate document)
In the event that a crisis is unavoidable, how would you like to be treated?
   1. Obtain extra medication to help me sleep
   2. Provide extra support from the team to help me cope, i.e. someone to talk to, go out with, distract me for a short while
   3. Home treatment with professional input from doctors and nurses
   4. Voluntary hospital admission if it is agreed by my care team that the risks identified in the risk assessment become too high and all of the above have been tried

5. Haloperdol as a last resort after other antipsychotics have been tried to control my behaviour *(in the scenario Joyce repeatedly said that she did not like the way this drug affected her)*
6. Do not contact my family until I am able to talk with them myself
7. In case I lose capacity my advocate is………..………………………………………………………………… and can be contacted on………………….……………….

Signed Client………………………………………..Care Coordinator……………………………………….
Date………………………..

For more information on early intervention in psychosis and crisis planning, visit the IRIS website http://www.iris-initiative.org.uk/

Psychological/spiritual

Service User Need/Problem	Goals	Care Plan
1. Joyce lacks control over her illness and fears that she will not be able to cope in the event of a relapse.	**Short-term goals** Joyce will be supported in managing her illness. **Long-term goals** Joyce will feel equipped to manage her illness with little support.	Provide Joyce with the opportunity to discuss and become familiar with her relapse signature (see crisis plan). Help Joyce identify and develop her coping skills and strengths, e.g. distraction, mood diary, automatic thoughts, cognitive behaviour therapy (CBT). Refer Joyce to psychologist for assessment and support. **Rationale:** *Promoting recovery – The 10 essential shared capabilities (Department of Health 2004). NMC Standard A – Manage oneself, one's practice and that of others, in accordance with the NMC code of professional conduct: standards for conduct, performance and ethics, recognizing one's own abilities and limitations.*
2. Joyce lacks hope and confidence in her ability to recover.	**Short-term goals** Joyce will identify her strengths to help her recover. **Long-term goals** Joyce will feel confident in her ability to manage her illness and be working towards her own recovery with little support.	Provide Joyce with the opportunity to take risks and develop her skills through social networking/activities. Help Joyce to review her progress and care by full involvement in the care planning and evaluation process. **Rationale:** *Identifying people's needs and strengths – The 10*

Service User Need/Problem	Goals	Care Plan
		essential shared capabilities (Department of Health 2004). NMC Standard D – Engages in and disengages from therapeutic relationships through the use of appropriate communication and interpersonal skills.

Sociological

Service User Need/Problem	Goals	Care Plan
1. Lack of significant relationships leading to feelings of loneliness and isolation.	**Short-term goals** Joyce will explore opportunities available within her local community to develop social networks. **Long-term goals** Joyce will be confident in attending local groups/activities without support.	Mental health worker to encourage Joyce to visit local groups resources to identify opportunities available. Mental health worker to help Joyce to manage her relationships through developing her communication and assertiveness skills in either a one-to-one or group situation. **Rationale:** Challenging inequality – The 10 essential shared capabilities (Department of Health 2004). NSF Standard 1 – Mental health promotion (Department of Health 1999b).

● Discussion point: Stigma and mental health

Stigma is a growing concern amongst people who use and work in mental health services. Stigma can be very destructive and may be considered a form of abuse if it manifests in some of the areas defined as abuse above (Department of Health 1999b, 2000, 2004). Facing stigma and helping the client to deal with it can be a significant factor in aiding their recovery. While the main focus of the mental health professional will always be on helping the person to recover their mental health, the social side of recovery is often neglected or not considered to be part of the job. If, however, you are truly committed to a holistic person-centered approach, the social needs of the client may be just as important in their recovery as their bio-psycho-spiritual needs. You may want to consider and discuss with your colleagues how the multidisciplinary team can aid the client to:

- Develop social networks independent of the mental health services.

- Access local community groups to develop social networks.

- Maintain contact with local services such as housing officer, welfare rights advisors, education providers.

- Access vocational or recreational activities and/or courses.

- **Personal strengths model** – focuses upon the person's ability to manage areas of their lives that might be strengthened by the involvement of mental health services.
- **The rehabilitation model** – encourages the independence of the client by helping them to identify goals and needs that will help them to recover and to develop individual coping skills to manage their illness.

Planning: The community mental health team

Community mental health teams provide full Care Programme Approach (CPA) care plans, which may be based around the clinical and/or brokerage model of case management. Current policy guidance suggests that other forms of case management should be provided by separate teams (Department of Health 2001a), although guidance from NIMHE's (2004) report suggests that all mental health practitioners should follow a strengths model. Joyce's care will be provided in the community as soon as she is discharged from the hospital. Joyce's care coordinator will need to have a care plan in place as required under CPA and Section 117 of the Mental Health Act 2007. The care coordinator should ensure that Joyce's needs are being met and alert other professionals to failures to meet Joyce's needs in the community.

The CPA has recently been reviewed and is now to provide care to people with complex needs only. The lengthy documentation a CPA care plan entails will no longer be required for people with less complex needs. However, people with less complex needs will still need to be provided with a care plan and a crisis plan, to ensure easy access back into services if their mental health relapses (Department of Health 2008; see also Chapter 5).

Implementation – the importance of the therapeutic relationship in discharge planning

Recovery from mental illness requires a person to develop the skills to overcome or manage the impairment that the illness creates in order to live as normal a life as possible by their own standards (Department of Health 2001a, 2006). Ron Coleman (2005: 3), a service user and advocate of recovery, suggests that:

> If people are the building bricks of recovery then the cornerstone must be the self. I believe without reservation that the biggest hurdle we face on our journey to recovery is ourselves. Recovery requires self-confidence, self-esteem, self-awareness, and self-acceptance; without this recovery is just impossible, it is not worth it.

The recent interest in mental health recovery has encouraged staff and patients to look for ways of restoring normal living patterns while at the same time helping the patient to cope with mental illness (Perkins and Repper 2004, Roberts and Wolfson 2004, NIMHE 2005, Department of Health 2006, see also Chapter One). *The 10 essential shared capabilities* guidance (Department of Health 2004: 15) suggests that staff should work towards promoting recovery by:

> Working in partnership to provide care and treatment that enables mental health service users to tackle mental health problems with hope and optimism and to work towards a valued lifestyle within and beyond the limits of any mental health problem.

However the nurse coordinates care, the empowerment and involvement of the service user and their carer is paramount in influencing the quality and effectiveness of the Section 117 community care plan. This ability to work collaboratively with clients is also referred to in the Nursing and Midwifery Council (NMC) (2004) Standard B, which states that the nurse must be able to:

> … practise in accordance with an ethical and legal framework that ensures the primacy of patient and client interest and well-being and respects confidentiality.

(See also Chapter 2.)

Student activity 10
In the final film:

🔊 www.oxfordtextbooks.co.uk/orc/clarke

and choose the video link
what attempts did the community mental health nurse make to:

- *Involve Joyce in the care planning process?*
- *Listen to how Joyce felt about her discharge?*
- *Collaborate with Joyce on developing her care plan?*
- *Help Joyce to develop hope and optimism in her recovery from mental illness?*

How could the community mental health nurse develop a trusting relationship with Joyce using the above skills?

Pilgrim (2005) suggests that coercive practice may be used to encourage people who suffer from mental illness to cooperate with their care/discharge plan. This can be avoided by developing an empowering relationship that encourages hope and involves 'being with' the client to share in their experiences and respect their concerns (Perkins and Repper 2004, Lloyd 2007). The community nurse in the final scenario did not demonstrate these skills as she gave very little time to listen to Joyce, was more concerned with coercing Joyce to take her medication, and did not show respect for Joyce when she gave the reason for her discharge as being a shortage of beds. This approach to developing relationships with clients demonstrates an imbalance in power, where value is placed upon the knowledge of the nurse rather than the knowledge and feelings of the client. While nurses do need to take responsibility for their decisions, they should be able to demonstrate attempts to share that responsibility through positive risk taking and good teamworking and communication skills (Lloyd 2007). Barker (1999: 119) also suggests that:

> We do not empower our patients; the person with mental illness empowers the professional. The only way we can be of real service is to *learn from the patient*. Having learned what to do *for* the patient *from* the patient, nurses often gain some understanding or insight which changes them – however imperceptibly.

Evaluation using the recovery approach

When evaluating the care that was planned and provided to help Joyce return to the community, it is important to note that this is a crucial time to listen to how Joyce is feeling about her recovery. The Chief Nursing Officer, in her report on mental health nursing (Department of Health 2006), suggests that mental health nurses must respect diversity and choice of individuals in order to encourage recovery. The recovery approach to mental health is based upon the experiences of people who have suffered from mental illness for many years. Whereas once it was believed that people who suffer from serious mental illness could only be 'maintained' in the community, evidence is emerging that people are able to recover from even the most severe forms of mental illness (Perkins and Repper 2004, Roberts and Wolfson 2004, Spence 2005, and see also Chapter 1).

Principles of the recovery approach

- Recovery begins when the service user decides.
- Practitioners should work to reduce, not foster, dependency.
- Recovery is aided when hope, spirituality, and culture are respected and understood and services users are supported to develop these areas of their life through education and meaningful occupation.
- Diversity and individual differences must be considered.
- The therapeutic approach is holistic.
- Integrated approach across bio-psycho-social–spiritual spectrum.
- Practitioners develop trusting relationships based upon hope.
- Practitioners operate from a strengths model.
- Recovery wellness/action plan is developed.
- Family and friends are involved as defined by service user.
- The community is involved in the recovery process.

(NIHME 2005)

While it is important to measure improvements in client outcomes, clients will only be willing to take responsibility for their own mental health care when they have a full understanding of their needs and how these might be addressed. Mueser *et al.* (2002: 1273), in their review of illness management and recovery research, suggest that:

> Enhanced coping and the ability to formulate and achieve goals are critical aspects of rehabilitation and are in line with the recent emphasis on recovery in the mental health self help movement.

It is important therefore to develop a sense of shared learning as suggested by Barker (1999) and Lloyd (2007) in order to avoid misunderstandings between the client, their carers, and professional staff (Roberts and Wolfson 2004). Whitehall (2003: 49) suggests that:

> Above all mental health nurses must be the bearer of hope and believe in the 'recovery' of service users no matter what particular path they have had to follow.

For more information on the recovery approach and to see Mary Ellen Copeland talk about the Wellness Action Recovery Plan (WRAP), go to the Care Services Improvement Partnership website: http://www.csip.org.uk.

Cutcliff *et al.* (2001) suggest that clinical supervision helps the practitioner develop their practice in a supportive environment (see also Chapter 10). Developing your skills in clinical supervision also supports the achievement of the Nursing and Midwifery Council (2004) standards for proficiency, and is a recommendation for good practice from the Chief Nursing Officer (Department of Health 2006):

> Manage oneself, one's practice and that of others, in accordance with the NMC code of professional conduct: standards for conduct, performance and ethics, recognizing one's own abilities and limitations.

Service user feedback

When evaluating the care plan, discuss with clients how involved they have been in their care planning when they were discharged from hospital. The following questions might be used as an aid:

- Were they asked to sign a pre-prepared plan or offered the opportunity to discuss their needs in any detail?
- How was the carer involved and were they given the opportunity to contribute to the care plan?
- Do they know what happens to their care plan and do they have their own copy?
- Do they know when the care plan will be reviewed?
- Did the nurse write the care plan in the client's own words?

Summary

This chapter has provided an overview of the discharge planning process including the Care Programme Approach. The sample care plans provided are typical of initial community care plans under CPA and Section 117 requirements but these plans will become more refined as the client becomes known to the community mental health team. The importance of involving the client in the whole process to aid their recovery has been emphasized. Recovery is a set of principles *in* practice rather than a prescription *for* practice. The skills of the mental health nurse are the tools that will implement the care plans effectively and clinical supervision has been highlighted as a way of developing those skills.

References and other sources

References

Baguley I and Dulson J (2004). Psychosocial interventions. In M Harrison, D Howard and D Mitchell, eds. **Acute mental health nursing: From acute concerns to capable practitioner**, pp. 198-218. Sage, London.

Barker P (1999). **The philosophy and practice of psychiatric nursing**. Churchill Livingstone, London.

Callaghan P and Waldock H, eds (2006). **Oxford handbook of mental health nursing**. Oxford University Press, Oxford.

Care Services Improvement Partnership (2006). **10 high impact changes for mental health services**. Department of Health, HMSO, London.

Coleman R (2005). Stepping stones to recovery. **Scottish Recovery Network** [online] <http://www.scottishrecovery.net/content/mediaassets/doc/0501_ron_coleman.pdf>

Cutcliff JR, Butterworth T, and Proctor B (2001). **Fundamental themes in clinical supervision**. Routledge, London.

Davidson L (2003). **Living outside mental illness. Qualitative studies of recovery in schizophrenia**. New York University Press, New York.

Department of Health (1994). **Butterworth Report: Mental health nursing review team. Working in partnership: a collaborative approach to care**. HMSO, London.

Department of Health (1999a). **Code of Practice Mental Health Act 1983**. HMSO, London.

Department of Health (1999b). **National Service Framework for mental health: modern standards and service models**. HMSO, London.

Department of Health (2000). **No secrets: Guidance on developing and implementing multi-agency policies and procedures to protect vulnerable adults from abuse**. DH, London.

Department of Health (2001a). **The journey to recovery: The Government's vision for mental health care**. HMSO, London.

Department of Health (2001b). **A practitioners' guide to carers' assessments under the Carer and Disabled Children Act 2001**. HMSO, London. [available online] <http://www.carers.gov.uk/pdfs/practitionersguide.pdf> accessed 20/07/2007.

Department of Heath (2001c). **Safety first: Five year report of The National Confidential Inquiry into homicide and suicide by people with mental illness**. HMSO, London.

Department of Health (2004). **The 10 essential shared capabilities – a framework for the whole of the mental health workforce**. HMSO, London.

Department of Health (2006). **Best practice competencies and capabilities for preregistration mental health nurses in England. The Chief Nursing Officer's Review of mental health nursing**. HMSO, London.

Department of Health (2007a). **Mental Health Bill, amending the Mental Health Act, Supervised Community Treatment, Briefing Sheet SCT A3**. HMSO, London.

Department of Health (2007b). **A positive outlook: a good practice toolkit to improve discharge from inpatient mental health care**. Care Services Improvement Partnership (CSIP) [online] <http://www.csip.org.uk/index.html>.

Department of Health (2008). **Refocusing the Care Programme Approach: policy and practice guidance**. HMSO, London.

Eldred DM, Brooks GW, Deane WM, and Taylor MB (1962). The rehabilitation of the hospitalised mentally ill – the Vermont story. **American Journal Public Health Nations Health**, **52**(1), 39-46.

James M and Mitchell D (2004). Measuring health and social functioning using HoNOS. In M Harrison, D Howard and D Mitchell, eds. **Acute mental health nursing from acute concerns to capable practitioner**, pp 29-50. Sage, London.

Kübler-Ross E (1969). **On death and dying**. Macmillan, New York.

Lloyd M (2007). Empowerment in the interpersonal field: discourses of acute mental health nurses. **Journal of Psychiatric and Mental Health Nursing**, **14**(5), 485-94.

Mental Health Act (2007). HMSO, London.

McCann G and McKeown M (2002). Risk and serious mental health problems. In N Harris and S Williams, eds. **Psychosocial interventions for people with schizophrenia**, pp. 205-11. Palgrave Macmillan, Basingstoke.

Mueser KT, Corrigan PW, Hilton TW, et al. (2002). Illness management and recovery: a review of the research. **Psychiatric Services**, **53**(10), 1272-84.

NIMHE (2004). **Emerging best practices in mental health recovery**. DH, London.

NIMHE (2005). **NIMHE Guiding Statement on Recovery. National Institute for Mental Health in England**. Department of Health, London.

Nursing and Midwifery Council (2004) **Standards of proficiency for pre registration nursing education**. Nursing and Midwifery Council, London.

Norman I and Ryrie I (2004). **The art and science of mental health nursing. A textbook of principles and practice**. Open University Press, Maidenhead.

Onyett S (2004). Functional teams and whole systems. In I Norman and I Ryrie, eds. **The art and science of mental health nursing. A textbook of principles and practice**, pp. 773-818. Open University Press, Maidenhead.

Perkins R and Repper J (2004). Rehabilitation and recovery. In I Norman and I Ryrie, eds. **The art and science of mental health nursing. A textbook of principles and practice**, pp. 128-153. Open University Press, Maidenhead.

Pilgrim D (2005). **Key concepts in mental health.** Sage, London.

Rayne M (2005). Early intervention in psychosis. In R Tummey, ed. **Planning care in mental health nursing**, pp. 69-85. Palgrave, Basingstoke.

Repper J and Perkins R (2003). **Social inclusion and recovery: A model for mental health practice**. Balliere Tindall, Oxford.

Roberts G and Wolfson P (2004). The rediscovery of recovery: open to all. **Advances in Psychiatric Treatment**, **10**, 37-49.

Short N (2007). Feeling misunderstood. In M Hardcastle, D Kennard, S Grandison and L Fagin, eds.

Experiences of mental health in-patient care: Narratives from service users, carers and professionals pp. 23-26. Routledge, London.

Spence W (2005). Rehabilitation and recovery: Evidence based care planning for enduring mental disorder. In R Tummey, ed. **Planning care in mental health nursing** pp. 86-107. Palgrave, Basingstoke.

Thornicroft G (2006). **Shunned: Discrimination against people with a mental illness**. Oxford University Press, Oxford.

Whitehall I (2003). The concept of recovery. In P Barker, ed. **Psychiatric and mental health nursing: The craft of caring**, pp. 43-9. Arnold, London.

Williams S (2002). The nature of schizophrenia. In N Harris, S Williams and T Bradshaw, eds. **Psychosocial interventions for people with schizophrenia. A practical guide for mental health workers**, pp. 3-17. Palgrave Macmillan, Basingstoke.

Wilson I (2002). Case management. In N Harris, S Williams and T Bradshaw, eds. **Psychosocial interventions for people with schizophrenia. A practical guide for mental health workers**, pp. 53-67. Palgrave Macmillan, Basingstoke.

Wing JK, Lelliot P, and Beevor AS (2000). Progress on HoNOS. **The British Journal of Psychiatry**, **176**, 392-3.

Zubin J and Spring B (1977). Vulnerability – a new view of schizophrenia. **Journal of Abnormal Psychology**, **86**(2), 103-24.

☾ Useful links

You may find it helpful to work through our online material, intended to help you to consider and actively work through issues raised by the cases in this chapter:

ⓦ   www.oxfordtextbooks.co.uk/orc/clarke

and choose the online resources for this chapter.

2007 Mental Health Act
For more information on the different sections of the 2007 Mental Health Act go to this link at thew Department of Health:
http://www.dh.gov.uk/en/Healthcare/NationalServiceFrameworks/Mentalhealth

Chapter 7
The nursing care of older people with mental health problems

Catharine Jenkins, Glyn Coventry, Linda Playford

Learning outcomes

After reading this chapter and interacting with the accompanying resources you will be able to:

- Place the problems faced by older people in their personal and social contexts.
- Recognize the impact of ageism on the lives of older and younger people.
- Relate how the experiences of common mental health problems can affect older people.
- Describe some common physical health problems that can affect older people, and discuss the impact they could have on mental health.
- Analyse the consequences of these problems for the older person and their family.
- Take part in an assessment of an older person with mental health problems.
- Outline the nursing interventions that contribute to recovery and support.
- Write a care plan that is evidence and values based.
- Recognize different types of elder abuse, and contribute to relevant team discussions and decision-making.
- Enhance your trans-cultural nursing knowledge and skills.
- Challenge your own values about ageing and older people.

Introduction

In this chapter you will learn about working with older people with mental health problems. The aim is to clarify your understanding of the issues that more often affect older people, and guide your learning about the process of placing these difficulties in context, and of assessment and care planning. Of course, older people can experience the same problems as younger people, such as low mood, hearing voices, substance abuse, and worries due to the problems of life. In this chapter we will concentrate on some of the difficulties felt more often by older people – memory problems, depression related to loss and the stress of caring, and emotional distress following the difficulties of growing old in a second homeland.

Nursing older people is both challenging and rewarding. The lifetime's experience of an older service user, together with a combination of physical, social, spiritual, and emotional factors mean that individuals' situations will be different, complex, and at times, confusing. Diagnostic labels do not always 'fit', which means the holistic assessment carried out by the nurse within a multidisciplinary team (MDT) is even more crucial for planning personalized and sensitive care.

In this chapter you meet three service users. The first two are Albert and Vera, a married couple, who have been together through thick and thin, but are facing a serious threat to their relationship caused by Albert's increasingly poor memory. Vera is struggling to make sense of it, and cannot understand why Albert is changing. She faces the gradual loss of the man she knows and relies upon, while Albert himself is distressed by the feeling of not knowing what is going on, and the frustration he senses in his normally kind and cheerful wife. The third service user, Mrs Bibi, is an older woman from Pakistan, who is saddened by the separation from dearly loved members of her family, and despite strong support from her family in this country, still struggles with the pressures of growing old – she has arthritis and diabetes. Mrs Bibi does not speak English, and does not really understand the health and social care system nor the advice she has been given so far.

People are living longer, and consequently the elderly population is increasing (Cantley 2001). Working with older people with mental health problems is therefore a growth area, and there are opportunities in specialized areas in both inpatient and community settings that demand commitment and specialized skills to support the care of this group.

The approach taken in this chapter is to consider our three service users from a holistic perspective and to take an anti-oppressive stance. The most common form of oppression affecting older people is ageism, a societal force that excludes, devalues, and reduces the life chances of older people (Thompson 2003: 102). This means they are both more likely to experience mental health problems, and less likely to be able to get the help they need. Unfortunately there is a danger that as nurses we can become more ageist than other people, because we tend to see older people more when they are mentally or physically unwell, thus confirming some of the stereotypes. Working with older people means that we as practitioners need to examine our own feelings about getting older, so that we can challenge discrimination towards older people and ensure the service we provide does not contribute to it.

Clinical scenario: Albert

At this point, please look at the films of Albert, Vera, and their son Mark.

📼 www.oxfordtextbooks.co.uk/orc/clarke

and choose the video link

First of all, notice how they make you feel; what aspects of their stories do you find interesting? Do some aspects make you feel sad, or angry? Do you think your feelings about Albert, Vera, and Mark could influence the way you interact with them? Make brief notes – later on you might like to come back to them to see if your first impressions have changed as you have worked through the chapter.

You have probably noticed that we are using Albert's and Vera's first names. Most people have strong preferences about how they like to be addressed, and sometimes people from older generations object to the assumption that their first names can be used without asking (Department of Health 2006). The simple solution is always to ask, and then continue with this form of address unless you are invited to change it. Our first two service users have asked to be called by their first names, Albert and Vera, while our third service user has asked to be addressed as Mrs Bibi.

Albert and Vera's problems began about two years ago when Albert first thought he 'was losing it' (his words at the time). He remembered that he had lost his sister, Mabel, about that time and that he had taken the news of her death badly, since they had been very close. Although he had mourned her death for a period, according to Vera he was never the same after that.

Albert had always been a hard-working man. He had enjoyed his job as a postman but was forced to retire, much against his will, at the age of 65. He found retirement difficult in the sense that he felt he had no status or purpose in his life. Perhaps to compensate, he would spend long periods in the bookies pursuing his hobby of horserace betting. He hadn't realized how much money he had been spending until Vera confronted him one day after she had discovered he had lost most of their life savings. Albert said it had been like a dream: he simply hadn't realized how much he had spent and now felt he had let Vera down. Following this revelation Albert stopped betting but instead appeared to become more self-absorbed. He tearfully told Vera that he was losing his confidence and found everyday life to be 'difficult'. At this stage, Vera was unsympathetic and told him to pull himself together.

Over the following months, Vera noticed Albert wasn't bathing and shaving as often as he used to, which (at least at first) she put down to 'laziness'.

Albert couldn't understand what the problem was and only saw Vera's prompting as unnecessary nagging. A number of arguments resulted from this that put a strain on their relationship.

Life, for Albert, appeared to be getting more complicated. He found he couldn't sleep at night and then would get confused as to the actual time of the day and night. On various occasions he confused a.m. for p.m., not noticing the darkness or light outside.

Increasingly, Albert would recognize in himself that he was forgetting things. This usually made him frustrated, irritable, and argumentative. On other occasions he would become really frightened because he couldn't make sense of anything and would start shouting for help. As the months went by, Vera began to suspect the worst (her father had died with dementia) but told herself that so long as she had her health she would be able to cope. Thankfully for Albert, Vera was usually on hand to reassure and give words of comfort. However, matters came to a head one day when Vera had gone shopping and Albert decided to make a cup of tea. Although they had an electric kettle, Albert thought he needed to put the kettle on the gas stove. He did this and went to look for some matches in the living room. When he got to the living room he noticed horseracing on the TV and was immediately spellbound.

Meanwhile the gas continued to pour out into the kitchen, so that when Vera came home she was frightened to breathe, and didn't dare even turn on a light. She bundled Albert out of the house and struggled with him to the neighbours, from where she phoned the emergency services.

Later, Albert couldn't make sense of all the people around him. He heard the word 'doctor' but he thought it was about Mark having chickenpox. He thought there was nothing to worry about since Mark was eight years old and all kids get such illnesses. He said to his family 'Well, Mark can stop in bed and I'll take the other two to play on the swings.' He couldn't understand what all the fuss was about!

The GP, having examined Albert in his home and discussed the situation with Vera, later referred Albert to a psychiatrist for assessment. The opinion of this doctor was that Albert was possibly in the early stages of Alzheimer's disease. He recommended that a community mental health nurse (CMHN) should visit once a week for support and monitoring, and that Albert should also be referred to a day hospital for two days a week.

You may find it very interesting to go online and look at Activity 1 – Albert: The care of people with physical problems in psychiatric settings.

 www.oxfordtextbooks.co.uk/orc/clarke

and choose the online resources for this chapter.

This additional information and the associated activities (including an online quiz) will assist you in developing your knowledge about the physical health problems someone like Albert could experience. It also offers the opportunity to consider the nurse's role and care planning priorities. Meanwhile the chapter text will continue to assess Albert's mental health problems.

👥 Assessment

The purpose of assessment is to gather thorough, appropriate, and relevant information on which to base your plan of care. Much can be gleaned through gathering together historical data, interviewing Albert's relatives (Vera and Mark), having discussions with other professionals involved in the case, and of course, the actual contact time that staff spend with Albert (which enables observational and interaction skills to be used to help staff form an opinion). Making sure that Albert is wearing his hearing aid, glasses, and dentures will ensure he is able to communicate as effectively as possible. Albert should be at the centre of the assessment, and should be asked what he believes his strengths to be, as well as his problems, and what he would like to happen as a result (Adams 2008: 128).

In interacting with Albert, a subtle observation of his physical demeanour, his non-verbal body language, and his 'facial talk' and eye contact should all be noted. The content of his speech and his affective (emotional) state will elicit further important clues. Specifically, look for evidence of a decline in:

- **Memory.** Has Albert forgotten that he mentioned things previously in the discussion? Is he repeating himself?

- **Speed of performance.** Are his responses slower than you would expect? Any thought block?

- **Language.** Assess his verbal fluency.

- **Executive functioning,** i.e. higher level skills of planning, problem solving, and flexible thinking.

- **Perceptual abilities.** How does he perceive his reality? Is there any evidence of psychosis?

- **Behaviour.** Is this appropriate to the social situation? Are there excesses or deficits in the behaviours observed? How does he react to various stimuli?

- **Level of functioning.** What is the level of self-care ability? Does he now require help with daily living compared to previous patterns of behaviour?

Another important aspect of Albert's assessment is about formulating a view with regard to the degree of risk with which Albert presents. Recent observation and historical data can obviously provide us with a lot of relevant information (see Chapter 2, p. 27). Indeed, the process of risk assessment involves linking these two in order to anticipate possible future change (Morgan 2000a: 2). Also remember that as well as the items listed above, formal assessment tools may be used to further add to the information gathered. In Albert's situation the Mini Mental State Examination, for example, may be routinely used. Please read Box 7.1 and then identify those aspects of Albert's behaviour that pose a risk to his well-being.

Student activity 1

Have a look at the Mini Mental State Examination (see link below) and familiarize yourself with its content and the process of this assessment. How would you get on if someone asked you these questions? Practise asking the questions sensitively, using a friend or colleague, and ask for constructive feedback.

http://www.alzheimers.org.uk/factsheet/436/

Albert may be tired or 'feeling off' when he is assessed. He may also display a degree of anxiety if interviewed outside his normal living space (known as 'admission anxiety'). His true, current level of functioning may

---

- Presentation:

  – appears disorientated in time, place, and person.
  – no longer argumentative, rather placid.
  – misinterprets people's identity – mistakes Vera for own mother, thinks eldest son is father.

- Can talk:

  – loosely based on triggers from environment.
  – minor echolalia, e.g. knife/wife.
  – or words by association, e.g. points to bread and calls it butter.
  – can tell stories – confabulations, based on past, e.g. 'I went to work this morning …'
  – also makes words up or strings together in (apparently) nonsensical sentences.
  NB some memories fade in and out – relates to time as a postman.

- Behaviour:

  – wanders around – looking for things.
  – doesn't necessarily recognize everyday objects, e.g. has to be shown how to use a cup.
  – occasionally shouts for mother if distressed.
  – needs to be prompted to sit, walk, eat, etc.
  – sits in chair at times, looking blank.

- Emotions:

  – sometimes incongruent – laughing/crying for no apparent reason.
  – labile – crying/laughing easily – suddenly stops.

- Insight:

  – appears occasionally to show some understanding of what's going on.

Box 7.1 An example of some observational notes following a day in the day hospital

therefore be skewed. What can be done to overcome this?

Revisit the video clip of Albert.

📼 www.oxfordtextbooks.co.uk/orc/clarke

and choose the video link.

Make notes this time round in order to assess his mental health and social needs.

The language used by professionals to describe the problems experienced by people with dementia can be very confusing to service users and families. You may be called upon to 'translate' professional jargon into language others can understand. The following are common examples:

- **Dysphasia** – difficulties with speech. This may be 'receptive', so messages received are not properly understood, or expressive, where the person has problems saying what he or she means.

- **Nominal dysphasia** – forgetting the names of people or objects.

- **Aphasia** – inability to speak.

- **Agnosia** – inability to recognize objects.

- **Confabulation** – filling a gap in memory with a likely explanation.

Student activity 2

As you watched the film of Albert to assess his mental health and social needs, you may have noticed some of the above problems. Think about how you could explain one of these terms to Vera in ordinary language. How could you adapt your own speech and non-verbal communication to make it easier for Albert?

Care planning

The planning of Albert's care will be based on his assessment. There will be data from interviewing Albert and his family, observing his behaviour, and the collation of his nursing and medical history, as well as information gleaned from liaison with other professionals. It is worth stating that with illnesses such as dementia, the long-term prognosis is not good. Atrophy of brain cells means that the disease process is not reversible and that associated brain functioning will inevitably decline. However, following the work of the Bradford Dementia Group and the late Tom Kitwood (1997), it has been theorized

that this rate of cognitive decline can be slowed by changes to the social environment. Even so, it is inevitable that care plans will have to be altered over the time of the client's illness in order to meet their needs as the condition deteriorates and the plan is evaluated. A care plan drawn up in the initial stages of care can look very different from one in the moderate stage and again this will differ from one in the severe stage. Long-term goals may not be that helpful to identify in this care context.

John, a staff nurse at the day hospital, has compiled the following care plan.

👤 Service user's comment

Is it usual practice for people to be interviewed in unfamiliar, perhaps rather clinical and unwelcoming surroundings? This caused distress, adding to Albert's difficulty in giving answers to questions.

Whilst the interviewer had a very friendly and sympathetic attitude, sometimes the interview seemed more like a test than an exploratory conversation. Is it good to ask certain kinds of questions that the person is clearly going to have difficulty with, e.g. how long …? Is questioning someone in the framework they find difficult, i.e. remembering, trying to find words they've forgotten, a good idea?

It was noticeable that Albert hadn't forgotten the actions to go with what he was trying to explain, e.g. the wheel of a car. So, as in other areas of mental and emotional distress, is it equally important to pay attention to non-verbal communication?

One of the things this clip highlighted for me – as well as the other clips – was how difficult it can be for practitioners to elicit information to help them make an assessment of what is actually going on, e.g. trying to find out about the betting shop and what Albert's son was up to.

Marion Clark · Service user

Albert's care plan

Need/Problem	Goals	Action	Rationale
Declining short-term memory, leading to confusion.	To use existing cognitive ability to the maximum. To reduce the distress of confused episodes.	Attend memory clinic Nurse to give immediate support — simple explanations. Albert gets reassurance from his hand being held.	**1.** The belief here is that Albert can be helped to retain his current level of cognitive functioning by undertaking exercises that stimulate his short-term memory. There is some evidence to support this 'use it or lose it' theory (see Cassel 2002). **2.** Being confused can be anxiety-producing and distressing to any individual. Immediate intervention by giving an explanation of what's happening in a reassuring tone can help Albert, particularly at this early stage of his illness while he retains some cognitive capacity to understand. Particular regard should be given to environmental stimuli and how these can help or exacerbate Albert's perception (see Goudie and Stokes 1995). **3.** The use of therapeutic touch in this regard can further convey a strong non-verbal message of empathy. A useful chapter on 'Touch as Therapy' can be found in Pickering and Thompson (1998). A number of workers in this topic area are mentioned in this chapter.
Disorientation in time, place, and person.	To help Albert recall each of these	Nurse to use 24-hour reality orientation approach — regular reminders. Nurse to demonstrate to Vera the basic technique. Nurse to give advice about use of home environment to trigger memory.	**4.** At this early stage of Albert's condition, it is believed that by reinforcing the reality of the world about him — i.e. reminding him of his name, where he is, the date and time, the identities of people around him, and also giving explanations of life going on around him — this can help him to recall his short-term memory and to make sense of the here and now. There is some randomized control trial (RCT) data that supports its efficacy as an intervention (see Spector, et al. 2003). **5.** Vera should be aware of this approach while Albert is in the day hospital so that continuity of care is maintained by the family in the home environment. Relationships between day hospital staff and Albert's family should also be fostered in order to avoid misunderstanding. See Lundh et al. (2000) for some interesting insights gleaned from a Swedish study.

Low mood – possible reaction to diagnosis.	To explore Albert and Vera's responses to the diagnosis. To facilitate catharsis. To explore coping strategies and continued support.	Joint counselling support for Albert and Vera. Six 45 min. sessions over six weeks. Referral to a carers' education and support group.

6. Much work has been done over the last few years in designing care areas for people with cognitive impairment (see: Gibson 2003). Triggers such as the use of colour and lighting, the use of pictures and even signs, can all have some potential effect. Also, the use of TV and radio should be moderated so that Albert's sensory stimulation is not too great. By manipulating the living space in this way at home, it is hoped that Vera will not encounter problems that are avoidable. For example, Vera could be advised that when a room needs to be decorated, she keeps to the same colour scheme so that Albert can continue to recognize his home.

7. Albert and Vera have received catastrophic news: a diagnosis of Alzheimer's disease. They both know that it is a progressive, degenerative disease with no cure. From onset to premature death, an average survival span is ten years (Cantley 2001). Although Albert currently retains insight, he knows that at some point his condition will deteriorate further. He remembers Vera's father, who died with the disease some years before. John knows that the psychological trauma to Albert is therefore immense. Likewise, Vera will be witness to Albert's demise, seeing his faculties deteriorate, his behaviour change, and possibly also an alteration in his personality. She dreads the future and is perhaps overwhelmed by the present. In this terribly sad context, John seeks to give specific psychological support to the couple through structured counselling sessions. A useful text on counselling older people is Scrutton (1999).

8. Catharsis is about releasing emotion. John knows that Albert and Vera have not had chance to express their true feelings with regard to what's happening to them. It's believed that by allowing the free expression of emotions, individuals can better face the challenges before them. See Junaid and Hedge (2007).

9. Towards the end of this scheduled programme of counselling sessions, it's important that the couple have a chance to talk about how they will cope with Albert's illness.

Need/Problem	Goals	Action	Rationale
			The emphasis of the counsellor here will be to move to practical suggestions around support in the family home and practical tips for managing activities of daily living. Part of the approach is to empower the couple by giving them some options and facilitating them to choose a particular course of action. Much depends on the facilitator style. In the NHS, Egan's (2002) counselling model tends to be familiar, as does Heron's Six Category Intervention Analysis (Heron 1975). Some of the choices made by the couple will entail John referring either or both to other agencies, such as support groups in the voluntary sector.
			10. As part of Albert's condition he is experiencing dysphasia. This is defined as 'difficulty in speaking as a result of a brain lesion' (Bailliere's Nurses' Dictionary 2007). In particular, John has observed that Albert has difficulty in recalling the names of objects (nominal dysphasia). At this point in Albert's illness he is still able to recall these words, perhaps with a little prompting, but simply needs time to do so. John wanted to bring this to the attention of the care team, therefore, so that rushing Albert is avoided. Kitwood (1997), called this phenomenon, 'outpacing', which is: 'providing information, presenting choices etc., at a rate too fast for the person to understand; putting them under pressure to do things more rapidly than they can bear.'
Finds it difficult to communicate at times – some motor dysphasia.	To make it easier for Albert to express himself.	Albert responds with prompting. Allow time for answers. Long-term memory good – ask him to talk about life as a postman. Nurse to advise Vera on the approach.	**11.** Although the deterioration of short-term memory (STM) is implicated in Alzheimer's disease, long-term memory (LTM), tends to remain intact. John knows that Albert has problems with his STM and may feel foolish and embarrassed in front of other people. By writing into the care plan a change of emphasis from the present to the past, e.g. for nurses to prompt Albert to recall his job as a postman, John is hoping to facilitate a situation in which Albert feels comfortable and competent. Indeed, he (Albert) is given permission to talk about what he did well in his life, to recall happy memories and to share positive emotions. There is some (though rather limited) evidence to show that such reminiscence is therapeutically worthwhile. (Woods et al., 2005). Moreover, such interactions with staff give staff a pretext to share in the positive emotions expressed by Albert and to comment on his achievements. Such interchanges serve to raise the value Albert places on himself; in other words, John is trying to help raise Albert's self-esteem.

Problem/Need	Goal	Intervention	Rationale
			12. John's note here emphasizes Vera's continued involvement with Albert's care and the need for continuity in approach. The nurse will explain the reason for getting Vera involved is to help her understand the difficulties that Albert has. It's possible that some carers living in close proximity with relatives can come to believe that the person is 'being awkward' deliberately, or even 'playing games'. John's approach is to assist Vera to gain insight into Albert's condition by helping her to view the world from Albert's frame of reference. Family education should involve all facets of educational support, which may overlap conventional therapeutic support. The NICE 2006 Guideline places emphasis on such education (see NICE 2006 Guideline, pp. 27–8).
Potential harm with kitchen appliances.	To keep Albert as safe as possible.	Refer to occupational therapist (OT) about assessment of home kitchen. Nurse to give Vera information about assistive technology.	13. Keeping Albert safe is a priority for Vera and the care team. The OT assessment will flag up any actual and potential areas of concern and recommend changes to the home environment, if required and feasible. The obvious rationale here is that if problems can be 'factored out' by making physical changes to the home, then the potential for problems developing will be lessened. In addition, the OT will advise on aids to help keep Albert safe. Assistive technology is 'any item, piece of equipment, product or system . . . that is used to increase, maintain or improve the functional capabilities of individuals with cognitive, physical or communication difficulties' (Marshall 2000). In Albert's case, a device to support safe use of the gas cooker could be installed. Also, devices to support his memory recall could be installed, such as calendar clocks, medication reminder devices, and locator devices. John thought it useful to spend time with Vera explaining what is available to assist her in her home with Albert.
Need for education about condition and care (Albert and Vera).	To help Albert and Vera understand Albert's illness and care responses.	Psycho-education on: 1 Nature of condition. 2 The care proposed. 3 Guidance on coping.	14. Educating both Vera and (to some extent) Albert about his condition and associated aspects of care can be empowering for both.
Need for carer support and monitoring.	To enable Albert and Vera to benefit from group support.	Refer to Alzheimer's Society Carers' Group.	15. User and carer support groups such as those run by the Alzheimer's Society can be therapeutic in several ways. Firstly, the couple can see that they are not alone; that in fact, there are a number of people experiencing similar life-changing experiences to them. Secondly, they can share their emotions with the people best positioned to empathize with them. Thirdly, they can garner tips on how to cope!

Need/Problem	Goals	Action	Rationale
Need to review state financial assistance.	To ensure that Albert and Vera are receiving their benefit entitlements.	Refer to social worker for a review of the couple's benefits. (Ascertain whether attendance allowance is being paid)	**16.** John is aware of the extra costs involved in Albert's care, such as taxi fares and easy-to-manage clothing. In hospital, the team social worker will usually be the person to deal with benefit issues, while in the community, the family may be advised to contact the local Neighbourhood Office or Citizens' Advice Bureau.
Need to review important issues before Albert's capacity declines further.	To ensure that Albert makes the choices he needs to before he loses his mental capacity.	Named nurse to meet with Vera and Albert to discuss this goal. Named nurse to raise issues with MDT at meeting.	**17.** Albert still retains some mental capacity but Vera and John know that this will deteriorate. While Albert can still make some decisions independently, he will be in a position to, for instance, make a will, make an advance directive, and perhaps, to request purchases. Moreover, he might wish to meet people (perhaps to renew friendships or even say goodbye), to visit places, or just to do the things he has been meaning to do for some time. These behaviours are traditionally seen as 'end of life' phenomena but may be equally appropriate in Albert's case, because while he has some capacity it can be argued that he has some control over his personal affairs. At this juncture, Albert's autonomy as a free individual is relatively intact and his free will is recognized within his family context and by professional carers. His mental capacity will need to be monitored through regular testing. The Mental Capacity Act 2005 has brought in a standard test for mental capacity, and so long as Albert retains capacity he can, under this Act, appoint someone (such as Vera) with Lasting Power of Attorney or (as mentioned above) could write an advance directive, both to be applicable should Albert be assessed as having lost mental capacity.
			John will need to discuss these issues with Albert and Vera, as well as liaising with members of the MDT. For more information about the Mental Capacity Act refer to
			http://www.dh.gov.uk/en/Publicationsandstatistics/Bulletins/theweek/Chiefexecutivebulletin/DH_4108436

Abuse and protection of vulnerable adults

Albert had been attending the day hospital for several weeks when on one occasion Vera, having accompanied Albert to the day hospital, asked to have a private word with John. Over a cup of tea in a small office, Vera, somewhat tearfully, related how Mark was, in effect, stealing money from them. She described how, to start with, Mark would ask for money to cover petrol costs and 'beer money' when he took his father out for a drink. Gradually, she noticed he asked for more and more until (in Vera's words) 'I put my foot down'. After this, she noticed that money was missing from Albert's wallet and 'money tins' (that is, the tins they used to hold saved coins). Mark claimed that Albert had either lost the money or had, in a confused state, given it away. Mark couldn't explain, however, why Albert's bank account was now overdrawn. Recently, Vera also noticed money missing from her purse and so had confronted Mark about this. He denied taking the money, although Vera could not explain its loss in any other way. She knew Mark was still gambling and drinking and suspected that he was taking advantage of Albert's position (as well as her own). Since Mark lounged around the house all day, the atmosphere at home was often tense, leading to minor rows. Vera was now at the end of her tether.

Naturally, anyone would feel stressed in Vera's position, but do you feel Mark's behaviour could actually be categorized as abusive? Sometimes it is difficult to know when a situation has tipped over from one involving very difficult relationships into one where we have a responsibility to liaise with other professionals about adult protection issues. Read the information in Box 7.2, which lists types of abuse, and identify those that are occurring in Mark's behaviour toward his parents.

Student activity 3
Note that Mark also appears in Chapters 5 and 6 – if you have already read these chapters, do you think that access to the above information would have influenced the way earlier situations were handled in those chapters (i.e. with Joyce)?

They also point out that people who have financial problems due to use of drugs and alcohol, and who are financially dependent on the person they care for, are more likely to be abusers.

Student activity 4
Which types of abuse can you identify in Mark's behaviour towards his parents?
How would you describe Mark's relationship with his parents?
Consider how John might help Vera and Albert.

Whether or not Mark sees his actions as abusive, however, is an issue that John or another professional may wish to explore with Mark. Vera is adamant that no one outside her family group and the day hospital staff should know about this abuse. When John suggested to Vera that if Mark doesn't stop stealing she should contact the police, Vera was (somewhat surprisingly to John) most defensive of Mark. She made it apparent that under no circumstances should Mark 'get into trouble'. In fact, this maternal defence may be quite common because of various considerations that may motivate the abused to keep the authorities from knowing the true situation (Biggs 1994). This, coupled with a united 'family silence' around the issue, helps to explain why abuse is perpetuated in families, sometimes for generations (Biggs *et al.* 1995). Certain situations increase the risk of abuse. Biggs *et al.* (1995) suggest that people in poor health, living with another person and with no one else to turn to, are more vulnerable. Perpetrators may gain from abuse financially, through having a feeling of control over the other person, or as a means of communication

---

Papadopoulos and La Fontaine (2000) identify five types of abuse:
1. **Psychological** – causing mental anguish, for example through verbal abuse.
2. **Physical** – causing harm, injury, or restraint to the body, including through sexual abuse.
3. **Material** – taking a person's money or belongings without permission.
4. **Active neglect** – intentionally refusing or failing to carry out care, or deliberately neglecting an older person.
5. **Passive neglect** – unintentionally failing to carry out care or neglecting the older person.

Box 7.2 Types of abuse

👤 Film clip of Mark – a service user's view

This clip shows again how difficult it can be for practitioners to make an assessment. Whilst Mark takes care of his father, his motives for wanting to keep the problems within the family, and for not wanting professionals to interfere, are suspect. He points out that people do take advantage of his father, but doesn't mention the betting shop.

Marion Clark · Service user

and stress reduction (Papadopoulos and La Fontaine 2000).

Student activity 5

Consider Vera's motives in wishing to cover up the abuse. What does Vera opening up to John tell you about John's professional standing in Vera's eyes?

Having had his discussion with Vera, John held the view that both Vera and Albert were being financially abused by Mark and that the abuse was unlikely to stop without intervention. Following the Department of Health policy document on abuse in older people, *No Secrets* (Department of Health 2000), all statutory care agencies are required to formulate multi-agency guidelines for the protection of vulnerable adults. These guidelines detail the principles and procedures to be followed by professional staff where abuse is suspected (see Box 7.3). Following his meeting with Vera, John referred to his Trust's Adult Protection Reporting and Safeguarding Protocol, which, in this case, required him to complete an Incident Form and notify his line manager (the day hospital manager) on the same working day. After subsequent discussions within the team, involving the day hospital registrar and social worker, it was decided to hold a multidisciplinary meeting the next day. Vera was in agreement with this action and accepted an invitation to attend with Albert. She stipulated, however, that Mark should not be allowed to attend. The day hospital team was in full agreement with this request because it was felt that Albert and Vera needed to offer their version of events without being intimidated by the presence of their son.

Student activity 6

Consider some of the options that may have been discussed at the meeting in order to help Vera and Albert. The next section provides a list of different models of intervention for such a situation. Which model do you think John and the team would find the most suitable for Albert and Vera's case?

- Aims to provide a framework for action for all relevant agencies to develop a coherent policy for the protection of vulnerable adults.
- Agencies should aim to prevent abuse or, if this fails, to have in place 'robust' procedures.
- Stresses need for partnership and interdisciplinary working.
- Local authority social services departments to take lead coordinating role.
- Advocates a multi-agency administrative framework.
- Advocates the development of inter-agency policies and strategies and formulation of inter-agency operational procedures.
- Offers broader guidance for staff, users, carers, and members of the public.

It is possible that Albert would be put on the Adult Protection Register, so that the situation can be assessed, planned for, and regularly reviewed.

(Department of Health 2000)

Box 7.3 The highlights of the *No Secrets* paper

Models of intervention (applied to Albert and Vera's case)

- Strengthen the family network – ask Steven (the other son) and Sandra (the daughter) to become more involved in daily family life (the **network** model).

- A lead worker takes on the role of advocate for Vera and Albert with Mark (the **mediation** model).

- Possibility of asking Mark to leave the family home, or removing to a refuge both Vera and Albert. Perhaps introduce them to a support group (the **protection** model).

- A lead worker works with the whole family to consider dynamics and relationship issues (the **professional carer** model).

- Possibility of taking out an injunction that forbids Mark to enter the family home (the **legal protection** model).

(See Biggs *et al*. 1995.)

Clinical scenario: Vera

In this section, we discuss how the nurse can assist Albert's wife, Vera, in coping with the stressful situation of looking after her husband. When working in the clinical setting (either within a hospital or the community) with people like Vera, it is important to consider how you would engage with her and develop a therapeutic relationship. Vera would need to trust you sufficiently to work in partnership with you. As you will have already seen throughout this textbook, mental health nurses adopt a problem-solving approach to mental health, beginning with assessment. In assessing Vera, it's useful to recognize that we are offering her an individually tailored service while at the same time meeting Standard 6 of the *National Service Framework for mental health* (Department of Health 1999) in carrying out a carer assessment. This means that we have to consider Vera not only in her caring role, but also her own observable behaviour and emotional state.

Watch the film of Vera now – her observable behaviour suggests that she may be someone with high levels of stress who is not really managing, or who may even be experiencing the onset of severe clinical depression.

www.oxfordtextbooks.co.uk/orc/clarke

and choose the video link.

When we assess Vera, one of the approaches is to consider whether the feelings she describes, together with our observations, match with the recognized features of depression. Feeling low or sad is not the only sign of depressive illness. These are some other common symptoms, which are set out in NICE guidelines on the treatment of depression (National Collaborating Centre for Mental Health/NICE 2004):

- A feeling of sadness, depression, or being 'down' that is worse than normal sadness.

- A loss of interest in life – not being able to enjoy the things that usually give pleasure.

- Feeling tired even when not doing much. The simplest task seems a big effort.

- Poor appetite and often losing weight (increased appetite sometimes seen also; this includes so-called 'comfort eating').

- An inner feeling of restlessness, making it hard to rest or relax properly.

👤 Vera – a service user's comment

What isn't clear from the clips is how long Albert had been having problems. Vera seemed very confused about what was going on and did not appear to have been told what might possibly be wrong (or in her own distress has forgotten what she had been told).

Vera's distress indicated the possibility of becoming ill herself, a common problem for carers. She felt she could not talk about her husband's problems, even to a close friend (although her son said something different). She did not appear to know about carers' support groups where she could go and share her problems and concerns.

Marion Clark · Service user

- Worrying and feeling anxious. Some people have always worried more than others but if this is unusual for the person, it may be a sign of depression.

- Wanting to avoid other people. This may include feeling irritable and snappy when people are around.

- Poor sleep. Waking early in the morning (at least an hour or two earlier than usual) and then unable to get back to sleep again.

- Losing self-confidence. Possibly feeling useless or a burden to others.

- Poor concentration.

- Feeling panicky.

- Loss of sexual feelings.

- Feelings of being bad or guilty. This may include dwelling on the past and be totally out of proportion.

- Thoughts of suicide – at some point most people with severe depression will feel like ending it all.

These feelings should be taken seriously because they mean that help is needed. Sometimes these feelings become so strong that a person will work out ways of harming themselves, and even make preparations. This is a sign that help is urgently needed.

Loss and pain are inevitable parts of growing up and growing older. Sometimes people we care for reject us, we write bad papers, our stocks go down, we fail to get the job we want, people we love die. In Vera's case, she is losing her relationship with Albert because of his memory problems, and facing an uncertain and difficult future. Almost everyone reacts to loss with some of the symptoms of depression (McCarthy and Thomas 2004). We become sad and discouraged, apathetic and passive, the future looks bleak, and some of the zest goes out of living. A widely used mechanism to measure this in mental health services is the Health of the Nation Outcome Scale (HoNOS) for the over 65s (Box 7.4).

> **Student activity 7**
> *Have another look at the film of Vera speaking – do you think that she is showing any signs of depression?*

www.oxfordtextbooks.co.uk/orc/clarke

and choose the video link.

There is evidence that depression is under-detected in older people, especially those in residential and nursing homes (Department of Health 2001). This may be related to ageism. Older people themselves may internalize ageist stereotypes and believe that old age is a miserable time of life, and so not seek help. They might also believe that resources should be spent on younger people. Professionals too may believe that feeling low is a natural response to the difficulties of old age and so not consider the need to carry out an assessment (see Box 7.5). Vera herself might believe that a visit to the GP is risky because she would have to leave Albert in the house alone. She might also think that her problems are not anything the doctor could help with, or that Albert is the patient, so she should be concentrating on his needs rather than her own.

	No problem 0	Minor 1	Mild 2	Moderate 3	Severe 4
Mood disturbance (depressed mood and symptoms associated with depressed mood in any disorder)	Nil	Gloomy or minor or transient changes in mood	Definite depression on subjective and objective measures (e.g. loss of interest, pleasure, or self-esteem, lacking in energy or feelings of guilt)	Marked depressive symptoms (on subjective or objective grounds)	Severe depressive symptoms on subjective or objective grounds (e.g. preoccupation with guilt and worthlessness or withdrawn due to severe loss of interest; profound loss of interest or pleasure)

Box 7.4 Health of the Nation Outcome Scale (HoNOS) 65+, Scale 7: Problems with depressive symptoms

The situation of the older person may be contributing to depression, so before the assessment it is important to think about whether their recent or past experiences may be contributing factors. So, for example, we need to consider:

- Past history of depression.
- Significant physical illnesses causing disability.
- Other mental health problems such as dementia.
- Side effects of medication.
- The impact of the caring role, as approximately one-third of carers are depressed (<http://www.alzheimers.org.uk/Research/Care/supportingcarers.htm> accessed 24/07/2007)

Use two screening questions such as:

- 'During the last month, have you felt worried about feeling down, depressed, or hopeless?'
- 'During the last month, have you felt worried about having little interest or pleasure in doing things?'

Box 7.5 Assessment of depression

Care planning

The next stage of the problem-solving cycle is planning care. The reasons for a care intervention are known as the 'rationale'. This may arise from evidence (published research outcomes), values, or the need to follow government guidance documents such as *The National Service Framework for older people* (Department of Health 2001), which are themselves both evidence and values-based. *The National Service Framework for older people* directs that care should follow an identified care pathway where the multidisciplinary team collaborates in working together to provide a seamless service, with, and for the benefit of, the service user. The care pathway, which is a local guide for good practice, may vary between areas, so it is worth investigating the expected care pathway where you work. You would then be able to 'signpost' or direct a person to the right part of the service, and also explain to someone like Vera how her care and that of her husband would be likely to proceed. The NICE guidelines on treatment of depression (National Collaborating Centre for Mental Health/ NICE 2004) involve a stepped approach to care, or clear pathway as follows:

- Step 1. Recognition in primary care and general hospital settings.
- Step 2. Treatment of mild depression in primary care.
- Step 3. Treatment of moderate to severe depression in primary care.
- Step 4. Treatment of depression by mental health specialists.
- Step 5. Inpatient treatment of depression.

In Vera's case her care would probably take place at home unless the team were concerned about suicidal risk. Vera is worried about Albert, who would himself need to be looked after if she was admitted to hospital. The idea of this happening to him, being taken where he would not know anyone and no one would know him, would probably distress Vera even more. Vera's care plan takes into account her role as carer for Albert, as one of her goals is to be able to continue looking after him (see care plan).

Best practice guidelines from the Department of Health state that psychological therapies are part of essential health care and recommend that they should be routinely considered as a treatment option when assessing mental health problems (Department of Health 2004a). The guidelines specifically recommend that particular attention is given to the psychotherapeutic needs of older people. It has been demonstrated that the patient's age is generally not an important factor in choice of psychotherapy and should not determine access to psychotherapies (Department of Health 2001). There is good evidence for the effectiveness of psychological interventions with older people. It is not acceptable to deny people access to psychological therapy on the basis of age.

Vera's care plan

Service User Need/Problem	Goals	Care Plan	Rationale
1. Vera is exhausted and stressed because of the difficulties of caring for her husband Albert.	**Short-term goals** Vera to cope with Albert's care more effectively and have opportunities for a break. **Long-term goals** Vera to feel more in control of her life and be able to meet her own needs as well as Albert's.	Spend time with Vera, offering her the opportunity to discuss her experiences, worries, and feelings. Gradually establish a therapeutic relationship in which Vera feels comfortable in discussing personal issues. Take a person-centred approach to counselling. Take a problem-solving approach to the issues Vera raises about Albert's behaviour. Discuss, and if Vera agrees, arrange respite and day-care; this may require a referral to the team social worker. Encourage Vera to think about her own needs as well as Albert's.	Kitwood (1997). NICE Guidelines on Dementia (2006). NCCMH/NICE Guidelines on Depression (2004).
2. Vera is low in mood, and may be seriously depressed.	**Short-term goals** Establish the nature and extent of Vera's low mood, and discover Vera's goals for interventions **Long-term goals** Manage any depression through interventions discussed and agreed with Vera, so that she can balance the demands of her life effectively.	Carry out an assessment using a suitable assessment tool while also making informal observations. Be sure to ask sensitively but directly about suicidal intent. Encourage Vera to talk about her understanding of the present difficulties, and her views about what she would like to happen and how this can best be achieved. Offer interventions such as supportive counselling or CBT. Liaise with MDT colleagues about their roles. For example medication may be prescribed by the doctor, a home safety assessment be carried out by the OT, and care package and benefits be arranged by the social worker.	NCCMH/NICE Guidelines on Depression (2004). Refer to Tom Kitwood's work (1997).

Service User Need/Problem	Goals	Care Plan	Rationale
		If medication is prescribed, explain how long it will take to work, and possible side effects, and encourage Vera to ask questions about it. Monitor concordance and therapeutic response.	See Health of Nation Outcome Scales 65+ Depression Domain – accessible via the Royal College of Psychiatrists website.
3. Vera is sleeping very badly. This may be partly due to being disturbed by Albert, or concerns about what could happen should he wake.	**Short-term goals** Establish reasons for poor sleep. **Long-term goals** Vera will gain adequate rest.	Ask Vera to describe her sleep pattern and any concerns that prevent her from sleeping. Explain the principles of sleep hygiene to Vera, and discuss tactics so that she can also improve Albert's sleep. Arrange respite, with Vera and Albert's permission, so that Vera can re-establish and catch up on her sleep.	Morin (1993), cited in Chalder (2000), recommends this strategy for self-management of sleeping problems.
4. Vera does not understand Albert's condition; she sometimes misinterprets his behaviour and this causes her further distress.	**Short-term goals** Clarify Vera's understanding of Alzheimer's disease. **Long-term goals** Manage any depression through interventions discussed and agreed with Vera, so that she can balance the demands of her life effectively.	Ask Vera to tell the story of Albert's condition. Encourage her to share her explanations of the recent events. Offer Vera information on Albert's condition, in a form she finds useful. This may be leaflets or in DVD form. Educate Vera on Alzheimer's disease by explaining the reasons for his behaviour, referring back to the information given to her. Encourage Vera to ask questions. Model effective communication skills with Albert, for example through use of short sentences, use of words in his vocabulary, and body language congruent with the conversation.	Alzheimer's Disease Society UK advice and information to carers – see website. NICE Guidelines on Dementia (2006).

| 5. Vera has concerns about the input of their son Mark into Albert's care. | **Short-term goals**
Vera to feel safe in discussing her concerns.

Long-term goals
Mark's input into care to be limited to a form that Vera and Albert find acceptable. | Reassure Vera that issues will be kept confidential within the team and that no action will be taken without her agreement.
Establish the nature and extent of Mark's involvement in his parents' care, and Vera's concerns about his behaviour (there have been previous allegations of financial and emotional abuse).
Ensure staff are accompanied when in Mark's presence, and that full and accurate records are kept of any conversation or incident involving him.
If necessary, discuss Protection of Vulnerable Adults procedure in MDT meeting, and follow local guidelines. | NMC (2008) Code of Professional Conduct.
Dept of Health (1999) Standard 6 NSF Mental Health Carer's Assessment.
NMC Guidelines on Records and Record Keeping (2002).
Local POVA Guidelines – Because Albert may lack capacity the MHN may need to assess ability to consent, and dependent on the outcome of that assessment, an independent mental capacity advocate will need to be consulted and be available if POVA Guidelines are implemented to work with Albert (MCA 2005). |

It is possible that Vera would be offered a form of talking therapy such as cognitive behaviour therapy (CBT), together with an antidepressant. As an older person it is more likely that she would be prescribed a selective serotonin reuptake inhibitor (SSRI). When an antidepressant is to be prescribed in routine care, it should be an SSRI, because SSRIs are as effective as tricyclic antidepressants and are less likely to be discontinued because of side effects (National Collaborating Centre for Mental Health/NICE 2004). The role of the nurse is to answer Vera's questions about the tablets and give her information that will help her make a decision about whether to accept medication.

> ### Student activity 8
> *Consider how you could answer these common questions:*
> *Are they addictive?*
> *How long will I have to take them for?*
> *What are the side effects?*
> *I took one last night and don't feel any better, why aren't they working?*

Older people who are carers tend to be in poorer general health than people of the same age group who are not carers. In addition, people aged 50 and over, particularly those aged 50–59, are more likely to be providing informal care than any other age group (Department for Work and Pensions 2005). There is a range of policies to support carers, but the focus is often on supporting them to return to work. More attention should be paid to older carers, who are often providing care for other older people. Consequently, they merely identify themselves as 'wife' or 'husband' as opposed to a carer. This indicates that caring often takes place within the broader context of ongoing relationships. There is a need for greater recognition and understanding of these relationships in order to provide appropriate support for older carers.

In a mental health promotion context for Vera, we need to recognize and strengthen her existing positive relationships with friends, family, and 'significant others'. The nurse would also need to recognize the negative impact that family can have on mental health and well-being in later life. Vera and Albert's son, Mark, has already shown himself to be a cause of stress through his abusive behaviour towards his parents. However, it is possible that Albert also distresses Vera with difficult behaviour. He is very dependent on her, and because of the damage the disease is causing to his frontal lobe (Cantley 2001), he may be disinhibited (see Chapter 5), and show his emotions more quickly and obviously. This could mean that if he is frightened or angry he is more likely to lash out.

🔖 Pharmacist's view

Increasing age affects the action of drugs, since their metabolism by the liver and removal by the kidneys is less efficient after middle age. Liver enzyme activity declines slowly with age, but is very variable. The ageing body is also less efficient at adjusting physiological functions such as blood pressure control and temperature regulation. All these factors can lead to an increased incidence and severity of side effects.

Gut motility decreases with increasing age, as does secretion of gastric acid, so drugs are absorbed more slowly and have a slower onset of action. This should be taken into consideration when answering Vera's questions.

Treatment with an antidepressant is usually started with a low dose and increased slowly as necessary. Some have a lower maximum dose for the elderly than for other adults. If compliance is likely to be a problem, a longer-acting SSRI, like fluoxetine, could be prescribed as discontinuation/withdrawal effects are less likely if doses are missed.

The antimuscarinic side effects of the tricyclic antidepressants (dry mouth, blurred vision, constipation, and urinary retention) can be more serious problems in the older person, so the newer SSRIs may be preferable. The SSRIs have been associated with psychomotor restlessness, characterized by a need to move, or distressing restlessness, often accompanied by an inability to sit or stand still. If a patient were to develop these symptoms any increase in dose may be detrimental and it may be necessary to review the continued use of the SSRI. Some SSRIs may increase the risk of upper gastrointestinal bleeding, a risk that increases with age. Hyponatraemia (see glossary) is more likely to occur in the elderly and more frequently with SSRIs than other antidepressants. Be aware of the symptoms. (The *British National Formulary* (BNF), published by BMJ Publishing Group Ltd and RPS Publishing twice a year in March and September and available online is a useful reference).

Aggressive behaviour is more common among people with dementia than among older people who do not have dementia (Finkel *et al.* 1996). Clearly we need to be aware of the possibility of this situation in Vera's case and ask her appropriate questions about it. The reason for this is so that she has the opportunity to feel safe discussing it, but also so that we can start to look at preventative strategies and appropriate support mechanisms. Albert and Vera's relationship prior to Albert's illness would have a major influence on Vera's willingness to care for him now he has dementia.

A serious complication of dementia is the development of psychiatric symptoms or behavioural difficulties that are now known collectively as 'behavioural and psychological signs and symptoms of dementia' (BPSD) (Finkel *et al.* 1996). Behavioural signs include aggression, agitation, screaming, sleep disturbance, wandering, and inappropriate sexual behaviour. The presence of BPSD in Albert, in particular escalating aggressiveness, would highlight the gender differences experienced by carers: a wife coping with an aggressive husband will probably find it more physically difficult to manage than a husband coping with an aggressive wife. Having a co-resident carer is the best protection for the person with dementia against institutionalization (Banerjee *et al.* 2006). There is also evidence available to support the view that presence of symptoms of BPSD is a major factor leading to institutionalization (Hope *et al.* 1998).

In some areas, emotional support and practical guidance can be provided by admiral nurses, who are specialist dementia care nurses. Their work focuses primarily on the needs of carers and supporters of people with dementia. Their educative and consultative role also aims to improve the delivery of dementia services.

Generally speaking, it will be the nurse at the day hospital (or ward, were Albert to be admitted) or the CMHN who will support Albert and Vera. Balancing their different needs may be difficult; for example Vera desperately needs a break, but Albert feels desperate when he is separated from Vera. Respite care, where Albert could be admitted to a specialist unit for a short time, would allow Vera to have a break, but would probably be distressing for Albert. The skill of enabling Albert to understand other people's perspectives, when he has limited memory and language abilities, should not be underestimated. Useful pointers include having the conversation in the morning when he is fresher, being in a calm environment, and using straightforward vocabulary, short sentences, and non-verbal communication to reinforce rapport and understanding. Regular meetings with Albert will help him remember and trust the nurse. Albert will also need continuous reassurance and understanding when he is at day care or respite, while Vera might appreciate knowing that he is safe and settling down.

In the last section of this chapter, we meet Mrs Bibi. You will notice that she has some problems and needs in common with Albert and Vera.

Clinical scenario: Mrs Bibi

Mrs Bibi is originally from Pakistan. She does not know her exact age, but is able to tell us that she was a small child at the time of partition, in 1947. Mrs Bibi only had a minimal education, and cannot read or write in either English or her first language, which is Punjabi. Her husband fought for Britain in the Second World War, then emigrated here in the 1960s and worked in heavy industry. He sent money home, and Mrs Bibi brought up their three children with the help of her extended family. She eventually came to this country with her daughter when her husband was dying, to nurse him. She stayed, as most of her family are now here, and she became involved in supporting her daughter-in-law in bringing up her grandchildren.

She now lives in a small house in an urban area, which is shared with other members of her family: her daughter and daughter-in-law, and their husbands and young children. It is quite crowded and noisy, as you hear at times in the film. Mrs Bibi's area is very mixed, and there are many families from her cultural group living nearby. She is able to walk short distances and visit other women and families. She is well respected, partly due to her age and position as an older person, but also because back in Pakistan she was an informal health worker, delivering babies and giving support and advice to younger women on childcare. Mrs Bibi is not isolated; she has frequent supportive visitors, and within her community is included and respected.

However, this contrasts with her experiences in the wider world, where she has been subject to direct racism and ageism, in the form of derogatory remarks. She is also aware that her religious group is viewed negatively by some of the non-Pakistani community. The triple jeopardy theory, first described by Norman (1985), suggested that older people from black and minority ethnic (BME) groups are more vulnerable because of a combination of difficulties related to poverty, ageism, racism, and lack of access to services, a theory confirmed many times since (Innes 2003). The experiences, changes, and challenges of migration are outlined in Box 7.6.

Now view the film of Mrs Bibi.

📹 www.oxfordtextbooks.co.uk/orc/clarke

and choose the video link.

Mrs Bibi describes not feeling well, but does not immediately clarify what the problems are, other than 'aches and pains'. It is clear that she is a frequent visitor to her GP because she has a bag full of a variety of prescribed drugs. However, she is vague about what they are for and how they should be taken.

Student activity 9

What are the potential risks of polypharmacy in this situation?

There is a stereotype that somatization is a process that is common in south-Asian cultures (Holland and Hogg 2001), meaning that emotional distress is expressed through bodily aches and pains. You can probably identify a similar process in yourself, perhaps a form of 'Monday-morningitis', when a depressing prospect seems to bring on a physical feeling of illness, such as a headache with nausea and lethargy. Emotional distress can be communicated in different ways. You may find it interesting to have a chat with your colleagues and see how many you can suggest.

Possibly Mrs Bibi's frequent visits her GP led the doctor to consider that there were underlying factors

that needed more time, and specialized conversations, to explore. However, Mrs Bibi does have serious physical problems that would have an impact on her mood. Lack of understanding of diabetes, suitable diet, and medication mean that Mrs Bibi's blood sugar is not properly controlled. She complains of poor eyesight and recurrent infections, including cystitis and thrush. She often sleeps badly, but it is hard to work out whether this is due to pain, aggravating itchiness, anxiety, noise, or sharing a bed with her granddaughter. Mrs Bibi also worries about poor concentration and problems with her memory. In common with many older people, she can remember events from long ago easily, but struggles to recall what she ate for breakfast.

Student activity 10

What are the long-term risks of poorly controlled diabetes?

What signs might you recognize? (See also Chapter 4 for more on diabetes.)

Now watch the film of Mrs Bibi. Does she seem to have memory problems in conversation, as far as you can tell?

📹 www.oxfordtextbooks.co.uk/orc/clarke

and choose the video link.

Mrs Bibi has swollen joints and pain when walking. In the bag of tablets there were a variety of painkillers, but Mrs Bibi does not know which they are, nor how many or how often to take them.

Student activity 11

What simple steps could you take to make Mrs Bibi's medicines both safer and more effective?

Who in the family could you liaise with?

What would be the advantages of tackling the physical health issues first?

- Separation from family members.
- Poverty, exacerbated by the need to send back money to extended family.
- Overcrowded accommodation.
- Difficulties with language and literacy.
- Moving from a rural, traditional society to an urban, more secular society.
- Being stereotyped and exploited.
- Racism.

Box 7.6 The experiences, changes, and challenges of migration

In Mrs Bibi's case, it is clear she has many problems that combined would contribute to the anxiety and low mood she describes, but she also has significant strengths. One of these is the relationship she enjoys with her daughter-in-law. The taboo in western cultures about consanguineous marriage (within the family, for example to a cousin) does not take into account the advantages. Mrs Bibi's daughter-in-law is her sister's daughter, which means they share a double bond, and each is committed to the other's welfare, an important factor when many in the family network live on a different continent. She has a secure home within the family where everything is provided, including a diet of healthy, freshly cooked food.

Mrs Bibi finds her faith a huge support, and it is central to her life. As a Muslim, she believes in Allah (as the one God) and she tries to live her life as much as possible in accordance with the tenets and principles of Islam as revealed in the Quran (the holy scripture of Islam, believed to be the direct words of the one God). Prayer is a source of comfort and strength, and Mrs Bibi talks about her spirituality in the film.

Mrs Bibi does live with her extended family, a source of great support, and at times, stress. However, it is important to be aware that not all older south Asian people live with a built-in support network. Inaccurate assumptions about families and their ability to provide care can lead to unsuitable care packages or even the failure to carry out a proper assessment (Holland and Hogg 2001).

Nurses often find trans-cultural assessments stressful, and nurses from minority groups can find assessments of older people from their community of origin stressful too, though for different reasons. Black and minority ethnic staff have reported being expected by their colleagues to act as an interpreter as well as carrying out their own duties, and to be key worker for all the patients from their group (Culley and Dyson 2001). Patients themselves may expect special treatment because of the nurse's cultural understanding and a feeling of family obligation. The stigma attached to mental illness, and sometimes to being a mental health nurse, can mean both parties feel awkward within the relationship. Within small communities, patients may have concerns about confidentiality (Robinson 1998).

Staff from majority communities may worry about saying or doing the wrong thing, to the extent that sometimes patients say they feel ignored. In times of stress, or with a failing memory, English as a second language may be lost, so communication becomes difficult and an interpreter is needed (Jenkins 1998). Staff express concern about how to work with an interpreter, and also about the change in the therapeutic relationship in these circumstances. We will address these and other challenging issues in the next section, as we assess Mrs Bibi and plan her care.

👥 Assessment

A person who does not speak Mrs Bibi's first language would need to carry out the assessment using the services of an interpreter (see Box 7.7).

Student activity 12
What are your anxieties, if any, about working with an interpreter?
After watching the film from earlier, do these anxieties still exist? Do you have any new anxieties or observations?

The conversation you see in the film is a nurse trying to explore the background to Mrs Bibi's current situation. Mrs Bibi raises many different issues, and the conversation ranges from the family back home to religion, aches and pains, and the behaviour of her grandchildren.

Student activity 13
When you watch the film, is it easy to define Mrs Bibi's problems by diagnostic category?
Is it easier to think about problems and needs?
Do you think it will be possible to resolve Mrs Bibi's problems? What are your realistic goals?

We often talk about the idea of 'holistic health', while usually limiting our interventions to separate activities directed towards physical or mental health, or a person's social situation. Mrs Bibi, though, really does think of her spiritual, emotional, and physical self, her family, and her environment as totally mutually dependent and related.

Many authors (Holland and Hogg 2001, Ferns 2005) suggest that we can only become aware and sensitive to others' cultural values when we become

The following points are a very useful aide memoire.

1. Allow plenty of time – English is a language with a massive vocabulary, so some terms, such as dementia, may need to be explained in other languages. Also, everything has to be said twice.

2. Use a trained interpreter – family members may be helpful, but using them as an interpreter can damage relationships and lead to confidentiality breaches.

3. Be sensitive about gender – women tend to feel more comfortable with a female interpreter.

4. Check that the interpreter speaks the same language as the service user.

5. If the service user comes from a country where there has been a civil war, make sure the interpreter comes from the same group as the patient.

6. Explain the purpose of the conversation to the interpreter, and ask them to tell you exactly what the service user says. Sometimes people say things that appear strange, and the interpreter may be tempted to 'make sense of' what the service user is saying, and change the meaning.

7. Remind the interpreter of the duty of confidentiality. In a small community, the interpreter may know the service user's family.

8. Introduce yourself, with the interpreter's help, and explain your role. Make it clear that both you and the interpreter will keep all matters discussed confidential.

9. As far as possible, seat yourself so that you, the interpreter, and the service user are equally distanced.

10. Ask the interpreter to introduce themselves and have a brief conversation to build rapport. The service user may feel more comfortable if they know a little about the interpreter.

11. Ask the service user what they would like to be called.

12. Direct your conversation towards the service user, make eye contact with them, and use positive non-verbal communications to convey interest and support.

13. At first it can be difficult to trust the interpreter; remember that English translates into fewer words so the answers can be shorter than expected.

14. However, if this happens repeatedly, it is okay to remind the interpreter to tell you exactly what the service user says.

15. Debrief the interpreter afterwards – they may have found aspects of the conversation upsetting and need reassurance. The interpreter may wish to tell you things that they could not at the time – for example with dementia the service user could have word-finding difficulties.

16. Book the same interpreter again, if all went well, as this will save time in building rapport and explaining the situation next time.

Box 7.7 How to work with an interpreter

aware of our own. Culture is often thought of as an 'iceberg' – we can see the tip, in visible aspects like food and dress, but beneath the surface lie deeper issues such as our assumptions and values. Culture is something we take for granted, and unless we meet someone with a different set of beliefs, it is easy to assume that everything we do and believe is 'normal' and 'natural'. It is useful to step back and consider our own values, but this is difficult without the prompt of 'difference'.

Student activity 14

Try the exercise in Box 7.8, from Ferns (2005), to see how cultures can vary and what your own values are. It would be interesting to compare your results with a friend's. If you come from a similar background, does that mean your responses are the same? If your background is different, do you have values in common? If you compared yourself with an older person from your cultural group, would your values be the same?

This exercise is based on the idea that cultures have different 'dimensions' that can be used to highlight similarities and differences. Answers can be plotted on a continuum.

1. Feelings – would you say you are 'expressive' or reserved'? For example if you met an old friend, would you hug them enthusiastically, or shake their hand, or maybe say hello, smile, or nod?

Expressive...Reserved

2. Rules – do you believe that rules should always be followed, or that the situation and needs of the person should be taken into account?

Flexible...Standardized

3. Individuality – if you were making a decision, would you decide what is best for you, then let family and friends know, or would you consider your role in your social group before making a decision?

Group...Individual

4. Problems – when you have a problem, do you ponder on it, maybe pray or meditate or 'sleep on it', or would you be more likely to write a list of 'pros' and 'cons'?

Intuitive...Analytical

Box 7.8 Personal Cultural Profile Exercise. Adaptation of Exercise from Ferns (2005) 'Personal Cultural Profile'.

MMSE
Can you tell me the date?
Examiner names three objects (e.g. apple, table, penny) and patient is asked to repeat them.
What is this (point to a watch, then a pen)?
Can you tell me the names of the three objects I asked you to remember?

GDRS
Are you basically satisfied with your life?
Have you dropped many of your activities and interests?

Box 7.9 Example questions from MMSE and GDRS

Trans-cultural assessments

Sometimes you may want to use a formal assessment tool. These have various advantages, for example you can compare a person's results over a period of time, and assess the severity of a problem in a way that makes it easy to discuss with colleagues. As Mrs Bibi is complaining of low mood and a poor memory, you might decide to carry out a MMSE (Mini Mental State Examination) and Geriatric Depression Rating Scale (GDRS). Examples of questions from these are shown in Box 7.9.

> ### Student activity 15
> *What problems can you anticipate in using these tools with Mrs Bibi, even if translated into Punjabi?*

If Mrs Bibi did have a memory problem such as Alzheimer's disease, what might be the consequences of an inaccurate assessment?

Informal assessments include observations of appearance, tone of voice, content of speech, relationship with family and friends, level of rapport, and any other observations made during conversations and activities. What do you think may be the advantages and disadvantages of formal and informal assessments?

Ferns (2005) suggests that sensitive trans-cultural assessments can be based around a series of straightforward questions (see Box 7.10, the ABCD model). These questions centre on the service user's understanding of the problem, and their wishes for dealing with it.

1. **Account of the situation**
What's happening for you at the moment?
What are the most important factors in your situation?

2. **Beliefs about causes**
How has the current situation come about?
What things have caused your worries to grow?

3. **Consequences of mental distress**
How have you and others been affected by your distress?
What are your greatest fears?

4. **Dealing with distress**
How have you coped in the past and what has helped you the most?
What help do you most want now?

Box 7.10 The ABCD model (Ferns 2005)

The assessment process, based on what Mrs Bibi says and the nurse's observations, might reveal the problems and needs outlined below:

Emotional problems

- Feeling sad.
- Feeling worried about possible memory problems.
- Feeling worried about money problems, over-crowding, living with young children, family back home.
- Disturbed sleep.

Multiple physical health problems

- Diabetes – poorly controlled, leading to further problems such as blurred vision and repeated infections.
- High blood pressure.
- Pain caused by arthritis.
- Polypharmacy.
- Lack of understanding about **antibiotics**, diabetes medication, and painkillers.
- Lack of access to health care and advice – Mrs Bibi's understanding of English is negligible, so she is excluded by language.

Care planning

Mrs Bibis care plan is shown on pp. 172–5.

Implementation and evaluation of the care plans

The care of Albert, Vera, and Mrs Bibi demands a wide variety of skills, and a positive, sensitive attitude towards older people and their problems. In placement your mentor will guide you on how to convey warmth, genuineness, and unconditional positive regard when the service user has particular communication problems (see also Chapter 2). Vera may be feeling low and anxious, and her concentration would be poor, especially if she had had a bad night. Albert might be disorientated and upset, and Mrs Bibi might be worried that you may not be able to look past the stereotypes and see the real her. Your assessor will welcome your input if you can show sensitivity, respect, and interest.

Listen to the service user's description of the situation and use skills such as reflection and open questioning to clarify your understanding. Aim to be clear

(Continued on p. 176)

Mrs Bibi's care plan

Service User Need/Problem	Goals	Care Plan
1. Physical health problems. Mrs Bibi has diabetes and arthritis. She does not understand these conditions or the treatment suggested by the GP. Her blood sugar is not controlled, making her vulnerable to further health problems. Mrs Bibi often has painful joints. At present she has a wide range of medication, including antibiotics, which she is not taking as prescribed.	**Short-term goals** Mrs Bibi will understand the medical approach to her problems, diabetes and arthritis, and collaborate with care and treatment. **Long-term goals** Mrs Bibi's diabetes will be managed effectively, improving her current and future health. Her pain will be controlled, allowing her to be more active, also contributing to a healthier lifestyle.	If you cannot speak Mrs Bibi's language, arrange an interpreter, being sure that they can speak the same language and dialect as Mrs Bibi. Explain the purpose of the visit to the interpreter beforehand, and ask them to tell you exactly what Mrs Bibi says. Set the seating positions so that you are equally spaced, and direct questions to Mrs Bibi, ensuring that your non-verbal communications match the content of your speech and convey warmth and supportive interest. Allow plenty of time. **Rationale:** The *National Service Framework for Older People* (Department of Health 2001) states that services should be accessible for those who do not have English as their first language. Spend time with Mrs Bibi, listening to her point of view on her illnesses. Explain the medical model approach. Negotiate a joint plan that Mrs Bibi will feel comfortable with, and which emphasizes her cultural strengths, such as a fresh healthy diet and the regular opportunity to walk short distances to visit friends. Ensure that Mrs Bibi, and the people in the family who cook, understand the need for a diet high in fresh vegetables and complex carbohydrates, and low in fat, salt, and sugar. Review Mrs Bibi's medication with the GP, and arrange for tablets to be administered in a medipack. If the family member responsible for prompting medication does not read English, make labels in their first language with the help of the interpreter. Monitor use of the medipack, checking that the system is working and that the medication is effective at current dosages.

Service User Need/Problem	Goals	Care Plan
		Liaise with the GP over changes.
		Rationale: Complies with Standard 2 of the *National Service Framework for Older People* (Department of Health 2001).
2. Low mood. Mrs Bibi describes often feeling tearful and hopeless. She relates this to separation from family members. Relocating to a second homeland is very stressful (Norman 1985) and this may be contributing to Mrs Bibi's emotional state.	**Short-term goals** Mrs Bibi will feel more optimistic about the future. **Long-term goals** Mrs Bibi will gradually come to manage the difficult feelings associated with her situation, and settle into her role in the family in this country. Alternatively, she may decide that she would feel better it she returned to Pakistan.	Ask Mrs Bibi if she would like to talk to you alone, or with members of her family. Offer Mrs Bibi the chance to talk through her worries. Encourage her to ventilate her feelings. Encourage her to use the strong support network that she has. Mrs Bibi has a role in supporting younger women. Encourage her to maintain this as it promotes her self-esteem. Mrs Bibi may like to join a day centre for older women from her background. Here she will be able to share problems with other women experiencing similar difficulties. Mrs Bibi's religion is a source of spiritual strength. Encourage her to discuss the benefits she gains from this, so as to promote ongoing recognition of its value to her. Knee pain can make kneeling difficult, which means the position for prayer is uncomfortable. Liaise with her main carer about giving painkillers 20 minutes before prayer times. Rationale: *National Service Framework for Older People* (Department of Health 2001) Standard 7.
3. Poor sleep. This may be connected to low mood, discomfort from physical health problems, or sharing a bed.	**Short-term goals** Establish reasons for poor sleep. **Long-term goals** Mrs Bibi will gain adequate rest.	Discuss the reasons for poor sleep with Mrs Bibi, and what she hopes for. Ask whether she is in pain at night, or uncomfortable. She may need a painkiller before bed. Discuss whether an alternative bed could be found for her granddaughter. Mrs Bibi may be sleeping in the day – advise her to keep awake, and to take a little exercise every day.

● Discussion point: Promoting independence

Independence is seen as a positive factor for mental health, for example in the *National Service Framework for Older People* (Department of Health 2001) and recent report on dignity in care (Department of Health 2006). However, it may be that Mrs Bibi values 'interdependence' more. According to Ferns (2005), the extent to which we value independence is culturally determined. Mrs Bibi's goal might be to live together with her family in relationships where she both gives and receives care.

4. Poor memory and concentration.

Short-term goals
Establish whether these problems are related to depression or a form of dementia.
Long-term goals
If dementia is indicated, discuss with the MDT, and plan accordingly.

Ongoing informal assessment, for example monitoring repetitiveness and orientation in conversation, should clarify this. (In the film, you may notice whether these problems exist.)
Reassure Mrs Bibi that poor concentration and memory are probably connected with her low mood, and will gradually improve.
The Alzheimer's Society produces useful resources, such as videos and leaflets in community languages. Mrs Bibi and her family may like to watch a video and discuss whether they feel she has this type of problem.
Continue to monitor; Mrs Bibi is at risk of vascular dementia due to her diabetes.

Rationale: *National Service Framework for Older People* (2001) Standard 7.

5. Mrs Bibi does not understand the health and social care system, so is unable to access help and advice and the benefits she is entitled to.

Short-term goals Mrs Bibi will get the benefits she is entitled to.
Long-term goals Mrs Bibi will feel more in control of her situation and have the skills to contribute to the management of future difficulties.

Mrs Bibi may feel disempowered by the experience of being an older woman from a minority ethnic group, and by lack of spoken English.
Explain all intentions clearly and negotiate interventions.
Ensure she and her family know how to contact the nurse and other professionals involved in her care.

Service User Need/Problem	Goals	Care Plan
		Introduce Mrs Bibi and her family to community support groups.
		Arrange a benefit review with the local neighbourhood office, informing them about language requirements.
		Mrs Bibi may be interested in learning to speak English. Women-only classes may be available locally; this would be a social outlet, and potentially empowering.
		Rationale: The 10 essential shared capabilities (Department of Health 2004a).

● **Discussion point: Assessment tools**

Assessment tools such as the Mini Mental State Examination (MMSE), as seen in Albert's assessment, may not be suitable for Mrs Bibi. What problems can you anticipate in trying to use the MMSE with Mrs Bibi?

● **Discussion point : Antidepressants for Mrs Bibi**

You may have noticed that no mention of psychotropic medication has been made in Mrs Bibi's case. This is because there are so many factors involved in her low mood, and because there is already a problem with polypharmacy. Adding another tablet may make things worse; initially it is important to get a clearer picture of the situation. It may be that with the interventions described above, Mrs Bibi's mood will lift. If this does not happen, the team would probably discuss the possibility of medication, and see what Mrs Bibi herself feels about it

on how the person sees the problem and what they hope for in a solution. You can then discuss ideas for how you can contribute to the plan of care with your mentor and the service user.

Student activity 16

Can you think of something you could do for each of Albert, Vera, and Mrs Bibi? Make notes on potential suggestions that you could adapt for your placement situation.

When you have got to know the service user, you might be able to initiate an activity based on reminiscence. Talking about the past can be relaxing and puts the service user in the position of being the expert. Kitwood (1997) tells us that the needs of people with dementia are attachment, inclusion, identity, occupation, comfort, and love. Reminiscence can help address all of these, not only for people with dementia, but for anyone who could benefit from reflection on the past. Reminiscence can be informal, where it develops in the course of a conversation, or may involve use of old photos or objects.

Evaluation of care should be carried out together with the service user, in a discussion about how they feel the service is meeting their needs and what still needs to be done. The family members will probably also have strong feelings about the person's progress and plans for their future support. Care plans will need to be updated regularly to reflect any concerns and plan for discharge. If the interventions on the plan are clear and measurable (you could use the 'SMART' acronym to test this), reviewing the plan and evaluating the care are straightforward (see Chapter 5 for discussion of SMART goals). You will also find it useful to look at the policies and guidelines listed in Box 7.11.

Good practice includes good trans-cultural care. The sensitivity and self-awareness you develop working with service users from different groups will help you avoid making assumptions about people from all groups, including your own. As cultures change over time, it is inevitable that you will meet people with cultural beliefs different from yours. These differences could be related to ethnicity or class, but will definitely include age.

Student activity 17 – Reflection

Working with older people can be challenging. Many of us find it hard to face the process of getting older – do you worry about grey hair (or no hair) or wrinkles? Sometimes it hurts us to think of people we love dying, and to contemplate our own deaths. Old age can remind us of the certainty of our mortality, something we might prefer not to think about.

Older people may also remind us of our own parents and grandparents. This can be used to prompt excellent standards of care, as students often say 'I try to look after people as I would like my family to be looked after.' This is sometimes known as the 'Golden Rule' (Rasmussen 1996). Not all families are the same though, so your understanding of what an older person needs, if you are Mrs Bibi's grandchild, may be quite different to Albert and Vera's grandchild's. The 'Platinum Rule' (Rasmussen 1996) suggests we should care for people as they would like to be cared for.

Whatever Albert, Vera, or Mrs Bibi tells us, there may be an element of their story that we find personally touching or difficult. Take some time to write a reflection on an aspect of their care that you personally would find challenging.

Raising the standard (2006) Royal College of Psychiatrists, http://www.rcpsych.ac.uk

Who cares wins (2005) Royal College of Psychiatrists, http://www.rcpsych.ac.uk

Everybody's business (2005) Care Services Improvement Partnership, http://www.csip.org.uk

HoNOS 65 (2002) Royal College of Psychiatrists, http://www.rcpsych.ac.uk

No secrets (2000) Department of Health, http://www.dh.gov.uk

Depression: Management of depression in primary and secondary care (2004) NICE, http://www.nice.org.uk

Promoting mental health and well-being in later life (2006) Age Concern/Mental Health Foundation, http://www.ageconcern.org.uk

Box 7.11 Useful policy and clinical guidelines for this chapter

Summary

In this chapter you have met Albert and Vera, their son Mark, and Mrs Bibi. Albert's situation illustrates how difficulties can arise for all the family when one member has memory problems. Vera is very stressed and as time goes on she too develops mental health problems. The ways in which Albert's family, and Mrs Bibi's family, deal with their problems are strongly influenced by their social and cultural contexts. As a nurse, it is part of your role to work together with the family so that they can use the advice and support you offer. Each care plan you design will reflect all of the above, as well as many personal factors, with the result that all care plans are unique.

A lifetime's experience leads to a strong personal identity; the challenge and satisfaction of working with older people with mental health problems is learning to work with the person, and their family, to support the sense of self at a time when society is valuing the person less, and mental illness may be undermining their identity.

Working with older people like Albert, Vera, and Mrs Bibi will help you practise all of the essential nursing skills. These include forming a therapeutic relationship, working in partnership and developing creative person-centred plans of care, and enhancing your ability to communicate effectively. Developing your self-awareness and sensitivity towards one excluded group, older people, will be an investment in your future ability to practise in an inclusive way where you demonstrate a positive, valuing outlook to all service users.

References and other sources

References

Adams T, ed (2008). **Dementia care nursing. Promoting well-being in people with dementia and their families**. Palgrave Macmillan, Basingstoke.

Bailliere's Nurses' Dictionary (2007). Bailliere Tindall, London.

Banerjee S, Smith S, Lamping DL, et al. (2006). Quality of life in dementia: more than just cognition. An analysis of associations with quality of life in dementia. **Journal of Neurology, Neurosurgery, and Psychiatry, 77**, 146-8.

Biggs S (1994). Failed individualism in community care: an example from elder abuse. **Journal of Social Work Practice, 8**(2), 137-50.

Biggs S, Phillipson C, and Kingston P (1995). **Elder abuse in perspective**, Open University Press, Buckingham.

Cantley C (2001). **A handbook of dementia care**. Oxford University Press, Buckingham.

Cassel K (2002). Use it or lose it: activity may be the best treatment for aging. **JAMA, 288**, 2333–5.

Chalder T (2000). Somatisation and inappropriate illness behaviour. In Newell and Gournay, eds. **Mental health nursing: an evidence based approach** pp. 225-42. Churchill Livingstone, Edinburgh.

Culley L and Dyson S (2001). **Ethnicity and nursing practice**. Palgrave, Basingstoke.

Department of Health (1999). **National Service Framework for mental health: Modern standards and service models for mental health**. Department of Health, London.

Department of Health (2000). **No secrets: guidance on developing and implementing multi-agency policies and procedures to protect vulnerable adults from abuse**. Department of Health, London.

Department of Health (2001). **National Service Framework for older people**, Department of Health, London.

Department of Health (2004). **The 10 essential shared capabilities**. Department of Health, London.

Department of Health (2006). **Dignity in care, Public Survey**. Department of Health, London.

Department for Work and Pensions (2005). **Opportunity age: Meeting the challenges of ageing in the twenty-first century**. Vols 1 and 2. DWP, London.

Egan G (2002). **The skilled helper: Models, skills and methods for effective helping**, 7th edition. Brooks-Cole, Monterey.

Ferns P (2005). **A holistic approach to black and minority mental health. The letting through light training pack**. Pavilion, Brighton.

Finkel SI, Costa E, Silva J, and Cohen G (1996). Behavioral and psychological signs and symptoms of dementia: a consensus statement on current knowledge and implications for research and treatment. **International Psychogeriatrics, 8,** (suppl. 3), 497-500.

Gibson F (2003). Seven Oaks: friendly design and sensitive technology. **Journal of Dementia Care, 11**(5), 27-30.

Goudie G and Stokes G (1995). **Working with dementia**. Winslow Press, Bicester.

Heron J (1975). **Six category intervention analysis, human potential research project**. University of Surrey, Guildford.

Holland K and Hogg C (2001). **Cultural awareness in nursing and health care**. Arnold, London.

Hope T, Keene J, Gedling K, Fairburn CG, and Jacoby R (1998). Predictors of institutionalisation for people with dementia living at home with a carer. **International Journal of Geriatric Psychiatry, 13**, 682-90.

Innes A (2003). Developing ethnically sensitive and appropriate dementia care practice. In Adams and Manthorpe, eds. **Dementia care**, pp. 202-12. Arnold, London.

Jenkins C (1998). Bridging the divide of culture and language. **Journal of Dementia Care, 6**(4), 22-4.

Junaid O and Hedge S (2007). Supportive psychotherapy in dementia. **Advances in Psychiatric Treatment, 13**, 17-23.

Kitwood T (1997). **Dementia reconsidered**. Open University Press, Buckingham.

Lundh V, Sandberg J, and Nolan M (2000). 'I don't have any choice': spouses' experiences of placing a partner in a care home for older people in Sweden. **Journal of Advanced Nursing, 32**(5), 1178-86.

Marshall M (2000). **ASTRID Project – A social and technological response to meeting the needs of individuals with dementia and their carers**. Hawker Publications, London.

McCarthy H and Thomas G (2004). **Home alone: combating isolation with older housebound people**. Demos, London.

Mental Capacity Act (2005). HMSO, London.

National Collaborating Centre for Mental Health, commissioned by the National Institute for Clinical Excellence (2004). **Depression: management of depression in primary and secondary care**. NIHCE, London.

National Institute for Health and Clinical Excellence (2006). **Dementia: Supporting people with dementia and their carers in health and social care**. NICE, London. [online] <http://www.nice.org.uk/cg42>

Norman A (1985). **Triple jeopardy: growing old in a second homeland**. CPA, London.

Nursing and Midwifery Council (2002). **Guidelines for records and record keeping**, revised edition. NMC Publications, London.

Nursing and Midwifery Council (2008). **The Code: Standards of conduct, performance and ethics for nurses and midwives**. NMC Publications, London.

Papadopoulos A and La Fontaine J (2000). **Elder abuse**. Winslow, Bicester.

Pickering S and Thompson J, eds (1998). **Promoting positive practice in nursing older people – Perspectives on quality of life**. Baillere Tindall, London.

Rasmussen T (1996). **The ASTD trainer's sourcebook: Diversity**. McGraw-Hill, New York.

Robinson L (1998). **'Race' communication and the caring professions**. Open University Press, Buckingham.

Roper N, Logan W, and Tierney A (1981). **Learning to use the process of nursing**. Churchill-Livingstone, London.

Royal College of Psychiatrists (2005). **Health of the Nation Scales** [online] <http://www.rcpsych.ac.uk/researchandtrainingunit/honos.aspx>.

Scrutton S (1999). **Counselling older people**, 2nd edition. Arnold, London.

Spector A, Orrell M, Davies S, and Woods B (2003). Reality orientation for dementia. **The Cochrane Library**, issue 1. Update Software, Oxford.

Thompson N, ed (2003). **Promoting equality. Challenging discrimination and oppression** Palgrave Macmillan, Basingstoke.

Wilson R, Bennett D, and Evans D (2002). Use it or lose it. **Journal of the American Medical Association**, 13 Feb.

Woods B, Spector A, Jones C, Orrell M, and Davies S (2005). Reminiscence therapy for dementia. **Cochrane Database of Systematic Reviews**, issue 1 [online] <http://www.alzheimers.org.uk/working_with_people_with_dementia/Primary_care/Dementia_diagnosis_and_management_in_primary_care/mmse.html> accessed 07/05/2008.

◯ Further reading

Diamond M (2004). The brain: use it or lose it, **Mindshaft Connection**, **1**(1) [online] <http://www.newhorizons.org/neuro/diamond_use.htm> accessed 17/05/2007.

Dudley D and Pringle A (2004). The use of timelines in dementia care. **Nursing Older People**, **15**(10), 18-20.

Holmes J Bentley K and Cameron I (2002). **Between two stools: Psychiatric services for older people in general hospitals**. Report of a I survey, University of Leeds, Leeds.

Chapter 8
Mental health nursing in the community
Andrew Walsh and Victoria Taylor

Learning outcomes

This chapter will assist you to:

- Understand the importance of constructive, partnership working with service users and their families and the need to negotiate achievable and meaningful goals.
- Demonstrate awareness of the need to provide care and treatment enabling service users to work towards a lifestyle within and beyond the limits of any mental health problem.
- Identify relevant knowledge and evidence-based practice in working with service users in a community setting, especially in the context of psychosis and anxiety-related problems.
- Understand how a comprehensive and systematic nursing assessment and care plan is formulated and documented, as well as how this might be evaluated.
- Consider the importance of working in ways that respect and value diversity.

Introduction

In this chapter you are introduced to two fictional characters, Paul and Molly, who need help with very different problems and who are intended to represent the wide range of emotional difficulties encountered by people referred to community mental health teams. Paul is a young man of Afro-Caribbean descent who has become isolated and withdrawn over a period of time. Paul's family are concerned and upset about his deterioration and he has been referred to community mental health services by his family doctor. Molly is a young woman who has been leading quite a stressful life; although successful in material terms, she has been experiencing anxiety and panic. This chapter demonstrates how practising community mental health nurses (CMHNs) might work with Paul and Molly in the process of assessing, planning, implementing, and evaluating the care planned alongside emerging mental health issues.

Clinical scenario: Paul

The first person we meet in this chapter is Paul, a young man who is referred to the community mental health team following concerns raised by his family about his changed behaviour. As well as being concerned for Paul's welfare, this section also prompts us to consider how we might work alongside his family, in this case, his mother Charmaine and his sister Caroline.

Student activity 1

Watch the films of Paul and his family and then read through the scenario here and the GP letter.

🎥 **www.oxfordtextbooks.co.uk/orc/clarke**

and choose the video link.

Paul's story

Paul is 21 years old. He lives with his parents, Joshua and Charmaine, and his 18-year-old sister, Caroline. Both Paul's parents came to the UK in 1971 from Barbados and they try to go back 'home' once a year to stay in touch with their extended family. They have lived in a three-bedroom house in Birmingham for the past 15 years. Joshua is 55 years old, a tool setter at an engineering factory, and Charmaine works part-time as a care assistant at a local nursing home. Caroline is currently doing A-levels and hopes to go to university. Joshua and Charmaine regularly attend at a Christian church, and are very proud of both their children, but would like them to be a little more respectful and attend the church more regularly.

According to his mother, Paul has always been a quiet person, and was quite shy at school. He did not make friends easily, but he stayed with the same friendship group throughout school and, until recently, kept in touch with those friends. His teachers described Paul as a studious, thoughtful, and gentle young man with excellent academic potential.

Paul completed three A-levels and started an electrical engineering degree at a local university when he was 19. However, he found the course increasingly difficult to cope with and decided not to continue after the first year. After withdrawing from the course, he said that he would like to undertake a modern apprenticeship but he has done little about this and has been unemployed and unoccupied for the last three months.

It was about nine months ago that Paul's family first noticed changes in his behaviour and character. These included him becoming withdrawn, less bothered about his personal hygiene, staying in his room more, associating less with his friends, and refusing to eat with the family. More recently he had started bolting his bedroom door, refusing to come out or talk to anyone and eating only by making night-time raids on the kitchen. On one occasion Charmaine had entered his room and found that Paul had been copying out parts of the Bible and then tearing up the paper. She often heard him shouting and ranting in his room but could not understand what he was saying.

Charmaine and Joshua sought help from their pastor, who came round to see Paul and try to talk to him. However, as soon as Paul knew the pastor was in the house he flew into a rage, screamed that the pastor was 'Evil, a false prophet' and would 'Kill them all.' Charmaine was very upset by this event, saying that she had never seen her son behave in this way and that he was 'Like some sort of wild man, his eyes staring, hair not brushed, dirty clothes and barefoot.' She then sought help from their GP who referred the case to a psychiatrist. A home visit was made and the psychiatrist concluded that Paul was probably in the early stages of schizophrenia. Hospital admission was indicated but there were no beds available. Paul was prescribed haloperidol 5 mg three times per day and an arrangement was made for a CMHN to make regular home visits for the two weeks or so until a hospital bed might become available (see Figure 8.1).

In the CMHN's first visit, Charmaine talked at length about the family difficulties. The pastor had persuaded Joshua that Paul's problems were spiritual in nature and that he would be best cared for by family and church members in Barbados. Charmaine thought that Joshua was trying to deny Paul's real problems and just wanted him out of the way. She knew that Joshua's own father had been a lifelong sufferer of mental illness and felt that this made the whole situation too difficult for him to deal with.

Charmaine said that she did not know what was going on. The psychiatrist had told her only that Paul was undergoing a 'stress reaction' and did not answer her questions about his likely progress. She had been unable to get Paul to take his medication. The CMHN tried to talk to Paul through his bedroom door but received no answer.

Schizophrenia

As you will see from reading the scenario, a psychiatrist has decided that Paul may be in the 'early stages of schizophrenia.' In recent years the medical categorization of schizophrenia has become increasingly disputed, to the point that it has become very difficult to sum this up without upsetting someone. Generally you would be advised to read this brief introduction and to familiarize yourself with the differing points of view about this area. Once you have done this, take the opportunity when you are on placement to speak with people who have been given the label/diagnosis of schizophrenia. You might want to talk about:

• How do *they* describe *their* lives?

• What problems do they have and why do they feel they have these problems?

```
Dear Community Mental Health Team,

Re: Paul Medford — DOB 13.03.1986  NHS No: 544986754

I would be grateful if you could offer an urgent assessment of this 21- year-old man
who I visited at home today. Since September of last year his mother reports marked
changes in her son's behaviour. In brief, he has become increasingly withdrawn and she
is very concerned regarding his lack of social interaction with family and friends.

Last week Paul resorted to locking himself in his bedroom, and was found copying out
parts of the Bbible and later tearing them up. He has also been heard by the family to
be 'shouting' and, 'ranting' and when visited by the local Pastor yesterday, 'flew into
a rage' and 'screamed' at him: 'evil, a false prophet' and threatened 'he would kill
them all'. Paul presents as withdrawn and unkempt with poor eye contact. It was dif-
ficult to establish rapport with him and I would welcome a diagnosis and management of
his symptoms.

I have prescribed haloperidol 5 mgs TDS and left this with the family, although Paul
was not keen on taking it. There is no past history of involvement with psychiatric
services and no medical history to note.

His mother, Mrs Medford, may be contacted on her mobile number to arrange an assess-
ment at your earliest convenience.

Thank you.

Yours sincerely,
M. Boulton
```

Figure 8.1   Referral letter for Paul

- What do they feel about the mental health services they have been exposed to; specifically what has been useful and helpful, and what has not?
- How do they feel about any treatments given? What has been helpful, and what has not?

You will no doubt be able to add questions of your own, but remember, if you really want to understand and to help people then there is no substitute for actually talking to them and most of all *listening*.

Medical descriptions

According to the *International statistical classification of diseases* (WHO 2007), schizophrenia generally has the following features:

" The schizophrenic disorders are characterized in general by fundamental and characteristic distortions of thinking and perception, and affects that are inappropriate or blunted. Clear consciousness and intellectual capacity are usually maintained although certain cognitive deficits may evolve in the course of time. The most important psychopathological phenomena include: thought echo; thought insertion or withdrawal; thought broadcasting; delusional perception and delusions of control, influence or passivity; hallucinatory voices commenting or discussing the patient in the third person; thought disorders and negative symptoms. "

Some medical terms that are commonly used to describe features of schizophrenia are defined in Box 8.1. Note that a very detailed medical description of

Medical term	Explanation	Notes
Delusional ideas	A delusion is usually described as being a false and fixed idea that does not correspond to the person's usual belief system and is held despite evidence to the contrary. In Paul's case he seems to have delusional ideas about the pastor, calling him 'evil' and a 'false prophet'. Other delusional ideas: Paranoia – Typically, the belief that people are talking about a person and possibly trying to harm them. Grandiose delusions – The person believes that they are special or different in some way, frequently having great, superhuman abilities or God-like powers.	Typically, medical approaches to the speech or voices heard by a person with schizophrenia would attribute no meaning to this experience. For example, you may hear the term 'word salad' to describe speech, implying that the person's words reflect a disordered mind and have no real meaning. More recently though, such ideas have been questioned. Nurses have been challenged to work with people who have these experiences rather than invalidating them. The aim of this is to try and help the person understand these experiences in the context of their own lives and to better manage or come to terms with this (see Romme and Escher 1993). Importantly we would not want to label as deluded someone whose beliefs are in keeping with their culture but not ours, e.g. some people in the Irish countryside may believe in 'the Banshee' – a wailing spirit that is heard before a death. Other ethnic groups may have similar beliefs. We may not share these beliefs but we cannot label them as 'delusional' because of this.
Hallucinations	Usually described as being 'sensory perception in the absence of sensory stimuli', or in plainer English this is when a person may see, hear, feel, smell, or taste something that is not really there. Visual hallucination – Seeing things that are not there. Auditory hallucination – Hearing strange things (usually voices).	

Affect	If you hear a psychiatrist talking about 'affect' then they are describing a person's apparent mood state. Therefore an 'affective disorder' is a state in which a person has an unusually high mood (mania) or is low in mood (depression). You may also hear the term 'incongruity of affect' – this means that a person's emotional reaction is not in keeping with the situation. An example may be seen in the person who laughs or cries when there is no obvious reason.
Blunted affect	Again, a term you may hear in practice. What is meant by this is that the person seems apathetic and unresponsive, indifferent to their surroundings and circumstances.
Thought insertion/ withdrawal	These terms describe characteristic problems with thinking that people may complain of. In thought insertion the person perceives thoughts as seeming to have come from an external source; withdrawal means that thoughts seem to have been taken out of one's head.
Thought broadcasting	The person feels that others can hear their thoughts, and that these have somehow been 'broadcast' out loud.
Thought disorder	Generally it is thought that patterns in a person's speech can reveal disorder in their thinking. An example of this is 'knight's move thinking' in which a person's speech may appear to lack logical structure (the knight's move in chess is unusual in that it combines both horizontal and vertical directions). In thought control or influence, the person has the experience that their thoughts and actions are being controlled by some external source. The term 'passivity' means that the person believes that thoughts have been inserted into their heads by external agencies/forces.

Critics of psychiatric practice would say that the medication given to people with mental health problems has a tendency to produce such behaviour.

| Negative symptoms | Schizophrenia is thought to consist of a range of 'positive' features (most of the above descriptions fall into this category, apart from blunted affect) as well as 'negative' features. Negative features of schizophrenia are described as follows: social withdrawal, poverty of speech (i.e. the person says little and does not initiate conversation), loss of motivation, self-neglect. |

Box 8.1 Medical terms used to describe schizophrenia

schizophrenia is outside the scope of this text; for more detail see WHO (2007).

Other descriptions

As a mental health nursing student it is important to recognize that most of these descriptions of schizophrenia have been disputed to a greater or lesser extent. It would be easy to fill an entire textbook with the arguments against established psychiatry, so the following summary can only indicate areas of further enquiry.

Schizophrenia – a medical diagnosis?

One of psychiatry's more prominent critics, Thomas Szasz, wrote about *The myth of mental illness* (Szasz 1972) in which he argued that mental illness has no objective reality. Instead it is an idea created by psychiatry and its practitioners. Szasz suggested that true illness must have a measurable physical cause and that what we call 'mental illness' is really a way of labelling behaviour that differs from the norm. There are arguments for and against schizophrenia having a physical basis. Some believe that there is clear scientific evidence for a genetic and physiological basis while others strongly dispute these findings.

In his book *Toxic psychiatry* (Breggin 1993), the author makes the case that not only is psychiatry misguided, it is also a dangerous and oppressive force in (mostly western) society. He argues that people who are labelled as schizophrenic are actually expressing confusion about identity or spirituality. Often this is a result of traumatic and (often sexually) abusive past experience. Breggin and many others believe that the medication given to such people is damaging (see Anthony's scenario in Chapter 4 of this book) and that rather than 'treating' an illness, it has the effect of disabling them.

Mary Boyle's (1990) work on the subject of schizophrenia states that there is no doubt that people do have strange and disturbing experiences and that sometimes these can be altered with medication. What is in question, though, is the whole concept of the diagnosis of schizophrenia (see also the Campaign to Abolish the Schizophrenia Label, CASL, http://www.asylumonline.net/). Boyle argues that the use of the label schizophrenia, for example in court cases or in scientific research, is misguided, obscuring the need to investigate other, truer causes of people's behaviour.

A good example of the different approaches to schizophrenia can be seen in the following references:

- Schizophrenia: Core interventions in the treatment and management of schizophrenia in primary and secondary care (NICE 2002).
- Schizophrenia: The 'not so nice' guidelines (Barker 2002).

The first was produced by the National Institute for Clinical Excellence and is intended as a guide to clinicians working with people who are diagnosed with schizophrenia. The second paper, by Phil Barker, takes a critical look at the official guidelines. You are also strongly advised to look at Romme and Morris's (2007) excellent critical appraisal of the concept of schizophrenia.

Ethnic issues and mental health services

If you look at the film of Paul's sister, Caroline, you will see that she has some reservations about him coming into contact with mental health services:

🎥 www.oxfordtextbooks.co.uk/orc/clarke

and choose the video link.

Although Caroline is sure that her brother does need help, she is worried about how he might be treated. As a nurse working with Paul's family you would need to understand some of the issues surrounding black people and mental health services. When one examines some of these issues it becomes clear why Caroline is so concerned for her brother:

- People from black and minority ethnic groups are more likely than white people to be referred to mental health services via the police, courts, or prisons.

- People from black and minority ethnic groups are less likely to be seen as outpatients, and once admitted to hospital they are more likely to experience compulsory detention there and to be housed in more secure settings.

- Many studies suggest that African-Caribbean people living in the UK are more likely to receive a diagnosis of schizophrenia than white people.

- There is evidence that African-Caribbean patients receive more medication and physical treatments and are less likely to be offered 'talking therapies'.

- There are ongoing suggestions that mental health services are perceived as culturally insensitive and racist.

This is a *very* brief overview of what is a large, complex, and important area, so you would be advised to consult the following:

- Fernando (2003), for a fuller account.
- *Breaking the circles of fear* (2002), published by the Sainsbury Centre for Mental Health.

- Delivering race equality in mental health care: an action plan for reform inside and outside services and the Government's response to the independent inquiry into the death of David Bennett (Department of Health 2005).

> **Student activity 2**
> *Look at the following report in Box 8.2 and consider the different points of view expressed in the articles. Note that the full text of the articles is freely available online via your place of study.*
> *Having considered these opposing points of view, reflect on the following:*

- What has been your experience of mental health services – do you agree with the above claims that they are institutionally racist or does Professor Singh's argument hold more truth?

- What do you think the patients with whom you are working might say on this subject?

- What would practising mental health nurses say on this matter?

- What do you think services need to do to improve the way that people are treated?

- What are services doing well?

> **Student activity 3**
> *Have another look at the films of Paul, his sister, and his mother.*

www.oxfordtextbooks.co.uk/orc/clarke

and choose the video link. Bearing in mind what you have read so far, think about what you have seen here.

- How do you think Paul, his mother, and his sister might be feeling?

- How would you feel if Paul was your brother/son/friend?

- What would you do if you were asked to see Paul as a community mental health nurse?

- What do you think would help Paul?

The 'Count me in' census published in 2006 (by the Health Care Commission, The National Institute for Mental Health in England, and the Mental Health Act Commission) showed that when compared to other groups, black people experience higher rates of admission to mental hospitals and are more likely to be admitted via the criminal justice system. The census also highlighted that ethnic minority groups were more likely to experience seclusion and restraint. This survey caused much comment and controversy, each with differing views.

The 'Count me in 2006' survey can be found online at:

http://www.healthcarecommission.org.uk/_db/_documents/Count_Me_In_2006.pdf

'Race and mental health: there is more to race than racism'
Writing in the British Medical Journal, Singh and Burns (2006) argued that high rates of admission and detention of black patients in mental hospitals are not a result of racism. Professor Singh goes on to question the basis for claims that services are racist and suggests that claims of 'institutionalized racism' actually damage services and their patients.

Read the full text of this online at:

http://www.bmj.com/cgi/content/full/333/7569/648

'Institutional racism in mental health care'
Writing in the same journal, McKenzie and Bhui (2007) argued that this census proves that mental health services are failing to meet the needs of a multicultural society.

The authors suggest that institutional racism in mental health services is responsible for the experiences of black people within the mental health care system.

The full text of this is available at:

http://www.bmj.com/cgi/content/full/334/7595/649

Box 8.2   Racism in mental health services?

👤 Paul – a service user's viewpoint

When you look at the person rather than the label of illness, as his sister did, he is not his usual self. His stressful situation and feelings of powerlessness seem to have manifested itself into unusual behaviour, which appears quite aggressive.

He is simply an angry and frightened young man, with real anxiety about his family's well-being, and frustrated at his sense of powerlessness. Paul seems very concerned about his family's welfare, but without any authority or control. They care about him but can offer him no solace, which only adds to his feelings of isolation – a 'them and us' type situation. But is this necessarily a sign of an emerging mental illness?

In his panic, he is possibly demonizing potential agents of control – for example the pastor. In his confusion and respect for his mother he does not realize she is actually the one with the power.

Using language like 'kill', etc. may simply mean he is frightened of losing his family if he gets sent abroad and in his intense distress he uses very powerful metaphors to try to communicate this devastating fear.

His only points of reference include family and religion. He takes on the pressures of worrying about his family, but has little control over things. However, he can control his voices/thoughts by shouting them down.

But **is** his unusual behaviour a danger to himself or others? Is it only unusual in terms of it being a little weird for onlookers to witness? He is in turmoil

» – but he is doing no more than wearing his heart on his sleeve. He is thinking his confused thoughts out loud – frustration leads to aggression, so he may appear a little aggressive on the outside – but he must be so frustrated by the competing 'voices'/characters/thoughts/points of view that he verbalizes them and translates them into visual images in his mind's eye in order to make sense of them – in order to give them an identity, in order to render them less confusing – maybe in a vain attempt to somehow distance himself from these distressing thoughts within a worried mind.

He switches from seeming quite in control for a second, quietly trying to describe how he feels, and then launches once again into confusion. He feels there is no hope and in his desperation to find a way out of his turmoil his thoughts are swirling.

He needs to be reassured that someone can actually help him and find practical solutions (other than medication), finding out whether he wishes to go to the Caribbean – I suspect no would be the answer – seems he's trapped with what his mum wants – what about **his** wishes?

It's all about his mum – the pastor – God – what about PAUL?

Tracey Holley, survivor

Nursing assessment

Presenting problems

Paul is a 21-year-old man referred by his GP on 22 May 2007 with a nine-month history of becoming increasingly withdrawn, with evidence of self-neglect. Recent history of locking himself in his room and shouting at family and visitors. Has taken to writing down extracts from the Bible and later tearing the paper up.

During first year of his undergraduate course suffered stress and difficulties with academic studies (non-completion of assignments and absenteeism).

Grandfather with mental illness?

Paul's perception of his problem

'I'm alright you know, I'm okay.'
'No need for medication, he needs medication not me, I'm alright.'
'Like to be on my own, don't have to be with people.'

Alcohol and substance use

Tobacco: Smokes average 20 per day (since age of 16 yrs).

Alcohol: Currently nil, previously approx 5 – 10 units per week.

Illicit drugs: No past/present use.

Family

Grandparents – Joshua's father suffered from mental health issues in the past but exact nature of this presently unclear.

Father – Joshua – age 55 yrs – tool setter – physical health: known diabetic (insulin controlled).
Mother – Charmaine – age 50 yrs – care assistant – no physical or mental health problems.
Sister – Caroline – age 18 yrs – A-level student – no physical or mental health problems.
Good relationships with family members.
Paul has a very close relationship with his parents and sister, and also with relatives back home in Barbados whom he visits yearly.

Personal history

Paul was born in UK.
No birth complications. Reached milestones.

Schooling

Junior School – Cottage Hill – age 5 yrs–11 yrs – mixed sex/state.
Secondary School – St Felix – age 11 yrs–18 yrs – mixed sex/state.
Relationship with peers good. Maintained contact with school friends up until recently.
Academic and social progress – shy at school and quiet pupil. Attained five GCSEs and three A-levels in maths, physics, and English language.
Relationship with teachers excellent. 'Studious, thoughtful, and gentle young man.'
No history of truancy or victim of bullying.
Attended university to study BSc in Electrical Engineering, completed only first year and left because of difficulties keeping up with work.

Social network

Has two close male friends from school days but has reduced contact in last few months.

Leisure

At present no leisure activities. In the past enjoyed reading and riding his bicycle. Described as quiet and a little shy but has always been outgoing and sociable with close friends.

Housing

For the past 15 yrs has lived with his mother, father, and sister in a three-bedroom house (owned by parents).

Finances

In receipt of jobseeker's allowance.
No known debts.

Activities of daily living

Usually self-caring. Currently needs prompting by family members to take care of his personal needs (hygiene/appearance).
Sleep has been disturbed in recent weeks, family report he is often up and about at night-time when others are asleep.
Eating at night, raiding kitchen.

Childcare responsibilities and child protection issues

No childcare responsibilities.

Past physical health history

No major physical illnesses.
No operations.
No known allergies.
Eczema as a child.

Spirituality

Christian – mother attends Baptist church and identifies her Christian faith as being very important. There is a possibility of some conflict here though.
Paul seems quite angry and hostile towards the church minister and has apparently been tearing up a Bible.

Clearly this is an area that will need to be explored further with the family.

Appearance and behaviour

Well built, average height.
Casually dressed.
Some neglect to personal hygiene observed (hair uncombed, long dirty fingernails).
Eye contact intermittent due to possible response to visual hallucinations.
Agitated throughout interview; fidgeting on chair, messing with clothing, rubbing head and neck, and frequently sniffing.
Poor rapport.

Mood

No episodes of mania or depression.
No diurnal variation in mood.

Sleep

Retires approximately 22.00 hrs, awakes early hours (to consume food) – later returns to bed. But some mention by family of disturbed sleep recently.
No early morning awakening.

Appetite

Eating patterns have changed over the last three months. He no longer eats with the family and helps himself to food at night time. Paul's family are unsure how much food he is eating.

Thought

Delusional ideas about the pastor, calling him 'evil' and a 'false prophet.'
'He needs medication not me.' 'Pastor tells nothing good.' 'Want to kill me and the whole family.'
Responding to what appears to be **visual/auditory hallucinations** (pastor), 'I don't like you, can't kill my family.'
'Don't come close don't touch, Jesus.' Observed as becoming increasing agitated at this point, staring.
Evidence of flight of ideas.

Speech

Content: Religious reference to Jesus and pastor.

Volume: Increased when experiencing hallucinations.

Negative symptoms

Isolation, self-neglect, and loss of motivation as described by family members.

Insight

Poor.

Consideration of risk

Suicide

No history of suicidal behaviour or threats to harm self; Paul quite clearly states that he does not want to harm himself. I have told Paul that we would like to be able to speak with him and also that we are concerned that he has isolated himself from others.

Harm to others

No history of harming other people although he is very angry about the church minister brought to home by mother. Paul states that he is 'evil' and a 'false prophet' and there is concern about the potential for harm if Paul decides to act upon these ideas.
Paul told me that he is trying to protect his family and himself from harm; clearly he feels vulnerable.

Neglect

Family have expressed concern about Paul because of lack of self-care; sister especially contrasted brother's present state with previous well-groomed, neat and tidy behaviour.

We do know that Paul is eating as family say that food is going from kitchen at night and there has been no weight loss.

Summary of initial assessment

Paul has been referred to the CMHT following a clear change in his behaviour. Over the past nine months there has been a gradual decline in his self-care and Paul has become increasingly solitary and withdrawn. This has culminated in Paul taking to his bedroom and only coming out at night to eat alone. Paul previously spent a lot of time with two particular friends but apparently over the last six months this has stopped.

Paul may be hearing voices and has expressed the idea that the pastor is 'evil' and may want to harm the family. Paul does not have a history of violent behaviour and there is no current suggestion of an intention to harm himself.

The family are very concerned for Paul; his mother identifies strongly with a spiritual element to his problems while his sister agrees that there has been a dramatic change in her brother.

Care planning

Paul's care plan is shown on pp. 192–200.

Family accounts

Charmaine's (mother) account of Paul's problems:
Reported her son Paul as having a few problems lately, often crying and keeping himself in his bedroom more than usual. Asked the pastor to come and see him 'to help him'. Discussed the need to take Paul back to Barbados as she believes there is 'nothing wrong' 'he's bright, makes no trouble', 'needs a bit of guidance'. Feels his return will make him 'alright'. Praying for her son daily. Very tearful on interview: 'I would be the first to know if anything was wrong.'

Caroline's (sister) account of Paul's problems:
Described her brother as not being the same and gave the example of Paul always being clean and tidy, but recently has 'not brushed his hair' 'messy, dirty, bare feet'.
'Like a wild animal.' 'Mum wants the pastor in the church to take away the evil spirits.'
Caroline acknowledges Paul needs treatment: 'want my brother back', 'needs help', but expresses her concerns. Fears if he goes into an institution he will not come out (crying at this point).

Paul's care plan

Based on the above assessment, the care plan is as follows:

Identified Need	Action	Responsible for action	Desired outcome	Review date
Mental health needs (1) Paul needs to feel safe, calm, in control. He needs to understand why he is having bizarre experiences. Paul is obviously distressed: • He is isolating himself from his family/friends. • Has been heard shouting. • Family identify that this is not his usual behaviour. • Family identify that Paul's speech content is unusual and disturbing. (See Evaluation section, p. 191)	(a) Nurse to introduce self to Paul, clearly stating who he/she is and why they are there. Ensure that clear language is used and that a positive and optimistic tone is used – ensure confidentiality. Give written material for Paul and family to refer to. (b) Encourage Paul to explain what he is worried about – ensure supportive, reassuring, and non-judgemental attitude and *listen to what he says*. Record this in progress notes. (c) Find out from Paul what is worrying him and what help he thinks would help him. (d) Encourage family to adopt similar approach (see Box 8.4 on 'High expressed emotion'). (e) Give Paul and family details of how to get support if needed out-of-hours.	Paul, CMHN, and family	• Paul is made aware that people are prepared to listen to and support him. • Paul is able to express fears freely and receive support. • Family is helped to support Paul. • CMHT will have a clearer understanding of his mental state. (Important that Paul is involved in what is done to help him and that a partnership approach to the situation should be adopted straight away.) **Rationale:** *This is based on the need to establish a relationship with the service user before proceeding with the intervention (see Chapter 2 p. 27). It is vital that we try to engage with the person rather than with an illness; therefore the above reflects an attempt to understand things from Paul's point of view (see 'Paul – a service user's viewpoint on p.188).* *The 10 essential shared capabilities (2004) also refer to 'Identifying people's needs and strengths'.*	One week
Mental health needs (2) Paul needs to feel safe. He needs to be able to control his desire to possibly	• Continue to monitor risk re self-harm. Arrange for prompt review if deterioration is noted. • Advise family that Paul is especially angry	Paul, CMHN, family, and other members of MDT	• Currently considered to be at relatively low risk of self-harm – aim is to continue to monitor this and to review as appropriate.	One week

Identified Need	Action	Responsible for action	Desired outcome	Review date
harm the family's church minister. Possibility of self-harm or harm to others? Assessment so far suggests minimal risk of self-harm but Paul has expressed anger towards church minister (although Paul has no past history of violent behaviour to others and has made no specific threats).	towards church minister. • Involve family in monitoring this area – encourage them to discuss with MDT if concerned. • Discuss with Paul his angry feelings – advise him that there is concern that he might harm the pastor – ask Paul about this. • Monitor as part of ongoing mental state assessment – ensure very prompt action in the event of deterioration in Paul's mental state. • Discuss and agree level of risk in first review.		• Some degree of concern about ideas and anger towards pastor. Aim is to explain concerns to Paul and involve him and his family in monitoring this situation. • Overall objective is to maintain safety of Paul and others while ensuring that care is conducted with the minimum level of restriction. • Discuss alternatives with the family – possibly asking that the pastor does not visit at the moment to minimize risk. **Rationale:** *See standards 1 and 7 of NSF (1999).* *Also 10 essential shared capabilities (2004) – 'Promoting safety and positive risk taking.'*	
Mental health needs (3) Paul needs to trust the CMHN so that he can be honest about his experiences. (Assessment has identified that Paul may be hearing voices.)	CMHN to work on developing relationship with Paul. Discover if Paul is actually hearing voices: • Ask him about this. • Does he have any past history of this behaviour? • Observe – i.e. does he appear to be hearing or responding to voices? • Have family seen him responding to voices? • If Paul is hearing voices, review care plan accordingly (see Box 8.3, Voices).	Paul, CMHN, family, and other members of MDT	• Important to firstly discover if Paul is actually hearing voices? • Ensure that physical illness is ruled out – therefore draw this possibility to attention of medical staff (see section on physical care). • Paul is either: (a) helped to reduce/eliminate this experience or (b) assisted to cope with it. • Paul should be given appropriate support. (Care plan will need to be reviewed depending on whether this experience is ongoing.)	One week

Identified Need	Action	Responsible for action	Desired outcome	Review date
			Rationale: *See Box 8.3 on Voices and Evaluation on p. 191.*	
Mental health needs (4) Medication issues – Paul needs to understand why medication has been prescribed and the indications for use. Paul needs to make informed consent to take the medication. Paul needs to be aware of the contra-indications and side effects of the prescribed medication. Paul has been prescribed haloperidol 5 mg TDS by GP.	Discuss with CMHT psychiatrist re immediate review of medication. *(It is recommended that people experiencing first episode of schizophrenia are not prescribed haloperidol – 'GP should consider starting atypical antipsychotic drugs at the earliest opportunity' – NICE 2002.)* Once medication has been reviewed, give information about medication and help Paul/family to understand this. Discuss with Paul and family possible benefits of taking medication: • If he is troubled by voices this may help to reduce these or make them less distressing. • If he is feeling overwhelmed by distressing ideas then medication may make him feel less distressed and able to cope with this/accept help from CMHT, family etc. • This may be a first step towards Paul resuming some of his previous activities. It is also important to discuss possible problems: • Discuss possible side effects (see pharmacist's view on p. 195 for more information on this).	Paul, CMHN, family, and other members of MDT	• Paul should be helped towards making an informed decision about taking medication. • Paul and family should know that medication needs to be taken regularly as prescribed. • Paul and family made aware of side effects and advised who to contact in order to discuss these/seek advice. • CMHN to participate in regular MDT review re medication. • Paul should receive maximum benefit from medication while minimizing possible problems. • Paul should receive smallest amount of medication for minimum possible period of time. **Rationale:** *Medical model.* *10 essential shared capabilities (2004) –Working in partnership.*	One week

Identified Need	Action	Responsible for action	Desired outcome	Review date
	Paul to be regularly monitored for effects/side effects of medication prescribed: • Monitor for effects/side effects on visits and give Paul and family contact details for advice. • Ensure that effects/side effects of medication are discussed and reviewed on a regular basis.			
General needs (1) Self-neglect (personal hygiene/appearance) – Paul needs to improve his personal hygiene/appearance to a socially acceptable level.	CMHN and family to encourage Paul to bathe/shower at least every other day and change his clothing at least every other day. Agree goals with Paul and gain support from family. CMHN to monitor on twice weekly visits.	Paul, CMHN, family, and other members of MDT	To encourage Paul to attend to his personal hygiene needs under supervision from family, until mentally stable enough to maintain by himself.	Two weeks

Pharmacist's view

People with schizophrenia are more likely to be overweight and at greater risk of developing hypertension, type 2 diabetes, cardiovascular disease, and dyslipidaemia than the general population. These potential problems can be worsened by side effects from antipsychotics. Visible side effects such as weight gain could affect compliance. Extrapyramidal side effects, which include tremor, dystonia (abnormal face and body movements), akathisia (restlessness), and tardive dyskinesia (rhythmic involuntary movements of the face, jaw, and tongue) are more common with the older antipsychotics than with the atypicals. They can be treated with antimuscarinic drugs, such as procyclidine. For further information on side effects consult the British National Formulary (BNF) section 4.2.1.

In discussion about side effects and the choice of therapy it could be useful to talk about treatment of a physical problem (Paul's father's treatment of diabetes with insulin) and compare it to treatment of a mental illness. Treatment should be started at a low dose and increased slowly every 1–2 weeks, depending on response. If Paul had been taking the haloperidol regularly, it would be wise to taper the dose down while increasing the new drug, to minimize side effects, as antipsychotics should not be stopped abruptly. Within 3–4 weeks some benefit should be seen, but if there is no response after 6–8 weeks consideration should be given to changing therapy.

MORECAMBE BAY HOSPITALS NHS TRUST

Identified Need	Action	Responsible for action	Desired outcome	Review date
General needs (2) Dietary intake reduced – Paul needs to have a daily calorific intake of at least 2000 calories.	CPN/family to monitor client's dietary intake. CPN and family to encourage Paul to eat regular meals with family – perhaps agree at least one meal per day? Discuss with Paul his feelings and beliefs about food and eating. What would Paul like to eat and how does he want this prepared? Are there any concerns/beliefs from Paul about possible tampering with food?	Paul, CMHN, family, and other members of MDT	Aim is to encourage Paul to eat with family if possible. Monitor/ensure that he is receiving sufficient nutrition. May require more long-term interventions if necessary, i.e. education on nutrition, healthy diet, food preparation etc.	Two weeks
General needs (3) Sleep disturbance – Paul needs to establish a pattern of sleeping at night between 22.00 and 09.00 for at least 6–8 hours.	Discuss with Paul re his sleep problems and ascertain his feelings about this. Discuss re usual sleep pattern? Encourage family to help monitor Paul's sleep pattern (where feasible) and discuss with CPN on home visits. CPN to educate Paul on sleep hygiene principles.	Paul, CMHN, CPN, and family	Monitor Paul's sleeping habits to establish a pattern of disturbance. Offer advice about sleeping (see Anthony's care plan in Chapter 4). Ensure this is included as part of case review **Rationale:** *Interventions are based on existing ill health diagnostic criteria and the medical model. Underpinned by and in accordance with national guidelines and policies.*	Two weeks
Specific cultural needs If nurse is from a different cultural background to Paul and family then need to be aware of potential for misinterpretation that may be caused by differences in values,	Try and understand from Paul and family what they see as important cultural needs from their point of view. Record this conversation and ensure this is reflected in any review.	Paul, CMHN, family, and other members of MDT	General aim is to ensure the following is achieved: • Care given by CMHT will reflect informed discussion with Paul/ family team.	This needs to be an ongoing process

Identified Need	Action	Responsible for action	Desired outcome	Review date
beliefs, and expression of distress. Family has strong spiritual beliefs and mother especially feels that nature of and possible solution to Paul's problems may be spiritual. *(NB Remember that Paul and family may or may not share views on spiritual beliefs.)* *(NB also – Paul may be rejecting his family's faith and the current difficulties could include the conflict this is causing – both internally for Paul and within the family.)*	• Try and understand Paul in context of his own previous lifestyle choices/behaviour, etc. Discuss his preferences and aspirations, and ensure that this is part of any ongoing care review. • Be guided by Paul and his family about what is 'normal' – don't jump to conclusions based on observations from different cultures. Again, need to document in ongoing care notes and ensure included as part of review. • Wherever possible CMHT staff should try to work alongside colleagues from a similar background to Paul. • Consider accessing support from any suitable local voluntary/NGO working with African-Caribbean community. Highlight any areas of staff uncertainty and discuss with managers.		• Care given by CMHT is culturally sensitive and appropriate and seen to be so by Paul and family. • Care given/interventions should reflect actual needs – should not reflect cultural misinterpretation/stereotyping. • Assessments and notes taken will reflect this ongoing discussion re appropriateness of care given. **Rationale:** *See Sainsbury Centre for Mental Health (2002) Breaking the circles of fear, and Fernando (2003).* *10 essential shared capabilities (2004) – Respecting diversity.*	
Concern about Paul's **physical health** because: • He has been neglecting his self-care i.e. diet, sleeping, hygiene etc. (see **General needs**). • Relatively sudden change in his mental state – possibility of physical	• Explain to Paul that there is concern for his physical well-being and involve him in planning to maintain his health. • Ask Paul how he is feeling, monitor/record apparent physical state as part of visit. • Attention to care plan areas as above (**General needs**).	Paul, CMHN, family, and other members of MDT	Aim is to ensure that Paul's physical health is monitored and a safe level of health is maintained. Paul and family should be involved and consulted in monitoring health. Ensure that full health check is completed and that physical health is monitored.	One week

Identified Need	Action	Responsible for action	Desired outcome	Review date
ill health or substance misuse needs to be considered. *(NB Paul denies substance abuse and has no history of this – this is a less likely but not impossible factor.)* Paul is in a distressed mental state therefore possible effect of stress on physical health.	• Discuss with medical staff re review of physical state. • Advise Paul and family re appropriate action if concerned about Paul's physical state. • Explain to Paul about importance of maintaining an adequate fluid intake – if he is going to stay in his bedroom for now, ensure that a suitable supply of drinks is available. Check with Paul and family re what is appropriate. • Check with Paul and family how much he is drinking. *Ensure prompt review if physical health appears to be declining. (Also, may need to consider more long-term needs –healthy lifestyle including exercise, diet etc. as part of future review.)*		**Rationale:** *NSF (1999) highlights the fact that people with mental illness have high rates of physical health problems.*	
Family are upset and concerned for Paul.	• Explain intention to work in partnership with family. • Although Paul may not want to join meetings etc. straight away, ensure he is asked to join in, and tell him what is happening. • Arrange to spend time talking to family. Encourage them to talk about their worries.	CMHN	Aims are as follows: • Establish principle of partnership, working with whole family as soon as possible. • Acknowledge family role as 'expert'. • Allow time for family members to express fears and concerns. • Provide support and facilitate outside support.	

Identified Need	Action	Responsible for action	Desired outcome	Review date
	• Ensure that family are given advice about how best to help Paul as well as maintain their own mental health.		• Provide information and advice about services/interventions and give honest answers to questions.	Two weeks
	• Recognize family role as 'expert' – need to ensure that their ideas are given prominence.		• Ensure family has appropriate out-of-hours service contact details.	
	• Discuss with family possible referral to appropriate local carer support groups.		**Rationale:** *NSF (1999) Standard 6 –'Caring about carers'.*	
	• Discuss openly with family ideas about 'expressed emotion' and family role in this (see Box 8.4 on Expressed emotion).		*10 essential shared capabilities (2004) – Working in partnership.*	
	Ensure that family members are helped to understand what local services are available and how to access these (including out-of-hours emergency).			

Reported experience of voice hearing may be an important factor in a person being diagnosed as having schizophrenia, as medically this is considered to be an important 'positive' symptom (see Box 8.1). As discussed previously, though, there is a lot of debate and controversy surrounding what exactly is being experienced by people hearing voices and a full description of this debate is outside the scope of this chapter. Some clinicians will take a very medical approach to this experience, others much less so. Certainly though the approach adopted if Paul were hearing voices would include some or all of the following:

- First rule out the possibility that voices are caused by physical problem, i.e. organic illness or from use of street drugs? (see physical care plan).
- Discuss with Paul what he is hearing and elicit his beliefs re this?
- How distressing does Paul find the voices heard?
- Is there any pattern, i.e. is it worse when he is in a noisy environment *(could this be why he isolates himself)*?
- Encourage Paul to make a note/diary of experiences and offer to talk about this with him.

Suggest to Paul that medication may help (see medication plan).

Box 8.3   'Voices'

The term 'high expressed emotion' (high EE) refers to the idea that patterns of family interactions might contribute to the development of schizophrenia in an individual. The suggestion is that a preponderance of 'over-involved', hostile, critical, and negative interactions within a family might have an effect upon a vulnerable individual. As with so many aspects of schizophrenia, this is an area around which there has been considerable argument.

- Research from the late 1960s onward has suggested that high EE could be a factor in the development of schizophrenia.
- There are consistent reports that high EE is an important factor in whether someone relapses once discharged from hospital treatment.
- If true, this would suggest that family interventions to reduce the emotional temperature within a family and to lessen negative/critical interactions while increasing social skills in the person with schizophrenia might be a useful intervention.

However, carers of people with schizophrenia have objected that these ideas set them up as being to blame for their relative developing mental health problems. For instance what does 'over-involved' mean – it is hard to use terms such as this and pretend to be a neutral outsider. Also, is it realistic to expect *any* family to live for years without occasionally becoming angry with each other? Certainly it would appear that:

- Family interactions must play some part in an individual's emotional life (in fact is it possible or even sensible to try to consider the individual as existing outside of their environment anyway?).
- Families who have a loved one diagnosed as schizophrenic will be in a state of shock and bewilderment – they will need and welcome empathetic support and advice from services.
- Therefore it is obviously important that we give consideration to our interactions with families as well as the individual client.

Whether the concept of high EE is a useful one or not is beyond the scope of this chapter but you may wish to read about this further (see below). You might also take the opportunity in placements to talk to people diagnosed with schizophrenia, their families, and your clinical mentors about this subject.

Suggested reading

Askey et al. (2007), Kuipers et al. (2002), Wuerker (2000).

Box 8.4 High expressed emotion and schizophrenia?

Care plan evaluation notes

One week later:

Mental health needs (1)

The CMHN has now made contact with Paul and explained to him who we are and why we have been asked to visit him. Although he was (and remains) a little unsure about whether he wants to talk to us, he is beginning to speak more freely to us and we feel we are making some little progress in developing a relationship with him.

The family have been encouraged to listen sympathetically to Paul and have been given details about where and how to ask for help and support if needed.

Mental health needs (2)

Paul has not expressed any intention to harm himself and denies that this is something he is considering. There is no apparent evidence of any plans to harm himself.

Paul is still expressing hostility towards the pastor – we have discussed our concerns with him but this remains a source of concern. There is no evidence of hostility being expressed towards others – indeed, Paul seems to want to protect people.

We have discussed with family re advising pastor not to visit for the moment.

Mental health needs (3)

(Re voice hearing) – Paul has told CMHN that he does hear voices coming from outside his head. These have been present for some time (unclear exactly how long) and have become much more prominent in recent times. At present, Paul is extremely reluctant to talk about this experience. We have been gently asking him about it but have told him for now that we are willing to try and help him with this experience when/if he wants us to.

Paul has now been seen by his GP at home, a general physical examination has been performed, and while no obvious problems were identified we have agreed to keep this under review.

Mental health needs (4)

Paul became angry and slammed the door shut when the subject of taking medication was raised with him – we have decided for the moment to focus our efforts on trying to build a trusting relationship with him but this is an area that may need to be revisited.

General needs (1)

Paul has agreed to bathe/shower on a regular basis and also to change his clothes – so far this remains a problem as he remains in quite an unkempt and dishevelled state, although he did allow his mother into his room to 'tidy' and he did change into the clothes that she put out for him. He is not as yet making any attempt to self-care and this remains an important goal of care.

General needs (2)

Initial fears that Paul was eating an insufficient amount of food may have been misplaced. Following the CMHN's first few visits, family were encouraged to monitor his dietary intake and it would appear that on Paul's night-time visits to the kitchen he is taking a very good level of nutrition. While from a long-term dietary point of view the foods he is eating are not ideal, this is perhaps an issue that can be revisited at a later date.

General needs (3)

In discussion with Paul, his sleeping patterns have been monitored for a week and it seems clear that his sleeping patterns are intermittent with long periods of wakefulness interspersed with sleep – there seems to be no particular pattern to this and this is unusual for Paul. Paul is not at all concerned about this and as he does seem to be getting an adequate amount of rest/sleep this is again something that can perhaps continue to be monitored and kept under review.

Specific cultural needs

So far we have had one discussion with family about care given – family at present are divided. Sister (Caroline) acknowledges that Paul requires help and she is pleased that we have been able to give some support and advice. She does however worry that it might become necessary to admit Paul to inpatient care and she is very much opposed to this because she is worried about the sort of care he might receive there.

Mother is ambivalent in that she has said that there is nothing wrong with Paul but is also obviously deeply distressed about the situation. We have told her that we are willing to talk about her fears but as yet she does not want to discuss these in any depth.

Concern about Paul's physical health

(See also General needs 1, 2, and 3.)
Have discussed with Paul our concern that we help him maintain his physical health.

We have started to generally monitor dietary/fluid intake etc. and this appears at present to adequate.

Paul is now denying feeling unwell.

GP has visited and done a general physical check-up – he could find no immediate cause for concern.

Agreed to monitor general physical health on an ongoing basis at the moment.

Family concern about Paul

We have explained to family that we want to work in partnership – as noted earlier, there is some concern that we might want to force Paul into an institution. We have explained that this would only be done if there was serious concern for Paul's well-being and that family would be involved in any such decision.

CMHN has been setting aside time to talk to family about their concerns and they have also been given details about how to contact out-of-hours support if needed.

Having examined how we may work with Paul and his family, you will have noticed the intensive involvement that this necessitated. Community mental health nursing involves working with a wide range of service user needs. Now we will move on to Molly, who requires a less intense, but no less important, set of interventions.

Clinical scenario: Molly

In this part of the chapter we focus on Molly, who has been referred to the community mental health team by her GP following a consultation in which she complained of feeling anxious. As a mental health nurse you will often encounter clients who are experiencing anxiety and it is important that you are familiar with this problem. You need to understand how anxiety affects a person as well as how we might help a person to deal with this feeling.

Anxiety

Sometimes, life is stressful. Psychologists have described anxiety as being the emotion we feel when external stressors begin to challenge our abilities to cope with these pressures. It has also been argued that chronic stress may have an effect upon the physical well-being both of individuals and society generally (Wilkinson 1996).

When our ability to cope is challenged then we are likely to begin to feel anxious; often this is a vague feeling of uneasiness but some people experience these feelings more intensely. All of us have felt anxious at some time in our lives and because of this there are aspects of this section that you will probably recognize from your own experience.

> **Student activity 4**
> *It might be useful at this point to reflect upon your own experiences of feeling anxious. Try thinking of a time when you felt anxious and consider the following questions:*

- What causes me to feel anxious? (Are there any particular situations, places, or people that cause me to feel like this?)
- How do I feel physically and emotionally when I become anxious? (Although our bodily responses may be similar, individuals tend to focus upon different things when anxious.)
- What is the effect of this feeling upon me? (Some people are aware that anxiety, to a degree, prepares them to respond well – for example actors before a stage performance. Others may feel that anxiety hampers their ability, i.e. 'I was so nervous I couldn't think straight'.)

- How do I look when I am anxious? (You may want to ask someone close to you about this – some people pace around, tap their feet, or fidget – are you aware of what you do?)
- How long does this feeling last? (Typically anxiety peaks and declines within us after a time – it can be useful to remind people of this when they are feeling tense and anxious.)
- What do I do to help me cope when I feel anxious? (Some people like to talk a lot, some prefer their own company, some drink alcohol or smoke.)

You might want to compare your answers to those given by someone else; you may find that another person gives very different answers to the same questions.

It is important that we are not too quick to label a person's feelings as 'abnormal'. Stress can be seen as the 'trigger' that causes us to adapt and to learn new ways of coping with these pressures. As Seyle (1956) put it: 'Complete freedom from stress equates with death.' Although anxiety is a common experience, there are times when people are identified as needing specialized care because of it. As mental health nurses we need to be aware that anxiety causes a great deal of distress and can become very disabling. Despite this, it is under-recognized and people may not receive proper help and advice. When we are faced with a stressful situation, our body responds by triggering physical changes that prepare us to react. This has been described as the 'flight or fight response', a reaction that has evolved in us that has helped us to survive as individuals and as a species. This physical response produces bodily feelings that may be uncomfortable – see Box 8.5.

Bodily response to stress

- Increased heart rate and force.

- Dilation of coronary arteries.

- Increased blood supply to muscles.

- Decreases peripheral blood supply.

- Reduces activity in digestive system.

How does this make you feel?

- Palpitation, tachycardia.

- Sweating.

- Tremor.

- Choking.

- Chest pain/tightness.

- Muscle tension.

- Nausea.

- Dizziness.

- Feeling 'unreal'.

- Fear of losing control, going mad, or dying.

(Adapted from ICD 10 WHO 2007 and Puri 2000.)

Box 8.5   Physical responses to stress

How do we help people who are anxious?

Generally our responses to a person who is anxious can be categorized as follows:

- *Personal interventions* – By this we mean reassurance, speaking calmly to a person, and just being there with them (see especially Barker 1999). Anxiety tends to peak and decline after a short while and in being with a person we can support them and help them to manage their anxiety. It is important that you are aware of your own feelings as another person's anxiety can make us feel uneasy too, and if they become aware of this it will not be helpful.

- *Relaxation therapy* – Helps people to understand the way the body responds to anxiety (see Box 8.5); the aim is to promote self-management of anxiety. Note though that relaxation may help *before* a person has become anxious; it is less useful once they have actually become anxious.

- *Confronting fears* – People who become anxious are often inclined to try and avoid anxiety-provoking situations, which has the effect of temporarily reducing anxiety. However, this is not a good long-

term strategy as the more someone tries to avoid situations, the less capable they become of dealing with them. This may result in the anxiety becoming a more chronic problem or perhaps even developing into agoraphobia or depression.

- *Education* – A central principle of mental health nursing is that we must help the person to manage their own feelings; an important part of this involves us in explaining to a person what is happening to them. For example, often people interpret the physical discomfort they feel as happening because they are actually dying. If we can educate them about how their body is responding and why, this can be very useful.

- *Cognitive behaviour therapy (CBT)* – Studies indicate (i.e. Hunot et al. 2007) that this is an effective approach to helping a person manage their anxiety. Certainly it has none of the disadvantages associated with some medications (see following section).

- *Bibliotherapy* – Use of written material to help people understand psychological problems (NICE 2007). This is an approach used with people experiencing mild to moderate stress and anxiety. (For a fuller account of this, see Reeves and Stace 2005.)

However, it is important to also consider:

- *Physical examination* – It is *critical* that physical symptoms must be investigated properly before we try to work with people. Has the person been adequately screened for physical ill health? Do not ever assume that symptoms are 'all in the mind' – a person may be found to have an underlying physical health issue. Therefore, in a community setting we would want to check that a referring doctor had first ruled out the presence of any underlying physical problems.

- *Co-morbidity* – Is the person depressed or are there substance abuse issues?

- *Use of medication?* – See next section.

Diazepam

Diazepam (also known as Valium) belongs to a group of drugs known as the benzodiazepines. These first began to be used in the early 1960s and soon gained a reputation as being almost a 'wonder drug'. They were enthusiastically marketed, prescribed, and consumed as a marked improvement on existing pharmaceutical interventions for anxiety. However, from about the 1970s onwards, it became apparent that many people were experiencing very significant problems due to their dependence on this medication. A public backlash directed at the pharmaceutical industry grew to the point that this was a common news issue during this time.

Withdrawal problems can include insomnia, anxiety, loss of appetite, tremor, perspiration, tinnitus, and perceptual disturbances; there may also be much more serious effects such as confusion, psychosis, or convulsions (BNF 2006). Short-acting lorazepam is associated with more problems on withdrawal than longer-acting drugs such as diazepam. With longer-acting benzodiazepines, withdrawal symptoms begin a few days after stopping and can continue for up to six weeks.

Diazepam is a very commonly abused drug because of its calming and relaxing effects; it also intensifies the effects of alcohol. There is evidence that a high proportion of people using other drugs of abuse may also be taking diazepam-like substances (you see this in Chapter 9 in Tracy's scenario, p. 237). However, it is important to remember that when carefully used ('*the lowest possible dose for the shortest possible time*', BNF 2006), drugs such as diazepam have a perfectly safe and valid medical role. For example

they are used to relieve anxiety prior to a surgical procedure, to help reduce the withdrawal effects of alcohol or in the use of rapid tranquillization, to control agitated and disturbed behaviour in patients who, left untreated, could cause harm to themselves or others. It is recommended that diazepam is only prescribed for short-term use; longer-term use causes dependency, and how long this takes to develop is very much dependent on an individual's reaction. NICE guidance (NICE 2007) on anxiety states that benzodiazepines are likely to be ineffective in the long-term management of anxiety and certainly should not usually be used beyond 2–4 weeks (see also the most recent edition of the BNF or Healey 2006 for a fuller account).

> **Student activity 5**
> *Now watch the film of Molly and read through the scenario and letter below.*
>
> 📼 www.oxfordtextbooks.co.uk/orc/clarke
>
> *and choose the video link.*

Molly's story

Molly J is a 30-year-old chartered accountant. Her home is a luxury flat where she lives alone. However, she is away a lot because her high-pressure job requires her to do much travelling about the country and, sometimes, abroad. She has a small but close group of friends, most of them successful professionals like herself. Apart from brief holiday romances, she is content to remain single and unattached. Her only relatives are her mother and a brother. Both of them live in distant parts of the country and contact with them is limited to occasional phone calls and get-togethers at Christmas.

Until a few weeks ago, Molly was very satisfied with her life and her engagement with the GP was minimal and routine. However, while on a business trip she had an experience that undermined her confidence. After an especially busy day she retired to bed in her hotel room. The room was stuffy and she found herself unable to sleep. By the early hours of the morning she was very worried about sleep deprivation preventing her from meeting the work demands of what was expected to be another busy day. She remained sleepless but nevertheless attended a business appointment as planned. This meeting turned out to be tense and unpleasant. In the course of it,

Molly found herself perspiring heavily and was conscious of her heart pounding. She then became dizzy and, when she stood up, she fainted. Molly's colleagues were very supportive and, despite her protests that she was feeling better, she was told to take time off and rest. One of them drove her home to her flat.

That night, Molly slept for only a few hours and woke early feeling un-refreshed. Not wanting to fall behind with her work commitments, she went to her office in the city. The lift wasn't working and she had to climb the stairs for three floors. When she got to the reception desk she had a repeat of the previous day's experiences and woke to find herself surrounded by a circle of concerned faces.

When she had recovered, Molly's boss insisted that she have a medical assessment and so, the same day, she attended a private clinic. A thorough assessment was conducted but, five days later, she was told that no physical abnormalities had been found. The doctor suggested that the symptoms were panic attacks and might be due to overwork and that what was required was a change in her lifestyle.

In the few days that Molly had been off work, she had not felt her normal self. She was jittery and unable to concentrate. Despite feeling exhausted most of the time, she was unable to sleep for more than a few hours each night. All of her former confidence had evaporated and her thinking was dominated by worries about being sacked from her job. She avoided receiving phone calls from her friends and work colleagues and went out of the flat only when she had to.

Because she was fearful of her employers finding out how incapacitated she was, Molly resolved not to use the private clinic and, instead, made an appointment to see her NHS GP. In the course of this and follow-up appointments, the original diagnosis was confirmed. As part of the plan of care, Molly was referred to a CMHN (see Figure 8.2).

Molly's evaluation of her implemented care plan

Anxiety management

Molly stated it had been very helpful to understand why she had experienced her panic attacks. She said she found it reassuring to learn about the links between her physical and emotional state, and to understand that her palpitations, rapid breathing, tingling in her fingers, and headaches were part of a 'fight/flight' response to stress.

She said she still needs to use the relaxation techniques regularly, especially when trying to get to sleep at night. She said they have helped her to feel she is regaining some control over her emotional and physical health but said she needs to keep practising them.

Sleep hygiene

Molly has given up caffeine altogether, and no longer reads or watches television while in bed. She said it has helped to have a bath before going to bed. Molly is sleeping better – she also puts this down in part to getting more fresh air and exercise.

Employment issues

Molly stated that her time away from work gave her the opportunity to re-examine her own values. She said that she has come to value her own health and happiness. Molly has decided to make a fresh start, and has found a new job with a smaller firm of accountants. The job will be less pressured and will allow Molly more free time. Molly has had some difficulty coming to terms with making her career less of a priority and has needed support, feeling that she is not living up to the expectations of others.

Social life and wider interests

Molly stated that her time out from work had given her the opportunity to remember the interests she had before she started her career. She has become involved in a local conservation project where she has made friends with a group of people from a range of backgrounds. She told me she has particularly enjoyed helping to clear weed from a local pond – wearing waders! This broadening of her lifestyle has softened the blow of changing jobs.

Initially Molly was reluctant to be discharged; however, she recognized how far she has come since starting to work on her anxiety. She has a range of self-help literature to help support her in continuing this work on her own. I have advised her to return to her GP in the unlikely event that she should experience any further problems. He would be able to re-refer her to the CMHT.

```
Dear CPN

RE Ms Molly Jones (aged 30)

I am referring this patient to you following her visit to the surgery today. She
describes a three week history of increasing anxiety in which she experiences panic
attacks and insomnia. On physical examination there is nothing worthy of note. I
have advised her that she needs to relax a little and recommended that she should
stop off work for at least two weeks and avoid anything stressful.
As you know, the surgery does not have access to counselling services and I was hop-
ing that you could assess this patient with a view to providing some help and
reassurance.


Thank you
Dr Smith
```

Figure 8.2 Referral letter for Molly

👤 Molly: a service user's view

She is very judgemental of herself and of how she, herself, appears in relation to others.

Her anxiety could be a sign that she is a perfectionist and presents herself with very high standards, which are sometimes impossible to meet.

She reminds me of myself when I was suffering from anxiety and clinical depression. She could be finding herself battling with depression, if she is not already.

She has what is described in cognitive behaviour therapy (CBT) as a very critical self, and may be harbouring the core belief, as I did, that she is inadequate or even a failure.

I know exactly how she feels when she describes the physicality of a panic attack and where these physical symptoms translate into anxiety.

When describing the trauma of such an attack we can identify with that emotion so well that we almost relive the panic attack and soon revert to a shrivelling wreck. It really is like seeing me on the screen!

The CBT techniques, however, have taught me how not to identify with such a relived emotion, to honour it, yes, but not to attach myself to it and to let it 'float' by. If Molly is offered CBT, she could learn to manage her emotions in a balanced way, and to recognize the emergence of any intrusive negative automatic thoughts before they render her helpless. CBT's tools for emotional competence (emotional intelligence) will enable her to challenge debilitating thinking patterns and to regain control over her life.

Although materially well off, she is emotionally impoverished. However, unlike Tracy (Chapter 9), she does recognize some of her feelings and is building a vocabulary for them. Having no emotional outlet, she puts all her energy into work in order not to have to face the fact she has no close relationship, except the one she has with her workload.

Isolation is a big problem for her well-being, having no one really to confide in. This may have been the first time she has spoken about her feelings, and she would benefit from solution-focused talking therapy.

Although she has friends, she feels alone amongst them, often comparing herself to them in a negative way. She feels isolated within her busy life. She has a lot of assumptions about her friends' apparent abilities to cope and sees them as ideal role models.

I suspect she spends no time just 'being' and never allows herself time to truly relax. Her constant sense of guilt pushes her further into mental turmoil. It is the physical sensations that highlight her mental turmoil.

Without knowing her gentle 'compassionate self', she is her own worst enemy. She would really respond to positive interaction, through talking therapy to rebalance her black and white thinking.

Her inspirational goals have not yet been met and she fears she will end up like her mother. She needs reassurance and hope that she can change the way she feels and that she will get back control of her life and her emotions.

Tracey Holley, survivor

👥 Assessment

Assessment date: 16 May 2008   **Assessment location:**   Team Base
Assessment time: 11:00 hrs   **Assessor(s):**   CMHN V Taylor

Presenting problem including person's perceptions of their problems

- Three weeks ago Molly experienced two incidents of fainting following what appears to be a panic attack
- Molly's physical health appears good and these episodes appear to be associated with stress at work
- She says she feels 'jittery' and unable to concentrate
- She reports that she is sleeping only a few hours each night – feels exhausted
- Molly says she has lost her self-confidence
- She appears to be preoccupied with worries about losing her job
- Molly tells me she has been avoiding contact with friends and colleagues
- She is also avoiding leaving her flat unless strictly necessary
- During the assessment Molly appeared anxious and agitated, she was noted to be wringing her hands, and appeared tearful at times

History

- Molly is 30 years of age
- She has a high-pressure job as a chartered accountant
- The panic attack and fainting three weeks ago was the first episode of this kind of problem
- The first incident occurred on a business trip: Molly slept very poorly and worried about work during the night before the first panic attack. Molly remembers the hotel room being particularly stuffy
- She attended a planned business meeting the next day, which is reported to have been very tense
- During the meeting Molly told me she could feel her heart pounding, and said she was perspiring heavily and feeling dizzy. When she stood up she fainted in front of her colleagues – Molly says she feels very embarrassed about this
- After sleeping poorly for a second night, Molly went into work the next day
- She climbed the stairs to her office on the third floor – this made her breathless, and she experienced the same symptoms before fainting again. This took place in front of colleagues at the reception desk of her office
- Molly has been signed off work for at least two weeks by her GP; however, Molly is concerned that her employers will conclude that she is not fit to do her job if they find out that these fainting episodes have been caused by stress

Summary of past treatment

- This is Molly's first contact with mental health services
- The doctor she saw privately through her employer suggested she was suffering from 'overwork' and thought that a change in lifestyle would help
- GP has signed her off initially for two weeks and has advised Molly to try to relax and to avoid stress

Previous mental health history

- No history of mental health problems reported by Molly or GP

Alcohol and substance misuse

- Molly tells me she has never used illicit substances
- She reports that she drinks only at functions relating to her work and then only moderately

Family history

- No reported history of mental health problems
- Molly's mother and brother live separately in distant parts of the country
- Molly speaks to them occasionally on the telephone, and they meet up for Christmas
- Molly lacks strong emotional support from her family – they are not aware of her recent difficulties, and Molly says she would be ashamed of telling them how she has been feeling

Personal history

- Molly is single and lives alone
- She describes having a small group of friends who are all 'successful professionals'. She says that they are all 'busy people' and see each other occasionally when work permits
- Molly is often required to be away from home, travelling in this country and overseas, as part of her job – this has an impact on her social life
- She told me she was happy with her lifestyle until 'things started to go wrong' a few weeks ago – now she says she feels she 'can't cope'. She told me that she feels she is a 'failure'
- She reported that she now feels afraid of what friends and colleagues will think of her, and ashamed of becoming agitated and fainting in front of other people
- She told me she feels alone in her flat – especially now that she has not been going to work – but says she feels she has lost all her confidence

Present circumstances

Carers/significant others/appropriate adults:

- Molly has not told anyone apart from health professionals about her current situation

Family/significant relationships:

- Molly has only occasional contact with her mother and brother. She is single and lives alone

Social network:

- Molly's social network is limited to a small circle of friends who are all in high-powered jobs. Her social network has also been limited by the fact that she travels a great deal in the course of her work

Employment/education:

- Molly is a chartered accountant and described years of single-minded study, which has led her into her current career

- Molly believes she would lose her job should her employers find out that she is suffering from stress and anxiety. This fear appears to be adding to her current burden of worries

Leisure:

- Molly has been focused on her work to the exclusion of leisure interests
- She is finding it hard to know what to do to occupy herself now that she has been signed off work

Housing:

- Molly lives alone in a luxury flat
- She tells me she has virtually no contact with her neighbours
- Molly is concerned about losing her job, and is worrying that should this happen she would not be able to keep up with her mortgage

Finances:

- Molly is concerned about her financial situation should she lose her job

Activities of daily living:

- Molly is sleeping very poorly at the moment
- She is finding it difficult to concentrate on simple tasks – told me she had recently left a meal she was attempting to cook to burn – only noticed what was happening when she set the smoke alarm off
- Molly says her appetite is very poor, and says she lacks motivation to shop for or prepare anything to eat
- Molly's self-esteem also appears to be suffering. She said she used to take a pride in her appearance; however she said her motivation to attend to her self-care has also deteriorated
- Molly's loss of confidence has also made her reluctant to leave her flat except when this is unavoidable

Childcare responsibilities and child protection issues:

- N/A

Physical health history

Smoking, blood pressure, obesity

- Molly has recently had a physical examination that did not highlight any health problems
- Molly does not smoke

Diversity issues

- Molly is from a white British background
- She is articulate and able to talk about her experiences clearly
- She is keen to learn about her condition and understand the relationship between her mental health and her physical experience of anxiety

Spirituality issues

- Molly says she does not have any significant religious beliefs

Mental status examination

- Molly appeared anxious and agitated during the assessment
- She described worries about her own competence and the possibility of losing her job – these appear to have become persistent concerns and interfere with her sleep
- Molly is avoiding feared situations: she is declining the opportunity to speak to friends and colleagues on the phone, is not leaving her flat unless strictly necessary, and at the moment is not at work

- In addition to this Molly has described two panic attacks with physical symptoms of anxiety: dry mouth, tight chest, shortness of breath, palpitations, 'butterflies' in her stomach, shaking, tingling in her fingers, and headaches
- Molly's self-esteem and confidence are also described as low

Physical status examination

- Carried out by GP – no evidence of any physical health problems

Outcome

- Education about the relationship between physical and emotional symptoms of anxiety
- Discussion about the limitations of using medication to treat anxiety
- Education and practising of relaxation techniques
- Discussion of how to promote better sleep
- Discussion of current lifestyle and vulnerability to stress, and ways to build up some support for Molly

Assessor

Name: VICTORIA TAYLOR
Signature:

Designation: CMHN
Date: 16 May 2008

Care planning

Molly's care plan

	Actions to be taken
Suicide:	No reported history of or current suicidal ideation. Discuss ways of making life meaningful and enjoyable.
Self-harm:	No reported history of or current thoughts to harm herself.
Violence/harm to others:	No reported risk in this area.
Risk to children: (including caring capacity)	No reported risk in this area.
Risk from others: (including exploitation)	No reported risk in this area.
Neglect:	No reported risk in this area.
Vulnerability:	Molly is vulnerable to stress due to her demanding job, and her lack of a strong support network and non-work-related activities. The care plan will include steps to broaden Molly's current social network and interests.
Substance misuse:	No reported misuse of drugs or alcohol. Continue to monitor this area as Molly currently lacks coping strategies for dealing with stress and anxiety. Care plan to include education on relaxation techniques.
Any other: (please specify)	No other reported areas of risk.

Identified Need	Action	Responsible for action	Desired outcome	Review date
1. Molly needs to be able to trust the nurse and to understand the purpose of interaction. She also needs to feel confident that the nurse will be able to assist her to resolve this crisis.	• Introduce self and explain role and purpose of interaction. • Discuss 'bounds' of interaction, i.e. how long, how often interactions will take place. • Encourage Molly to state what she is looking for from your sessions and jointly negotiate a strategy. • Encourage Molly to talk about her recent problems, listen using person-centred principles. • Be aware that anxiety can be 'catching'; consider your own demeanour and behaviour in order to maintain Molly's confidence. • Molly needs to be given contact details.	CMHN Taylor	*Molly should understand who the CMHN is as well as having an idea about what to expect.* *Molly should know practical details such as how to contact help.* ***Rationale:** This part of the plan covers the need to develop a relationship with Molly before trying to encourage her to talk about her problems. No doubt you would not want to discuss (possibly intimate) details of your life with a stranger – we should not expect our clients to do this either. It is also necessary for us to let people know who we are, why we are there, and what we are going to do, as well as discussing time limits and the boundaries of the intervention.* *This complies with NICE (2007) guidance on management of anxiety.* *You may wish to refer to Chapter 2 for a discussion of this (especially the section on assessment as well as Carl Rogers and the humanistic approach).* *See also the 10 essential shared capabilities (Department of Health 2004) – Working in partnership.*	Six weeks
2. Molly needs practical advice about how to manage her anxious feelings and the accompanying physical experiences.	Nurse should offer practical strategies:	CMHN Taylor	*Molly will be able to use identified strategies to cope with anxious feelings.*	Six weeks

Identified Need	Action	Responsible for action	Desired outcome	Review date
	• Try and do something that is distracting. It is better to try and do something simple and repetitive that doesn't require a lot of concentration. • Breathing – explain about breathing into a paper bag. Also explain about slowing her breathing down. • Try to find someone to talk to about experiences. • Advise Molly that anxious feelings will eventually diminish; staying in the situation will eventually help her to cope with the anxiety. • A gentle stroll may help but make sure this is safe. • Be aware of triggers for anxiety, but Molly should be advised that avoidance is not a helpful strategy. Nurse should also discuss with Molly and try to identify things she might do that she finds helpful. Nurse should also discuss with Molly about keeping a diary to record her anxiety. Molly should record when it happened, a brief description of what was happening at the time, what happened, and how she felt afterwards. Molly may also rate the anxiety on a scale of 1–10.		Molly will record and rate incidence of anxiety so that this information can be used as part of a reduction strategy. **Rationale:** *Mental health nursing is not something that is 'done' to a person. We should be trying to take a partnership approach towards helping a person to manage their problems. Part of this involves helping the person to understand what is happening to them while remembering that each person is unique and responds differently to difficulties. For this reason Molly would be encouraged to develop her understanding of what she is experiencing and how she might begin to manage this. NICE (2007) guidance on anxiety lists shared decision-making as a key priority in helping a person to manage anxiety.*	

Identified Need	Action	Responsible for action	Desired outcome	Review date
3. Mental health – Molly needs to feel calmer and in control of herself (Molly is suffering from anxiety and panic attacks).	Molly is to be offered six-weekly sessions with CMHN for anxiety management. The effectiveness of these sessions will then be evaluated. **Week 1** Education on anxiety and panic attacks to help Molly understand the relationship between her physical and emotional symptoms: Education and self-help material about the body's arousal reaction, how avoidance can increase anxiety, and how thoughts can increase anxiety. Education and self-help literature about relaxation techniques. Information about the parasympathetic responses, progressive muscle relaxation exercise, procedures for controlling acute hyperventilation, distraction techniques, and positive self-talk. Set homework to read through materials, practise relaxation techniques daily, and keep a diary and rating of anxiety. **Week 2** Revisit week 1 information and check for understanding. Review self-help/homework. Practise relaxation techniques.	CMHN Taylor	For Molly to regain her own sense of well-being, and for her to feel she has helpful methods of managing anxiety effectively for the future. **Rationale:** *NICE (2007) guidance on anxiety lists key strategies in helping a person to manage anxiety.* *Improving access to psychological therapies (Department of Health 2007) recommends a stepped approach to anxiety and promotes self-help strategies.*	Six weeks

Identified Need	Action	Responsible for action	Desired outcome	Review date
	Identify negative thinking – work with Molly to identify her beliefs about her past, present, and future (cognitive triad).			
	Establish Molly's hierarchy of anxiety-provoking situations (see box below).			
	Set homework – practise relaxation techniques daily, keep a diary of negative thoughts and rating of anxiety.			
	Week 3			
	Practise relaxation.			
	Review self-help/ homework.			
	Focus on negative thinking, encourage Molly to begin challenging her negative beliefs.			
	(An example from Molly's experience might be that she **must** succeed in everything – this is sometimes referred to as 'musturbation'. The nurse would work with Molly to reframe this. Examples might include thinking 'I like to be successful but it is ok if I sometimes fail.)'			
	Set homework – maintain relaxation practice and diary of negative thoughts and anxiety ratings. Challenge at least one negative thought each day and reframe it in the diary.			
	Week 4			
	Practise relaxation.			

Identified Need	Action	Responsible for action	Desired outcome	Review date
	Review self-help/homework.			
	Continue working on negative thinking and beliefs.			
	Start exposing Molly to anxiety. Encourage Molly to imagine herself in an anxiety-provoking situation while practising anxiety management techniques.			
	Set homework – as last week.			
	Week 5			
	Practise relaxation.			
	Review self-help/homework.			
	Continue working on negative thinking and beliefs.			
	Work with Molly through her hierarchy, step by step, practising relaxation and cognitive reframing at every stage.			
	Week 6			
	As week 5, but now nurse's role is confined to supporting Molly.			

Molly's hierarchy of anxiety-provoking situations

In discussion with Molly she revealed the following list of anxiety-provoking situations (note that this will differ greatly between individuals):
(Least first)

1. Looking at her briefcase.
2. Accessing her email at home.
3. Answering the telephone.
4. Driving to work.
5. Being at work.

Identified Need	Action	Responsible for action	Desired outcome	Review date
4. Insomnia – Molly needs to re-establish a reasonable sleep pattern based on around 6–8 hours sleep per night (Molly is sleeping very poorly at present).	Education about sleep hygiene: the avoidance of caffeine, refraining from doing daytime activities before going to bed or while in bed, having a warm bath and milky drink, doing progressive muscle relaxation in bed.	CMHN Taylor	For Molly to be satisfied with the quantity and quality of her sleep. *Rationale: This is based on a holistic assessment of needs assessed as part of nursing process as well as medical model criteria.*	Six weeks
5. Employment issues – Molly needs an appropriate work/life balance (Molly has a very demanding job and appears to be suffering from burnout).	To discuss Molly's current employment to see if changes to her workload or particular role could be made to reduce the stress this is causing her at the moment. To support Molly, and liaise with Workplace Occupational Health Department as appropriate.	CMHN Taylor	For Molly to feel empowered to make changes in her employment for her benefit. *Rationale: This is based upon the need for a holistic understanding of Molly's problems in which her anxiety is understood as having arisen from the stresses placed upon her. Research suggests that while individual stress reduction has its place, organizations must also consider the stress that they place on employees (Cattan and Tilford 2006: 154).*	Six weeks
6. Social isolation – Molly needs a supportive social network. **Wider interests –** Molly would like to broaden her interests to help her to relax and 'switch off' from work.	To support Molly in thinking of ways to make some new friends, or draw on her current relationships. To discuss groups and volunteer projects Molly may be interested in joining. To support Molly in thinking of new interests she would like to develop.	CMHN Taylor	For Molly to have a good network of relationships for support and encouragement. For Molly to develop interests to make her life richer, and to help provide broader interests as a defence against future stress. **Rationale:** *Specific policy directives e.g. NSF Mental Health (1999) Standard 1.* *See also discussion on social inclusion in Chapter 4 (p. 86).*	Six weeks

Summary

In this chapter you have been introduced to two service users who are experiencing very different problems. It is hoped that this will give an impression of the range of problems that may be encountered by mental health services. Obviously some problems encountered will require more intervention than others but accurate assessment is required before such a decision can be made.

Working with people who have been given a diagnosis of schizophrenia is an important part of the work of a mental health team; therefore we have looked at a brief summary of some of the medical descriptions of schizophrenia. As we have discussed, however, the term 'schizophrenia' has attracted a great deal of debate and although we have tried to reflect a small part of this debate in this chapter, we would encourage you to explore this area further in order for you to reach conclusions based upon your own thinking. The assessment, care planning, and evaluation of the plan of care developed for Paul has been included and we have tried to draw attention to areas in which you might work with families in these circumstances.

This chapter has also touched upon some of the issues surrounding the treatment of people from black and minority ethnic groups. Again, this is an area that could easily be expanded into a textbook of its own; we could not hope to do it justice here and would encourage you to spend some time reading around this issue.

The example care plans we have produced for the two fictional service users, Molly and Paul, are intended to be a starting point for you to consider how you might plan care with service users. We have not attempted to produce 'perfect' examples of care plans and we recognize that some readers might take issue with aspects that are included or left out of these. We hope this chapter has prompted you to consider how you would plan high quality care for community mental health users.

References and other sources

References

Askey R, Gamble C and Gray R (2007). Family work in first-onset psychosis: a literature review. **Journal of Psychiatric and Mental Health Nursing**, **14**, 356-65.

Barker PJ (1999). **The philosophy and practice of psychiatric nursing**. Churchill Livingstone, Edinburgh.

Barker P (2002). Schizophrenia: The 'not so nice guidelines'. **Journal of Psychiatric and Mental Health Nursing**, **10**(3), 374-8.

Boyle M (1990). **Schizophrenia: A scientific delusion?** Routledge, London.

Breggin P (1993). **Toxic psychiatry: drugs and electroconvulsive therapy: the truth and the better alternatives**. Harper Collins, London.

British National Formulary (2006). **British National Formulary**. BMJ, London.

Cattan M and Tilford S, eds (2006). **Mental health promotion: A lifespan approach**. Open University Press, Maidenhead.

Department of Health (1999). **National Service Framework for mental health: modern standards and service models**. DH, London.

Department of Health (2004). **The 10 essential shared capabilities**. DH, London.

Department of Health (2005). **Delivering race equality in mental health care: An action plan for reform inside and outside services and The Government's response to the independent inquiry into the death of David Bennett**. DH, London.

Department of Health (2007). **Improving access to psychological therapies**. DH, London.

Fernando S (2003). **Cultural diversity, mental health and psychiatry: the struggle against racism**. Brunner-Routledge, Hove.

Healey (2006). **Psychiatric drugs explained**, 4th edition. Churchill Livingstone, London.

Hunot V, Churchill R, Teixeira V, and Silva de Lima M (2007). Psychological therapies for generalised anxiety disorder. **Cochrane Database of Systematic Reviews**, issue 1.

Kuipers E, Leff J and Lam D (2002). **Family work for schizophrenia**, 2nd edition. Royal College of Psychiatrists, London.

McKenzie K and Bhui K (2007). Institutional racism in mental health care. **British Medical Journal, 334**, 649-50.

National Institute for Clinical Excellence (2002). **Schizophrenia: Core interventions in the treatment and management of Schizophrenia in primary and secondary care**. NICE, London.

National Institute for Clinical Excellence (2007). **Anxiety: Management of anxiety (panic disorder, with or without agoraphobia, and generalised anxiety disorder) in adults in primary, secondary and community care (amended version)**. NICE, London.

Puri BK (2000). **Saunders' pocket essentials of psychiatry**. W.B. Saunders, Edinburgh.

Reeves T and Stace JM (2005). Improving patient access and choice: assisted bibliotherapy for mild to moderate stress/anxiety in primary care. **Journal of Psychiatric and Mental Health Nursing, 12**(3), 341-6.

Romme M and Escher S (1993). **Accepting voices**. MIND Publications, London.

Romme M and Morris M (2007). The harmful concept of schizophrenia. **Mental Health Nursing, 27**(2), 7-11.

Sainsbury Centre for Mental Health (2002). **Breaking the circles of fear: a review of the relationship between mental health services and African and Caribbean communities**. Sainsbury Centre for Mental Health, London.

Seyle H (1956). **The stress of life**. McGraw- Hill, New York.

Singh S and Burns T (2006). Race and mental health: there is more to race than racism. **British Medical Journal, 333**, 648-51 (23 September).

Szasz T (1972). **The myth of mental illness: foundations of a theory of personal conduct**, Paladin, London.

Wilkinson R (1996). **Unhealthy societies: the afflictions of inequality**. Routledge, London.

World Health Organization (2007). **International statistical classification of diseases and related health problems**. WHO, Geneva.

Wuerker A (2000). The family and schizophrenia. **Issues in Mental Health Nursing, 21**, 127-41.

◐ Online Resource Centre

You may find it helpful to work through our short set of online materials, intended to help you to consider and actively work through issues raised by the cases in this chapter:

@ www.oxfordtextbooks.co.uk/orc/clarke

and choose the online resources for this chapter.

◐ Further reading

Cooper JE (1994). **Pocket guide to the ICD-10 classification of mental and behavioural disorders** Churchill Livingstone, Edinburgh.

Department of Health (2006). **Best practice competencies and capabilities for pre registration mental health nurses in England: The Chief Nursing Officer's review of mental health nursing**. DH, London.

Chapter 9
Additional skills for complex cases in mental health nursing

Nicola Clarke, Victoria Clarke, Sandy Fitzgibbon, Marion Johnson, Pam Virdi

Learning outcomes

The aims of this chapter are:

- To help the student gain the skills to 'combat discrimination against individuals and groups with mental health problems, and promote their social inclusion' (Department of Health 1999).

- To introduce the student to the additional skills required for the therapeutic engagement of those service users who are, through the complexities of their mental health problems, difficult to engage.

After reading this chapter you will:

- Recognize the importance of inclusion of all groups irrespective of illness/diagnosis/problem.

- Have knowledge of different therapeutic concepts.

- Have enhanced awareness of best practice, and areas of inclusion, encouraging excellence in the service provided for people with mental health problems based on evidence-based practice and research.

- Have enhanced awareness of how exclusion from services can impact upon the health and well-being of service users.

- Have gained a knowledge base, that promotes understanding of the different subjects under discussion in each section of this chapter.

- Have gained important skills of engagement.

Introduction

In this chapter we will focus on some service users and mental health nursing skills that are more specialized than many students may experience. However, in introducing these concepts it is hoped that the chapter will help to prepare students and encourage exposure to such areas. You will meet four different service users from four different areas of mental health: child and adolescent mental health (Sarah, who has the additional complexities of an eating disorder, p. 224), substance misuse issues (Charlie, p. 231), forensic involvement and personality disorder issues (Tracy, p. 237), and post-traumatic stress in a person seeking political asylum (Feodor, p. 246).

It is important to state at the outset that using the term 'areas' of mental health may lead students to believe that these are specialisms within the field of mental health nursing. The reality is the opposite. These issues and concerns are common for many service users that mental health nurses encounter in practice. While you may find that during your education you receive little formal teaching or experience in these areas, you will find some knowledge of these issues appropriate when, after-qualification, you are working with service users who are experiencing related problems.

It is important to understand the context from which many of these issues may emerge. There is recognition of the structured inequalities in Britain's health and social system, including for example substance misuse, ageism, unemployment, homelessness, poverty, sexism, and racism. For a variety of reasons, mental health service users may find themselves in situations of social disadvantage and economic hardship. The social effects of mental health problems can lead to individuals being effectively disabled, often with greater challenges than the mental health problem itself. The *National Service Framework for mental health* (NSF) (Department of Health 1999) encourages all mental health professionals to promote social inclusion. But how do we promote social inclusion of individuals who are ultimately excluded from services, potentially because of our lack of skills in these 'specialist areas'?

Engaging young people with anorexia nervosa

This section focuses on engagement with young people who are experiencing an eating disorder, namely anorexia nervosa. Young people often demonstrate a high state of ambivalence towards both recognizing that a problem exists and that clinical intervention is necessary. This is complicated by young people misunderstanding what constitutes a mental health problem, and by the stigma attached to mental health issues, which often prevents them from getting help (Vostanis 2007). The mental health needs of young people need to be viewed within the context of their development, family, peer group, education, and the social environment (Mental Health Foundation 1999). Most young people are greatly influenced by media messages and societal expectations, which include ideas on how we think, act, and look, and as dieting is now widespread in developed countries it is not surprising that this is having an impact upon their emotions and cognition. Surveys report that many young people have dieted at some time during their teenage years but only a minority of them go on to develop an eating disorder (Thambirajah 2007). The majority of young people who wish to or try to lose weight are often not a cause for concern, but a minority will develop more serious presentations that can become entrenched and difficult to resolve. Such young people often report that they feel better when they are losing weight, regardless of how underweight they are becoming.

When these problems are more entrenched the ambivalence about seeking help is exacerbated, because anorexia is an **ego-syntonic** disorder. This means that there are outcomes of their illness that are valued by the person, despite the fact that it may also be causing them physical, psychological, and social problems. They may understand that their way of being is ultimately limiting their life and is destructive, but they still feel an overwhelming compulsion to continue. In this respect parallels can be seen with someone who is addicted to drugs or alcohol. For instance it is not uncommon for worrying events such as 'passing out' to be viewed positively by a person with an eating disorder, who may view this as a sign that they are achieving their goal of 'getting seriously thin'. The person is therefore constantly in two minds about the benefits and ill effects of their behaviours. Denial is a major part of the illness and many young people coming for a first appointment may not even be able, or willing, to acknowledge that a problem exists for them at all. This state of ambivalence can remain with the person throughout their treatment and needs to be constantly evaluated and engaged with in a therapeutic way.

Imagine then the confusion experienced by many adolescents, but now with the addition of ambivalence brought forth by the illness. Then consider engaging this young person, particularly when they are often not the one who is seeking help, but rather someone else is demanding they get help. In addition, we must remember that young people are not children, but neither does our society consider them adults; thus some understanding of adolescent development, in addition to the anorexia disorder, will help with the engagement and assessment process.

Student activity 1
In Table 9.1 is a list of the developmental outcomes expected to be achieved through the adolescent years.
1) Consider when you achieved these stages and what or who helped you to achieve them – or have you yet to complete this transition?

Table 9.1   Developmental outcomes during adolescence

Developmental outcomes in adolescence	When did you achieve this?	What helped you to achieve this?
Forming a clear individual identity		
Accepting a new body image		
Attaining emancipation from parents		
Developing a personal value system		
Achieving financial independence		
Developing cognitive skills and the ability to think abstractly		
Developing the ability to control one's behaviour according to socially acceptable norms		
Taking responsibility for one's own behaviour		

2) Consider a young person with an eating disorder problem. What stages do you think may be difficult to negotiate?

Causes of eating disorders

Eating disorders are thought to be most likely to appear in adolescence due to the physical changes and psychological challenges that this transitional stage brings about (Kendall 2000). Anorexia nervosa has a higher incidence in westernized countries, where it typically affects more women than men (Hsu 1996, Tsai 2000). It is suggested that influences such as the westernization of cultures and the idealization of thinness amongst young women have a role in this. However, the exact role that socio-cultural factors play in the development of anorexia is not fully understood (Wildes *et al.* 2001). Other factors believed to be significant in the development of anorexia include low self-esteem, body dissatisfaction, dieting behaviours, family history of eating, and personality traits such as perfectionism, compliance, and dependency (Thambirajah 2007). Dieting is the pathway into

the illness. Feeling dissatisfied with your body and dieting to change it has become 'normal' behaviour in today's culture where thinness is idealized. Unachievable standards are perpetuated by the media and set the stage for widescale body discontent in young children, including a growing number of boys. Girls tend to desire thinness while boys desire a larger and more muscular appearance (Smolak *et al.* 2001). There have been numerous studies measuring body satisfaction or some related aspect of body image in young girls and boys. The findings are consistent across different countries, indicating that between 30 and 50 per cent of child and adolescent girls are dissatisfied with their weight (Thompson and Smolak 2001).

It is common for teenage girls to worry about weight and shape and a lot of young people who are not overweight strive to be thinner, but instead of a balanced diet and regular exercise they select to skip meals. For some, worries about weight can become obsessive, and it is often difficult for parents to know when something is going seriously wrong with their teenager's health. During adolescence most young people converse more easily with their peers than with their parents. Furthermore, the young person in the grip of the eating disorder will tend towards hiding their weight loss behaviours for fear that other people will intervene to stop them. This makes early detection even more problematic.

In February 2006, the Eating Disorders Association (EDA) highlighted that young people have problems in getting help with eating disorders. Their report, titled *Time to tell*, reveals that despite recognition of a problem, 45 per cent of young people feel they cannot tell anyone about it. The survey (EDA 2006) involved 1000 young people with personal experience of an eating disorder, and their parents. Forty per cent of the parents said they would recognize the early signs; however, only 21 per cent of young people said their parents had noticed the eating disorder. This may be because the young person had actively worked at hiding the signs until really obvious, for example by wearing baggy clothes and avoiding others seeing their body, or telling others they had eaten when they hadn't. This may also be a result of the ambivalence they feel, becoming more and more trapped, wanting someone to know but being terrified of having people intervening to take away their control over their cherished behaviours of not eating and over-exercising.

Anorexia nervosa is most likely to start in mid-adolescence, although Dawson (2007) has declared that she is beginning to treat girls as young as eight. Young Minds (2007) consider that eating problems are particularly common among teenage girls. Issues with weight and eating are not necessarily going to become an illness unless eating patterns are unhealthy, or worries about body size and eating become a constant preoccupation. So when is it an anomaly in the young person's developmental stage and when is it a serious problem? When do normal teenage dieting and body concerns become a disorder?

Student activity 2
Consider a young person who may have a serious eating disorder and have a go at identifying how you think they may present. Note your ideas down in Box 9.1. In particular think about the effects of starvation and persistent under-eating.

Psychological causes

Eating disorders are not about food, they are about feelings. 'Eating disorders are a way of coping with something that a person is struggling with, which yield feelings such as anger, sadness, guilt, loss or fear' (EDA 2002). People who develop anorexia are usually lacking in a cohesive and firm sense of self. Body and food control for such a person is a very effective way to enhance the fragile sense of self. The person organizes their life around non-eating and the pursuit of weight loss, maintaining control over this all-absorbing goal until it becomes prioritized over everything else. While it is important to understand the psychological origins of eating disorder, we must also be alert to the disabling and potentially lethal physical effects of starvation and other dangerous behaviours that the person may be engaging in. Follow-up studies show mortality figures up to 20 per cent (Palmer 2001), which is the highest of any psychiatric illness, and deaths do frequently arise from the direct result of starvation or suicide. In Table 9.2 are some of the symptoms of anorexia nervosa. How many were you aware of?

Young people with anorexia nervosa

A typical young person who may develop anorexia nervosa is one who is introverted, conscientious, and well behaved. They have an excessive need to please others and are very good at picking up moods and problems in others. However, they are often unable to identify and acknowledge their own needs and so rarely share much of their own inner world with

Physical signs	Behavioural signs	Psychological signs

Box 9.1   Signs of anorexia nervosa

Table 9.2   Some of the symptoms of anorexia nervosa

Physical signs	Behavioural signs	Psychological signs
Severe weight loss	Wanting to be left alone	Intense fear of gaining weight
Periods stopping (amenorrhoea)	Finding it hard to deal with the stimulation of being with other people – isolating self	Depressed mood
Hormonal changes in men and boys		Feeling emotional
	Wearing big, baggy clothes	'Fasting high' – state of euphoria that can kick in within 24–48 hours of fasting
Difficulty in sleeping	Excessive exercising	
Dizziness	Lying about eating meals	Feeling cut off, detached, and anaesthetized to feelings
Stomach pains	Denying there is a problem	
Constipation	Difficulty concentrating	Obsession with dieting
Poor circulation and feeling cold	Wanting to have control	Obsessive calorie counting
	Eating very slowly	Preoccupation with food
Decrease in body temperature, heart rate, respiration, and basal metabolic rate	Rituals around food, cutting up food into tiny pieces, mashing, spoiling food with spices, salt, etc.	Mood swings
		Distorted perception of body weight and size
Tingling in hands and feet		
Hair loss	Unable to cope with frustration	Reduction in the ability for complex thought
Loss of sexual interest and drive	Rigid and obsessive routines around food and daily functioning	Thinking becomes simple; no in-betweens
Feeling tired/exhausted		
The more the weight loss, the more disorientated and out of touch with reality the person will be	Every aspect of life needs to be totally predictable and organized well in advance	Strongly polarized perceptions (dichotomous thinking in extremes, for example: 'I am totally in control or I am completely out of control', 'I am thin or I am fat', 'I am good or I am bad'
	Laxative use	
	Vomiting after eating	
	Over-exercising	Lonely
	Taking over-the-counter herbal remedies for weight loss Abuse of diuretics	
	Avoiding social situations where they may be asked to eat	
	Weighing self numerous times a day	
	Body-checking behaviours for signs of weight change	

👤 What the service users say

The comments here are taken from the Beat (2007) report *Something's got to change*:

I was worried what people would think of me and whether they would think I was a bad person.

My dad thinks that I only have anorexia to get attention.

One teacher noticed, but she didn't speak to me she spoke to my friend. I could really have benefited from somebody acknowledging it.

My first GP put me off. I was told that lots of women have this problem and it doesn't make you any different and it will just be a phase.

I felt I had no right to help.

You need to know someone in the world cares or even notices that you are alive. I got so lonely and felt so worthless, I tried to kill myself.

---

others. Many young people present with a high level of scholastic achievement and traits such as perfectionism and obsessive behaviours are often evident. They take little pride or joy in their achievements, however, always trying to fend off crippling feelings of inadequacy and ineffectiveness, pushing forward to the next goal, which they hope will make them feel better about themselves but which sadly rarely does.

Clinical scenario: Sarah

In this section you will meet Sarah on her first presentation to the eating disorder unit. First, read the scenario of Sarah during the first stage of her assessment.

Sarah is a 17-year-old young woman who is in her first year of college undertaking AS-level study and who wishes to go on to university to become a psychologist.

As you read, try to identify some of the behaviours listed in Table 9.2.

History

Sarah first became interested in losing weight during the summer break prior to starting secondary school. She was worried about leaving her friends and going to a grammar school for which she had received tutoring. All her friends except for one acquaintance were going to other schools. At that time she recalls feeling worried about sitting her GCSEs even though they were some time away. She was highly anxious about fitting in and making new friends. She felt okay talking with people she knew but found it hard to interact with strangers. Sarah tried dieting but her mother was against it and she found it hard to avoid meals, so

she gave up on this at the time. However, she continued to feel that it would be better if she were fitter and healthier, even though everyone told her she was fine as she was.

At school, Sarah excelled in sports and was a high achieving academic student. Her teachers liked her and she was known amongst her friends for being the clever one. She did not like being boxed into this 'geek' kind of identity. Although not overweight, Sarah worried about her body becoming fat. As her body changed during puberty, she became more and more unhappy with how she looked. Feeling there was no one to share her feelings with, Sarah kept her worries to herself.

During Sarah's study leave to revise for her GCSE exams she vowed to 'get serious about getting fitter and healthier'. She reported that the thought of exams would 'make me panic' and she set very high standards for herself. She believed the only acceptable outcome would be to get all A's across her exams. Paralysed with anxiety and unable to study, she found the unstructured time hard to deal with. Focusing on counting calories was a distraction and as she started to lose weight she noticed that her anxiety lifted and she felt more in control of herself. Sarah felt much calmer and life appeared more manageable. She noticed that she felt happier and a bit distanced from all her usual worries. She was delighted to be achieving success in losing weight. Soon other girls at school started asking her for her secret for losing weight. It felt fantastic to be good at something other than homework and to be getting all this attention, especially from some of the more popular girls.

Sarah's dieting behaviour, which started as a bid to get fit and healthy, very quickly became a burning and all-consuming obsession. Nothing else mattered as much as getting those scales to show ever reducing numbers. Although she felt she was on the right path, other people started to be concerned. The gentle worry of her mother had now turned into a full-blown control fight. She felt her mother watched her constantly and this often caused rows between them. She felt trapped, she couldn't see why other people were on her back so much – if only they would leave her alone. At the same time, there was a niggling feeling in the back of her mind that something was wrong. But everyone was dieting, so there couldn't be anything wrong with what she was doing, could there? And she was good at it – so self-disciplined and in control. Everyone thinks that's a good way to be – don't they?

In addition to obsessively counting calories she wanted to exercise every day. Within a few weeks of starting this she was doing three hours exercise a day, getting up early to do an hour before school. She started to walk to school (three miles away) rather than getting the bus. She felt hungry and tired but each time she succeeded in avoiding food she got 'such a buzz'. Sarah felt she was winning.

Occasionally she would make herself sick but mainly chose to avoid eating.

It took at least six months for Sarah's parents to realize that something was seriously wrong. By this time she had lost a significant amount of weight and was now noticeably underweight. Her parents finally put pressure on her to go to see the GP, who referred her for assessment.

Student activity 3

Now watch the video of Sarah when she initially presented at the eating disorders unit:

📹 www.oxfordtextbooks.co.uk/orc/clarke

and choose the video link.
Try to answer the following questions:

1) *What important factors are raised in the initial interview?*
2) *What techniques does the nurse use to engage Sarah?*

Engagement

Engagement is considered here as the clinician's ability to enlist the young person's and the parents' cooperation by developing a rapport, reducing concern and/or blame, and developing meaningful goals for all parties. Engaging all parties is paramount to successful assessment and subsequent treatment, and a negative alliance at this stage is often difficult to reverse (Vostanis 2007). Few young people or their families want therapy, particularly when it means exploring difficulties and problems. Respecting and acknowledging everyone's point of view is an essential ingredient in engagement.

Resistant young people often cooperate more if the clinician pays attention to their goals and incorporates these into the process. A useful way to secure engagement with young people is to designate them as expert consultants in solving their own problems. They more often than not want parents and adults to 'get off their backs' and leave them alone. If this is the case, questions such as this one can be useful:

'If your parents were to get off your back tomorrow, what would you do or say differently, so that they would no longer be on your case?'

Often questions such as these will assist in fostering a cooperative working relationship by defining the young person as an expert who can solve their own issues in specific and concrete ways.

When working with young people, their parents and other family members should be involved in some way. Parents should be engaged to help support the young person towards some change. During the engagement process time needs to be made for the parents to voice their concerns, frustrations, and anger away from the young person. The video shows only Sarah in her first interview, but following engagement with Sarah, her mother, who accompanied her to the clinic, was given time to express her concerns and voice her frustrations and was engaged with the treatment approaches with Sarah.

Anyone coming to consult a clinical practitioner is likely to be anxious about the experience. It is usual for young people with eating disorders to be highly anxious about this meeting. In clinical experience many report worrying about it for weeks in advance.

Usually a young person will be brought to see the clinician by a parent who is at the end of their tether with worry and confusion about what is happening to their child. They may have gone down the route of looking for physical causes, investigating conditions such as irritable bowel syndrome and food allergies, not realizing that the young person is not telling them the full truth about why they have such problems with abdominal pain, diarrhoea, and constipation. Many of these symptoms are secondary to laxative abuse. They may have reached a point of not even recognizing the young person they once thought they knew, both physically and emotionally. Family life as they once knew it no longer exists.

When first coming for an assessment, the young person with the eating disorder will usually see a member of the medical team for a careful medical examination. Regardless of which professional they first meet, the meeting is a crucial one. Trying to help someone who at best is a reluctant participant is not an easy task and often they are terrified that their control will be taken away and that they will be 'forced to eat' and 'made to get fat'. However, the effects of undereating will usually have produced enough ill effects for the person to be willing, at least in part, to hear what you have to say about what might need to change to make their situation better.

Even so, one should remember that much of their motivation will still be weighted towards an anti-recovery position. They may be fearful and suspicious that you will want to dominate them and take away their control. Showing someone that you understand their uncertainty and that you are not there to push them in any direction is fundamental to starting the therapeutic alliance. You need to show the young person that you understand their dilemma of both wanting to keep the eating-disordered behaviours and wanting to get rid of the things that are becoming problematic for them.

Many sufferers do not like the fact that their hair is thinning and they are developing dry skin and brittle nails. This is something they are often motivated to change. Additionally, if someone is vomiting regularly, they may have noticed erosion on their tooth enamel and be worried about the longer-term effects of this. For young people particularly, these visible deteriorations in their physical appearance can be a motivator for contemplating change. The main aim of the first appointment is to get them back for a second one.

Motivational interviewing

Denial is an overwhelming feature of anorexia nervosa and the person often finds it hard to accept that anything serious is wrong with them. Neither do they generally accept that it is within their power to change. At best the person is highly ambivalent about moving towards change.

Motivational interviewing, which is part of motivational enhancement therapy (Miller and Rollnick 2002), is often the first line of intervention. This approach seeks to help the person to explore their reasons for continuing with their illness behaviours and also to find reasons for doing the work to move towards healthier ways of being.

The approach is based on a model of health behaviour that is commonly used in many areas of health psychology. Two factors need to be addressed to implement and sustain any behavioural change. Firstly, there needs to be recognition of the problem and a belief that change is needed. Secondly, the person must have some belief and confidence that it is within their ability to bring about the behaviour change successfully.

The model is based on a collaborative philosophy as opposed to the expert position often taken in medical models. In this model the service user is viewed as the expert on their own problem and the role of the therapist is one of facilitation. This model encourages clinicians to try to understand the private experience of the person, to empathize with their distress at the prospect of gaining weight, and to acknowledge the difficulty of change. This method is useful with this client group because it emphasizes collaboration, curiosity, openness, patience, and systematic inquiry and individual discovery.

Care planning

The initial assessment has already engaged with Sarah's wants and needs, which should act as a basis for the care plan. However, the risk factors acknowledged at this time should be identified.

Student activity 4

Watch the video again if you need to and try to answer the following two questions:

1) What has Sarah identified that she wants help with?
2) What risk factors can you identify?

 www.oxfordtextbooks.co.uk/orc/clarke

and choose the video link.

Risk

Assessing risk associated with eating-disordered behaviour is vital; remember, people can die. Consider their weight, for example: the more weight a person loses, the more physically compromised they will be. The average expected body weight (AEBW) is recommended by Duker and Slade (1994) as the quickest way of establishing the margins of safety around physical and psychological change. The average expected body weight is calculated on the basis of a person's age, sex, and height.

Assessing risk related to weight

Body mass index (BMI) is a number calculated using a person's height and weight. For adults with anorexia nervosa this is a commonly used method for ascertaining how much weight has been lost.

The formula for BMI is weight in kilograms divided by height in metres squared.

For example: if a person weighs 53 kg and is 1.6 m in height, their BMI would be:

$$\text{Weight } (53 \text{ kg})$$
$$\div \text{ Height squared}$$
$$(1.6 \times 1.6 = 2.56)$$
$$= \text{BMI}$$
$$53 \div 2.56 = 20.7$$
$$\text{BMI} = 20.7$$

If you want to calculate your own BMI, the following converter tool will assist you if you are moving from feet and inches to metric: http://www.simetric.co.uk/feet_to_metres.php

A BMI of 17.5 is required to meet the 15 per cent weight loss in the criteria for anorexia nervosa as defined in the DSM-IV (*Diagnostic Statistical Manual* produced by the American Psychiatric Association 2000).

For children and young people below the age of 20 years, BMI is calculated in the same way as for an adult but the interpretation of the BMI figure needs to be both age and gender specific. This is because children grow rapidly, and boys and girls grow at different rates. BMI growth charts should be used to translate the BMI number into a percentile for the child's gender and age. A BMI-for-age less than the fifth percentile is used as part of the diagnostic criteria for anorexia nervosa. The fifth percentile-for-age is equivalent to the DSM-IV weight loss criterion for anorexia of '85 per cent of that expected' (Selzer *et al.* 1995). For adults, BMI is interpreted through categories that are not dependent on sex or age.

If a person suffering from anorexia loses enough weight to reach the point where they are only 65 per cent of their AEBW, they will be at the point of being dangerously physically ill. The associated effects of starvation will also mean that they will have become extremely rigid in their behaviours, and communication problems will be severe. Keeping a track of changes in body weight on a regular basis is therefore vital to safety. This is not an easy task for someone with anorexia to engage with. The extreme over-concern they have about weight, and what it represents to them in terms of their self-worth, makes it a fearful and panic-evoking prospect. Skilful negotiation and engagement with this issue is necessary and sometimes the therapist may have to go so far as to make this a non-negotiable part of treatment. Rapid weight loss is likely to destabilize the body more seriously than a slower, steadier rate of weight loss, which gives the body time to adjust its homeostasis. It is important to assess the degree of weight loss and also over what period of time it occurs.

Risks associated with vomiting, laxatives, and diuretics

Many people use vomiting, laxatives, and diuretics as a means to try to control (via elimination) what is ingested. However, these behaviours are very risky as the abuse of laxatives and diuretics and self-induced

---

✎ Pharmacist's comment

The volume depletion caused by dehydration can cause low blood pressure and rapid pulse, along with dizziness. Long-term laxative abuse can also cause constipation because of decreased motility of the colon.

vomiting can all lead to electrolyte disturbance (Garner *et al.* 1985). Of particular concern is the lowering of potassium to critically low levels (hypokalaemia). This is associated with general muscle weakness, cardiac arrhythmias, and electrocardiograph (ECG) changes, which if not corrected (through supplementation and/or ceasing of the behaviour) can lead to sudden death. Therefore, it is vital to monitor these behaviours and provide education and support to help reduce them. It is useful to educate clients about the ineffectiveness of these methods for preventing the absorption of calories. For instance, laxatives work by emptying the large intestine; however, by the time digested food reaches the large intestine, calories from food have already been absorbed in the small intestine. The only effect of laxatives is the elimination of waste products that would have been evacuated anyway, but with additional unnecessary dehydration resulting in depleted electrolytes.

Vomiting only results in temporary weight loss and this will cease over time. In fact, vomiting does not get rid of all the calories eaten. What appears to happen is that over time the body learns to compensate for regular vomiting by capturing calories before they are purged. Remember, young people with eating disorders can die from starving themselves or suffer a range of health problems such as heart, kidney, gastrointestinal, and fertility problems. Anorexia nervosa presents itself as having one of the highest rates of mortality for any mental health condition (EDA 2002).

Risks associated with body image

We are bombarded daily through the media with strong messages of how we should look and cajoled into instant fixes for our body shape and what we perceive to be weight problems. Schilder, as early as 1950, highlighted the importance of our individual thoughts and feelings in the formation of our body image. You will have noted that Sarah is very aware of her body and engages with some risk behaviours when her perception is distorted following some meals in the evening.

Care plan for Sarah

Student activity 5
Now try your hand at completing a care plan for Sarah from the scenario information and the video. A version of this document is available online at:

 www.oxfordtextbooks.co.uk/orc/clarke

and choose the online resources for this chapter. If you like you can print it off, fill it in, and include it in your portfolio of learning.

An example of a care plan for Sarah is included as a guide; however, be aware that this is only part of the initial assessment, as interviews with parents and medical assessment will also help to develop a more in-depth care plan.

In addition, assessment is an ongoing process and constant review of care plans is essential in meeting the changing needs of the young person and their family.

Evaluation

As acknowledged previously, the care plan should be reviewed on a regular basis and this should be undertaken with the young person in order to evaluate the effectiveness of the therapeutic interventions, the therapeutic relationships, behavioural risks, and the needs of the young person and their family.

NICE guideline to standardize care

The NICE guidelines (2004) made specific recommendations for the treatment of young people with eating disorders in recognition of their unique needs, which are as follows:

- Effective assessment, which includes coordination of care, the involvement of patients and their carers, providing good information, moral support, and getting help early.
- Involving family members, including siblings, in the treatment of children and adolescents with eating disorders.

Summary

The difficulties of identifying that a young person is experiencing an eating disorder are complex and can easily be distorted by developmental outcomes and societal pressures. Body image is not just a cognitive construct but also a reflection of attitudes and interactions with others.

Student activity 6
As a final exercise before moving on to the next section, have a look at the following list and consider

Sarah's care plan

Needs/Wants	Risk behaviours	Short-term goals	Long-term goals	Interventions
To establish a safe, trusting therapeutic relationship.	Food restriction.	To establish a strong, trusting therapeutic relationship.	To maintain a strong therapeutic alliance.	Building a trusting and safe relationship. Motivational enhancement.
To be given psycho-education regarding the effects of starvation and eating-disordered behaviours.	Laxative abuse.	To educate Sarah on the medical consequences of starvation and eating disorder behaviours. To provide medical monitoring.	To assist Sarah in developing healthier, adaptive ways of coping with stress – learning how to problem solve.	Psychoeducation. Medical monitoring.
To be given support to understand the origins and functions of her eating disorder.	Vomiting after eating.	Education on the ineffectiveness of vomiting and laxative abuse as a means to lose weight. To advise Sarah on ways to prevent erosion of dental enamel.	To help Sarah view herself positively without solely over-valuing her weight and shape and her ability to control them.	Psycho-education.
To be given support to work out reasons to make changes or reasons to stay the same.	Self-harming due to body image distortion.	Use motivational interviewing enhancement methods to assist Sarah to explore her reasons to continue with illness and behaviour, and reasons to move towards health. To assist in making connections between thoughts, emotions, and behaviours.	To assist in improving her motivation towards making behavioural changes to her under-eating. To manage body image distortion without reverting to restricting foods or self-harm behaviour.	Motivational enhancement. Body image interventions to reduce image distortion.

how these examples of different people are portrayed in the media.

Women	*Men*	*Black people*	*Glamorous women*
Lesbians	*Slim people*	*Rich people*	*Teenage parents*
Older people	*Fat people*	*Mothers*	*Disabled people*
		Working women	*Single parents*

Substance misuse

In this section we will be considering the needs of an individual suffering from a substance dependency disorder (refer to the ICD 10, World Health Organization 2007, and the DSM-IV, American Psychiatric Association 2000, for criteria for diagnosis).

Around 4 million people in the UK use at least one illicit drug each year and around 1 million people use at least one of the most dangerous drugs (such as ecstasy, heroin, or cocaine). Many of these individuals will take drugs once, but for around 250 000 problematic drug users in England and Wales, drugs can cause considerable harm to themselves and others (Updated Drugs Strategy 2002).

As a future mental health nurse you will find that 22–44 per cent of adult psychiatric inpatients will use alcohol and/or drugs problematically, with up to half of them being drug dependent. In high security hospitals, 60–80 per cent of patients have a history of substance misuse prior to admission. It has been suggested that less than 20 per cent of those patients will receive treatment for their substance misuse problems (Department of Health 2006). Therefore it is very important that as a pre-reg student you make an effort to learn as much as you can about substance misuse. At this point in their training, most students do not feel equipped to help service users with substance misuse problems. However, this worry can be addressed by reading this chapter, looking at the further reading, and by having the motivation to attend post-registration courses on substance misuse. Bear in mind that specialist training is also often provided 'on-the-job'.

Student activity 7
Can you identify the drugs in Box 9.2 from their street names? Answers are included in Box 9.4.

The National Treatment Agency

In 1998, in recognition of the problems associated with drug misuse (i.e. lack of effective treatment, criminal activity, drug-related deaths, social factors, and stigmatization of drug users), the government decided to tackle the subject by the development of a ten-year drug strategy, *Tackling drugs to build a better Britain*, which was updated in 2002 (Crown Copyright 2002). The strategy sought to provide direction and coherence to initiatives undertaken separately across the government. Four overarching aims were developed:

- **Young people:** to help young people resist drug use in order to achieve their full potential in society.

- **Reducing supply:** to stifle the availability of drugs on our streets.

- **Communities:** to protect our communities from drug-related antisocial and criminal behaviour.

- **Treatment and harm minimization:** to enable people with drug problems to overcome them and live healthy, crime-free lives.

To support the strategy at a local level, 150 (drug action teams (DATs), comprising senior representatives from local authorities, health authorities, and criminal justice agencies, were given the responsibility and authority to develop and deliver local drug action plans in accordance with the four key aims above. In order to oversee plans at a national level and provide a structure that the DATs could be accountable to, in 2001 the government developed a special health authority, the National Treatment Agency (NTA). The NTA has a special remit of improving the availability, capacity, and effectiveness of treatment for drug misuse in England.

Brown, 'H', Benzos, Eggs, Charlie, Poppers, 'E', Special K

Hash, Speed, Brownies, Flash, Snow, Billy Whizz, Dexies, GBH

Box 9.2 Street names for drugs

The NTA's overall purpose is to:

- Double the number of people in effective, well-managed treatment from 100 000 in 1998 to 200 000 in 2008.
- Increase the proportion of people who successfully complete or, if appropriate, continue treatment.

In order to ensure that there are national standards in the field of substance misuse when it comes to the availability and accessibility of services, range of services, quality of care, and competency of staff, the NTA in 2002 (in conjunction with the Department of Health) developed a document called the *Models of care*. This document sets out national frameworks for the commissioning of drug treatment services (NTA 2006b). This is a document that has as much importance in the field of substance misuse as the *National Service Framework for mental health* (Department of Health 1999).

Student activity 8

As student nurses who may wish to work with those who suffer from a substance dependency problem, it is important to have knowledge of the NTA (and similar organizations if you study outside England). You may now wish to access the NTA website to review whether or not these targets have been met and what future targets have been set, as well as to browse through the Models of care document: http://www.nta.nhs.uk/

For students outside England, research the topic using the keywords: country name + national + drug + strategy + guidelines.

👤 What the service users say

Getting off is the easy bit. Staying off is what really tries you.

The only way to stay clean is to cut all contact with the old friends. Two died before I went to jail, three died while I was in jail, and two died since I've been out.

You do what you need to in order to get your fix, that's what being an addict is about.

From the Frank website (2008)

http://www.talktofrank.com

Clinical scenario: Charlie

In this section you will meet Charlie on her first presentation to services. You may find it useful to read the scenario first and then access the brief film of Charlie and her first contact with services.

Charlie is a 19-year-old woman who is having her first contact with services. She began using butane gas at the age of 11 and ceased doing so at the age of 16 when she was taken into hospital. The gas abuse had affected part of her brain. This has left her with some minimal cognitive impairment. At the age of 16 she started smoking cannabis and at 18 she had progressed to smoking heroin. She is now injecting, using approximately one £10 bag per day, slightly more at weekends. She has a heroin-using boyfriend who is in his 20s and he will often inject her as she is 'no good at it' herself. She reports that she was bullied at school, which is why

---

Heroin (medical name diamorphine) is one of a group of drugs called 'opiates', which are derived from the opium poppy. Opium is the dried milk of the opium poppy. It is converted to morphine and codeine in the body; both are effective painkillers. Heroin is made from morphine and in its pure form is a white powder (Drug Scope 2006).

Heroin can be smoked (chasing the dragon) or injected. You may wish to research heroin in more detail to fully understand the effects it has on the human body, physically and mentally. A good place to start the research process would be the National Institute on Drug Abuse: http://www.nida.nih.gov/NIDAHome.html.

Box 9.3 Heroin

she started using gas, in order to 'fit in' with a particular crowd. There is a possibility that she may have been raped but she never discusses this. She tends to spend nights away from home without telling her parents where she is; she has received a caution for shoplifting.

She presents as a passive, quiet woman. She is not abusive to her parents, has never stolen from them, or spoken back to them. She has aspirations to be a model. Her appetite is very poor, but this is a symptom of heroin use, not of an eating disorder. Her boyfriend abuses her verbally and sometimes physically but she doesn't speak ill of him and she says she loves him. It could be suggested that she is easily led, never really expressing her own opinion. She tends to go along with the crowd just for an easy life, and the damage that the gas abuse has done does not help. Charlie carries a lot of guilt regarding her younger sister as she feels that her sister is 'following in my footsteps'. Charlie feels that she should set a better example. She doesn't really think that the drug use is doing her any real harm. She also believes that she should have done more to help her dad overcome his alcohol dependency. Charlie is naive about her drug use and does not perceive it to be an issue. She cannot quite understand why her parents are so worried about her.

Charlie has never been in contact with services for treatment regarding a drug problem. She never received treatment specific to gas abuse apart from the stay in a general ward for medical problems associated with this.

> **Student activity 9**
> *You should now watch the video of Charlie meeting the nurse for the first time.*

🔖   www.oxfordtextbooks.co.uk/orc/clarke

and choose the video link.

Engagement

The most important jobs you will have as a substance misuse nurse are to engage your service user and retain them in treatment. In order to do this you will need to have an excellent working relationship with your service user from the first time you meet. It is important that the key worker builds a therapeutic relationship with the client. To do this, the key worker needs to be non-confrontational, listen reflectively, and encourage the client to identify and talk through their problems and needs (NTA 2006b). You will notice from the video that the nurse was non-confrontational and open, and conducted the interview in a genuine and warm manner. The main aim here was to create an atmosphere of acceptance that would allow the service user to talk about issues she felt were important to her. Certain techniques were used to achieve this. As a substance misuse nurse you will need to have a 'tool box' of techniques from different models of working that you can use to help the service user achieve their ultimate personal goal. The main techniques used by the nurse in the video were taken from two different models of working, are the first being the humanistic approach (client-centred). Carl Rogers (1996, see also Chapter 2, p. 26) talks about how individuals have within themselves vast resources for self-understanding, for altering their self-concept, attitudes, and self-directed behaviour. Rogers felt that the individual could tap into these resources if the right climate, conditions, and relations were provided. In order for this to happen, the nurse would need to be genuine/congruent, and demonstrate unconditional positive regard, warmth, and empathic understanding. The nurse for the most part would need to be non-directive in their approach (Rogers 1996).

The second is a model called motivational interviewing. This was developed in order to help individuals build that intrinsic motivation to make a change in their life, strengthen their commitment to change, and then develop a plan to accomplish that change (Miller and Rollnick 2002). A key component in the spirit of motivational interviewing is its collaborative nature, working in partnership with the service user. It relies upon methods of exploration and support rather than persuasion and argument. When things go well in motivational interviewing there is a 'sense of moving together, like two dancers gliding across a dance floor' (Miller and Rollnick 2002).

The responsibility for change lies completely with the service user. The nurse will use techniques that confront the service user with the idea of need for change without being argumentative. The model works with ambivalence, drawing out and eliciting information from the service user that allows them to ultimately present their argument for change (William and Miller 1994).

Both of these models helped the nurse in the film create a climate that allowed for the formation of a tentative working relationship from which the service user felt that she wished to have a further meeting. There is a lot more to the underpinning ideology of motivational interviewing than can be presented here. It is important that you follow up on this model of working and learn as much as you can about it by reading about the topic (you may find it useful to begin with the texts on motivational interviewing that are listed in the reference section of this chapter).

> **Student activity 10**
> *Having reviewed the film, can you:*

1) Identify some client-centred techniques used by the nurse?

2) Identify motivational interviewing techniques used by the nurse?

Care planning

Care planning is based on assessed need and actively involves the service user (NTA 2006a). Care planning needs to be delivered within a framework that focuses on the service user's treatment journey (NTA 2006a). There are important factors to take into account from this initial meeting with Charlie when formulating a care plan with her. The first is her level of risk, and the second and subsequent factors are to identify:

1) What is it that Charlie wants to aim for regarding her drug-using behaviour?

2) What does Charlie wish to achieve from the work that she will do with you?

3) What are Charlie's aims and objectives for her treatment?

> **Student activity 11**
> *1) Identify Charlie's risk factors.*
> *2) What do you think she wants to achieve from her sessions with the nurse?*

There are a number of risk factors for Charlie at the moment and there are also a number of things that she wishes to achieve for herself. Both of these subjects will have an impact upon the care plan that you and Charlie put together.

Risk
- Injecting behaviour.
- Boyfriend injecting her.
- Cannot be certain that the needles are clean, fresh, and that her 'works' are not being used by anybody else, or being shared by the boyfriend with anyone else.

- Abuse from others.
- Overdose.
- Possible mental health issues.
- Irreversible damage from the gas abuse, heroin use impact upon this?
- Lack of appetite and appears to be quite underweight.
- Naivety regarding her drug use.

Wants
- A better relationship with her mother.
- To not feel guilty about her father and sister.
- To continue using heroin.
- To remain with her boyfriend.
- To move out from home.
- To be a model or work in the fashion industry.
- To see you again.

As you can see from the video and the above, Charlie does not at this point wish to cease using heroin. There may be concerns from her perspective that if she stops using, her boyfriend will leave her. This is an assumption made from her discussion of the boyfriend in the video. Therefore the care plan that is developed will need to take into account this very important factor.

> **Student activity 12**
> *Have a go at developing a care plan for Charlie, based upon what you have read from the scenario and what you have seen in the film. To help, you may wish*

Brown = heroin, 'H' = heroin, Benzos = benzodiazipines, Eggs = tranquilizers, Hash = cannabis, Speed = amphetamine sulphate, Brownies = ecstasy, Flash = LSD, Snow = cocaine, Billy Whizz = amphetamine sulphate (speed), dexies = dexamphetamine, GBH = gammahydroxybutyrate, Charlie = cocaine, Poppers = alkyl nitrites, 'E' = ecstasy, Special K = ketamine

Box 9.4 Identifying drugs from their street names: answers

Charlie's case plan

Needs/Wants	Short-term goals	Long-term goals	Interventions
Engagement with services.	Development of therapeutic relationship.	Maintain therapeutic relationship.	Nurse uses techniques to engage Charlie in a meaningful, collaborative, working relationship.
To continue using heroin.	Inject herself safely. Ensure use of clean, new injecting equipment.	Cease injecting behaviour. Constant monitoring of the impact heroin use is having upon her physical and mental well-being.	Nurse will advise her on how to inject safely and properly, and maintain constant assessment of injection sites. Nurse will advise on where and how to gain clean, new injecting equipment, i.e. nearest needle exchange scheme. Nurse will advise her on how to prevent and manage accidental overdose. Nurse will use motivational interviewing techniques to help her move from injecting to smoking heroin. To plan in accordance as the need arises: urine screens, GP appointments to monitor physical health, relapse prevention.
Mental health.	Enable her to be mentally healthy.	Restoration of self-confidence.	Nurse will monitor mental health and help her to gain tools to prevent and combat low mood. Nurse will use techniques to allow her to tell her story, and help her to build her self-esteem.

Needs/Wants	Short-term goals	Long-term goals	Interventions
			Possible referral for counselling should this become a 'want' for her.
			Help her to work towards gaining some of her career aspirations.
Physical health.	Gain healthy sleep and eating patterns.	Maintain a healthy attitude towards eating and sleeping.	Nurse to assess and discuss her eating and sleep patterns. Assess for areas of concern.
			Nurse to advise on healthy eating and sleep hygiene.
			Nurse to use client-centred techniques to help her maintain this goal.
	Hep B vaccination.	Possible referral to the genitourinary medicine clinic for Hep C and HIV test.	Referral to GP for check-up, Hep B vaccination, and sexual health advice.
			Nurse to advise and support her in this area should the need arise.
To become heroin-free.	To have the contact numbers for self-help groups such as Narcotics Anonymous. (http://www.ukna.org/)	To attend a self-help group.	The nurse will help her to access self-help groups in the area and take her to them if necessary.
			The nurse will use motivational interviewing techniques to help her move towards wanting to no longer use heroin.
		The nurse will advise her of treatment options to achieve this.	Options include detox from heroin using suitable medication such as buprenorphine (Subutex) or methadone treatment, and then detox at a later stage.

Needs/Wants	Short-term goals	Long-term goals	Interventions
			The nurse together with Charlie will develop a further package of care that addresses relapse prevention to help her maintain her new drug-free status. This may include a referral for counselling, and rehabilitation.
Better relationship with mother and sister.		To support her in gaining her idea of a healthy relationship with the rest of the family.	Inter-professional working with other services involved with the rest of the family, with permission from Charlie. To develop a separate care plan for family interventions – this may include family therapy.
Social aspirations.	Gain information on careers in the fashion industry.	Live independently.	Advise and help Charlie on where and how to access this information, e.g. colleges etc. To help her to gain the information required to achieve this and ensure that she is in touch with the right services to help her achieve this goal.

to read the *Care Planning Practice Guide* developed by the NTA (2006a).

From the initial meeting Charlie has made it clear that she does not want to stop using heroin, and therefore you will need to work from a harm reduction standpoint. In their broadest sense, 'harm reduction polices, programmes, services and actions work to reduce the health, social and economic harms to individuals, communities and society that are associated with the use of drugs' (UK Harm Reduction Alliance 2005).

Important note

You will complete an initial assessment and then a comprehensive assessment. You must always remember that substance misuse is very rarely static, so assessment and review must be an ongoing, continual process that changes in accordance with the needs of the service user. Constant review of the care plan must occur to ensure that it meets the changing needs of the service user. The example care plan on pp. 234–6 is just to offer you an idea of the kind of work involved.

Evaluation

Remember, to be effective, you will need to review the care plan on a regular basis, monitor the effectiveness of interventions, and ensure that both you and the service user are clear on what to expect from each other and what each can bring to the therapeutic relationship (NTA 2006a).

Working with people with a diagnosis of personality disorder

The focus of this part of the chapter is working therapeutically with marginalized mental health service users, who are not just likely to be rejected and excluded by society in general, but are also likely to experience this exclusion within mental health services. An example of this exclusion is the unfortunately typical reaction from many mental health professionals when hearing a diagnosis of personality disorder; their tone becomes dismissive and their responses to service users are often rejecting. Successive governments have recognized a range of factors that are linked to social exclusion such as unemployment, poor education, poverty, family breakdown, poor housing, custodial sentences, disability, and experiencing mental health problems. Interrelated to exclusion are issues of stereotyping, prejudice, and discrimination. These are all demoralizing to individuals or groups that are targeted and ultimately prevent people from reaching their full potential in life, denying their right to contribute to society. In an effort to address these issues, the Labour Government of 1997 established the Social Exclusion Unit.

Student activity 13
Take some time out to visit the social exclusion website at http://www.socialexclusion.gov.uk and review the materials provided there. Specifically focus on issues around exclusion and the mentally ill.

Exclusion in mental health services

The *National Service Framework for mental health* in England (Department of Health 1999) sets out seven standards, one of which specifically addresses mental health promotion and social inclusion. In order to address and achieve this standard, several guidelines have been issued.

Some of the most marginal people within the service tend to be those with a diagnosis of personality disorder. However, the National Institute for Mental Health in England in their 2003 document, *Personality disorder: No longer a diagnosis of exclusion*, are seeking to suggest otherwise and to promote more inclusive practice with this client group. This document does acknowledge some positive changes and provides examples of good practice but there is also recognition that difficulties for people with this diagnosis in mental health services still exist. Some of the attitudes, beliefs, and values that you will come across in clinical practice may be prejudiced, excluding, and damaging to people with this diagnosis. So why does this diagnosis tend to generate such intense responses from people, and what are the particular issues that you need to be aware of? Our next fictional service user is Tracy – some mental health professionals would suggest that Tracy has a diagnosis of personality disorder. At this point it's useful to look at Tracy first before we make any decisions about her or her life.

Student activity 14
Take a look at the film of Tracy now and then consider the points below:

www.oxfordtextbooks.co.uk/orc/clarke

and choose the video link.
In the first two chapters of this book you carried out work on your self-awareness. Take some time out now and jot down your answers to the following questions.

- *Do you feel sorry for Tracy? Would you like to help her?*
- *Do you feel annoyed by Tracy? Do you think Tracy is being honest?*
- *Do you think Tracy is wasting Doug's time and doesn't really want help?*

Once you've watched the film and completed the activity, read the scenario available to you here and then view the film again.

Clinical scenario: Tracy

Tracy is a young single woman. She is without a home of her own but usually manages to find accommodation by moving between the homes of friends, squats, and night shelters, occasionally having to sleep rough.

She left her family home, a council house on a run-down estate, when she was 14 but continues to live in the vicinity. She left home because of physical abuse from her stepfather. She now has little contact with her parents or her six siblings. Tracy consistently refused to attend school from the age of 12. Prior to this she was identified as someone with minor learning difficulties and serious conduct problems. Her ability to read and write is very limited.

Shoplifting and burglary offences led to her coming to the attention of the juvenile courts and she has had periods of detention in youth treatment centres. Between the ages of 14 and 16 her problems were compounded by her habit of solvent abuse.

When she was 17 she gave birth to a child. Tracy had no permanent home and the father of the baby girl was unknown. The child was taken into care and Tracy has had no further contact with her.

Tracy's only experiences of legitimate paid employment was a paper round when she was a schoolgirl and occasional attempts to sell the *Big Issue* in the local shopping centre.

Over the past year Tracy has increasingly abused benzodiazepines (oral use) and alcohol and is now dependent on them. The benzodiazepines are obtained illicitly. She has been financing her habit by petty crime and, more recently, prostitution.

She has accessed mental health services on a range of occasions but never engaged effectively with them. She is still registered with a GP from the time she lived with her parents but had previously made little demand on his services. However, a recent combination of events led to her presenting herself with a request for assistance: Tracy told the GP that one of her prostitution clients beat her up, and then, soon afterwards, her drug supplier cheated her out of the little bit of money she had. She was then forced to steal from the friend who was accommodating her and this led to him throwing her out. After sleeping rough for three nights she developed pneumonia but she got herself admitted to hospital via the casualty department. For the five days she was in hospital she had the chance to review her life and came to the conclusion that 'it was time to get things sorted out'.

With the help of a social worker she was living in temporary accommodation. She was struggling to control her consumption of benzodiazepines and alcohol and, so far, had avoided resorting to prostitution or crime. She asked for assistance in breaking her dependence on these substances.

At first, the GP was suspicious that Tracy was trying to trick him into simply feeding her drug habit. However, after making some investigations, he was satisfied she was genuine and agreed to help her by prescribing a diminishing dose of diazepam. He subsequently sought the involvement of a community mental health nurse.

In the video you've seen that Tracy has been arrested for shoplifting and assault while drunk. You will have seen her being interviewed by a community mental health nurse who is assessing Tracy in order to determine whether she should remain within the criminal justice system or be referred to mental health services.

♟ Tracy – a service user's point of view

Her basic human needs are not being met. She has no shelter; she is homeless and is sleeping rough. Her environment is not conducive to good health; neither is her past. She is probably not eating properly and is grieving over losing her child.

The environmental factors and drugs notwithstanding, she has so much stress from her grief and her lack of autonomy and is not necessarily aware of this. She has little self-insight or respect, often hiding her real emotional distress through nervous laughter. Her only points of reference are an abusive partner and her alcoholic friends; **she has lost her identity**, probably from a young age.

She had received inappropriate treatment by doctors but seems to blame herself and has a 'them and us' view of medical intervention. This only confirms her loss of self-worth, which she had already learned from her abusive childhood.

Her core belief is that she is worthless in relation to the rest of the world.

This would emphasize her feeling ostracized from society; she does not realize how the isolation impacts upon her sense of self-worth, and of course upon her mental health.

She has had very little shared 'humanness' in her life; she needs another human being to believe in her, that she has **potential**.

She does seem to rely upon the medical model of medication and is trying to self-medicate with alcohol, not realizing it is her environment which affects her thoughts, feelings, and emotions.

She needs someone to reach out to her and to supply her soul with a sense of **hope**. She has lost her way and has no insight into what her feelings are telling her, or, indeed, what feelings are. She is used to a daily barrage of disdain and recrimination. She is a human being doing the best she can with the knowledge she has at this point in time.

She needs to be empowered to honour her emotions and to realize that she has indeed suffered. She deserves non-judgemental and solution-focused support; to be shown that there is an emotional outlet other than despair and drugs.

She needs someone to explain the physical and mental effects of the drugs she is taking and how that affects her thought processes, and indeed what thought processes are. For someone who has rarely enjoyed the exchange of positive human emotion, all this would seem alien to her and she has been alienated enough.

Although she is vulnerable and downtrodden she has the motivation of wanting her baby back, of getting out of an abusive relationship, and of feeling physically better. She just needs to be shown **how** and to be reassured that all this is a possibility.

Knowledge is power. She will feel empowered by knowledge and insight into her own emotions and medication, and with the knowledge that there is a positive solution and that she is worthy of love and respect from her fellow man.

Tracey Holley, survivor

Tracy – a pharmacist's view

Although the withdrawal programme is managed by the doctor, it is important to ensure that Tracy takes an active role so that it will be more likely to succeed. She has a personality disorder, which gives her a greater likelihood of developing dependence on benzodiazepines, and her alcohol intake adds an additional problem.

When using the care plan, consideration should be given to the timing of the introduction of an antidepressant in relation to the withdrawal programme. The central nervous system (CNS) depressant effect of the alcohol, diazepam, and the antidepressant must be taken into consideration.

For further information on benzodiazepines, refer to Chapter 8, and for more about alcohol withdrawal read the scenario on Feodor later in this chapter, p. 246.

Assessment

We have provided you with the opportunity to observe a simulated assessment interview. This is only a little over ten minutes when in fact actual service user assessments take considerably longer. We feel it is useful to analyse the process and outcomes of what you have seen to promote your learning by showing you an example of a possible practice environment.

In the interview you will notice how defensive, even angry Tracy is, but over time how Doug helps her to begin to relax and communicate with him. Doug (who is not an actor) is a skilled and experienced community mental health nurse and you will notice that his non-verbal communication mirrors how he wants Tracy to feel; he uses himself to demonstrate to her appropriate communication. You can learn from this strategy that if you seek to keep calm and relaxed in interactions with mental health service users, this can show them how to be. Also look at the physical environment, how he has positioned the chairs; he ensures that they are equal and not too close together. It is possible to suggest that the desk could be a barrier to communication but Doug has to consider his own personal safety, and in light of what we find out during the assessment interview, it may well enable Tracy to communicate more if she feels it offers her some distance and protection.

Doug also makes sure that there are no police in the room; this helps him to establish that he is separate from the police and not seeking to punish or control Tracy. Also consider how he engages Tracy in eye contact; he regularly seeks out contact to ensure that he understands what she has said but also to check for her meaning. We often talk about congruity in communication; this means that emotional expression and non-verbal communication match verbal communication. We can all send mixed messages, for example the person who says 'take me seriously', while laughing. Doug seeks out eye contact with Tracy to ensure that he is reading her meaning correctly.

Doug sets out the purpose of the interview very early on and makes Tracy aware that he will ask difficult questions but will seek to keep her answers confidential where he can. His assessment strategy is very much focused on her understanding of how she got to be in her current predicament. Initially, Doug focuses upon how Tracy got arrested but quickly recognizes that there is more to her than just being a 'shoplifter'. He begins to explore her social and psychological history, which helps him to provide a context to her behaviour. Doug also picks up verbal and non-verbal cues around those areas that are particularly difficult for her. You may well have felt uncomfortable at times watching the video. You will have noticed that Doug expresses his own discomfort and acknowledges Tracy's discomfort at sharing intimate and traumatic experiences with him. This self-disclosure can help to establish a common bond between the nurse and service user. However, Doug remains very calm and controlled and continues to instil confidence in Tracy, showing that despite feeling uncomfortable, he is not going to reject her or disbelieve what she is saying.

Tracy reveals a very fragmented life. She feels she was rejected by her mother as she entered puberty, and that her mother chose her stepfather over her. Tracy eventually tells Doug that her initial experimentation with drugs and alcohol was to deal with the pain, both psychological and physical, of being physically abused by her stepfather and sexually abused by her grandfather. There are also hints that Tracy physically self-harms and continues to abuse alcohol and tranquillizers.

Student activity 15
Tracy has a history of self-harm. Make a list of aspects of Tracy's life that could reduce her risk of self-harm. Now make a list of the issues that could increase her risk of self-harm. Discuss your findings with both your colleagues and your clinical assessor to ensure that you haven't missed important issues.

Assessment summary

During this assessment Doug has pieced together the significant problems that Tracy has. He identifies:

- Her drug and alcohol abuse.
- Her anger and aggression.
- The fractured family relationships and Tracy's experiences of abuse as a child.

In terms of her drug and alcohol misuse, you can consider the care planning materials provided under Charlie's scenario earlier in this chapter as a useful example. It is essential that we respond to Tracy's misuse of both alcohol and drugs to ensure that she is able to work towards recovery. While Tracy's anger and aggression is directed at others, it is also internally directed when Tracy self-harms. Doug recommends Tracy access mental health services, offers a positive, supportive outcome, and leaves her with an offer of help.

Care planning

Please note that the following examples are a sample only, and are not intended to be a complete guide.

Important note: Staff need to be mindful, in any interaction with Tracy, of her history of abuse, particularly if they touch her. Something as simple as a pat on the shoulder can become significant and disturbing for a mental health service user with a history

of trauma and abuse, and within certain cultural contexts is considered inappropriate. There are several areas on a person's body that it is always unacceptable for nurses to touch except in the context of a specific medical investigation, before which we must get the appropriate informed and written consent. In Tracy's case the best answer may be to negotiate whether she is comfortable for staff to make physical contact with

Tracy's care plan: anger

Service User Identified need	Goals	Prescribed mental health nursing care
Tracy needs to learn how to express her anger, aggression, and frustration through appropriate channels of communication.	Tracy will approach her identified mental health worker and ask for time to discuss her feelings before she reacts angrily or aggressively to any situation. Tracy will not directly self-harm. Tracy will, in partnership with her mental health worker, identify and analyse the following: A. **Antecedents** to her aggressive outbursts. B. A daily record of the frequency, intensity, number, and duration of episodes of her aggressive **Behaviour**. C. **Consequences** of her behaviour. (This is often referred to as an ABC analysis in correlation to antecedents, behaviour, and consequences, alongside a FIND assessment.)	For Tracy's identified mental health worker to discuss access to manage her aggression at the beginning of every shift. Establish alternative behaviours to cutting, for example negotiate with Tracy the use of ice instead of a razor. Negotiate with Tracy the potential need for supervised, limited, and sterile cutting. A. Having identified trigger factors, review with Tracy changing typical daily activities so there are fewer antecedents (events including people and thoughts that may trigger a behavioural response) occurring. Consistently monitor aggressive outbursts. B. As Tracy shifts towards communicating her feelings rather than acting impulsively, show her how she is improving. Accept that at times Tracy will respond inappropriately. Encourage her not to feel overwhelmed or a failure but to focus on how much she is achieving. C. Typical consequences of aggression include increased attention and concern. Ensure that Tracy gets attention and time on appropriate request. If she does become aggressive, indicate that she will get positive attention and time when calm and in control. Staff need to be aware that when Tracy is aggressive it is important that they: 1) Do **not** not take this as a personal attack. 2) Be effective, calm role models in all interactions.

Tracy's care plan: relationships

Service User Identified need	Goals	Prescribed mental health nursing care
Tracy needs to learn how to develop appropriate emotional attachments and boundaries within her existing relationships.	Tracy will acknowledge her traumatic childhood experiences and their ongoing impact on her life and behaviour. Tracy will become aware of how unhealthy, damaged, and damaging her current relationships are and recognize the repeating nature of her relationship patterns. Tracy will develop realistic emotional attachments in her relationships. Tracy will recognize and establish what acceptable boundaries in her relationships are. Tracy will become aware of how she seeks to encourage people to reject her. Tracy will develop her ability to trust other people. Tracy will become aware of how she encourages people to see her in a victim role/life position (see discussion point). Tracy will develop positive self-belief, self-value, self-esteem, and self-worth.	A simple example of the care that mental health nurses could deliver is outlined below, alongside some suggested additional responses. To promote Tracy's ability to trust, we need to use our relationship with her as a key example as follows: • Develop a therapeutic relationship. • Establish, maintain, and consistently apply appropriate professional boundaries. • Demonstrate acceptance, warmth, and genuineness. • Demonstrate commitment and a belief in her potential as a person. • Be a positive role model by demonstrating effective functioning of personality through a 'stable self system; satisfying interpersonal functioning and social/group relationships'. (British Psychological Society 2006). Johnson (2007, unpublished) recommends the application of the following acronym: H – holistic approach O – opportunity to talk P – progress as an individual through motivation E – emotionally release the fast and fears for the future
		What mental health services will offer in the way of care will vary depending on the model underpinning practice and what is available where Tracy lives, but might include the following: Psychodynamic models. Individual therapy based on a range of possible approaches, but typically

Service User iIdentified Nneed	Goals	Prescribed mental health nursing care
		with the emphasis on the relationship between the patient and the therapist. There is very definite use of the process of transference. The patient is involved in a process of learning and personal development. The therapist–patient relationship provides the opportunity to learn how to develop full and satisfactory relationships with others, while becoming self-aware and having successfully worked through previous unhealthy or destructive patterns of relating (see the work of Dryden 2007). The patient is given the opportunity to test it out in the real relationship between them and their therapist.
		Group therapy strategies seek to recreate the primary group or family group so that they can encounter and work through transference and countertransference issues, sibling rivalry, and competition. Arguably this process is much closer to reality in that we are expected to live within groups within society. There are specialist services available for people with severe personality disorder who need intensive in-patient care, and an incredibly useful model of practice is seen at therapeutic communities.
		Cognitive behavioural approaches may be used and dialectical behaviour therapy is currently one of the most recommended strategies for people with personality disorders. and It is based on the work of Linehan (1993) in the USA.

her. Ideally we would draw up a specific care plan that would detail the agreements.

Often, dealing with this real and not uncommon problem is seen as beyond the ability of general mental health services and frequently it will not be responded to. Tracy may be advised to seek support externally to the service or she could be referred to a specialist therapy service offered by the trust. However, the *Chief Nursing Officer's Review of mental health nursing* (Department of Health 2006) stipulates that mental health nurses need to become increasingly skilled and capable practitioners in these types of psychological interventions. Some possible examples are provided below.

● Discussion point

Some people will adopt certain roles in their lives that are not always healthy.

You will see in Figure 9.1 three specified roles that people can play: rescuer, persecutor, and victim. If you think of a person in a 'victim' role, they often feel that things just happen to them; they have little control over their lives, and they find everything threatening. Early experiences of trauma can lead to patterns of behaviour that are linked to recurring risk of further traumatic experiences; as Van der Kolk (1996: 199) states, 'Once people have been traumatized, they are vulnerable to being victimized on future occasions.' But of course the 'victim' role only allows you to respond from either a rescuing position or a persecuting role. It is essential that the mental health nurse does neither. It is our purpose to explore what earlier traumatic experience is being revisited by the service user and avoid participating in any re-enactment of this, otherwise we risk recreating the original abusing relationship.

Implementation

The initial focus of implementing Tracy's care needs to be on ensuring effective boundaries are maintained with her, so that she can feel safe, learn to live acceptably with other people, and manage her risks effectively and differently.

Evaluation

Specifically measurable goals such as reducing aggressive outbursts are very easy to evaluate. Simply put, has Tracy had fewer aggressive outbursts, have they been less intense, of shorter duration, and occurring less frequently over time? The same could be said of direct self-harm behaviours; however, helping Tracy develop adequate emotional bonds is a much more nebulous concept. In this case we would specifically need to focus on Tracy's perception of change and improvement in the evaluation process, alongside that of the team involved in her care.

Student activity 16

Reflect back on the answers you jotted down immediately after watching the film about how you felt about Tracy. Think for a moment about your friendships. Are you the person everyone phones for advice, help, and support, or are you the person they come to for a sound telling off when they've messed things up, or are you the person constantly seeking advice or messing things up? In this discussion point the reason for considering what role you tend to play, and how you feel about others who also play this game, will hopefully become apparent and help to develop your own self-awareness.

Tracy's reaction to her perceived threat and position as a victim who is expecting someone to persecute her has led to her becoming violent and aggressive. It is likely that both the shop and the security guard will prosecute and the evidence that Tracy used a dangerous weapon will probably lead to her appearing in court. In those circumstances Tracy may be placed on a Section 37, without restriction, of the Mental Health Act (2007).

Student activity 17

It is vital that mental health nurses are familiar with mental health law. Visit the web link below and make notes on what Section 37 of the Mental Health Act (2007) is. Include in your notes what having restrictions/no restrictions means in relation to this section.

http://www.dh.gov.uk/en/Healthcare/ NationalServiceFrameworks/Mentalhealth/ DH_063423

Forensic mental health services are intended for individuals who have committed a criminal offence while suffering from a mental illness. The court will usually place the person on a section of the Mental Health Act and order treatment in a psychiatric unit. This is usually dependent on the seriousness of the crime and the potential risk to the public. As you will see from Tracy's care plan, this is based to some extent within an inpatient forensic unit, as in all likelihood Tracy will be placed initially into this sort of facility. It is important to be aware of Horne's (2004) estimate that 90 per cent of all prisoners have a mental health problem. The alternative to Tracy going into a forensic unit is prison. The Corston Report (2007) highlights the vulnerabilities that women who have mental health problems face in the criminal justice system.

Student activity 18
For a brief review of this report, visit this web link: http://www.homeoffice.gov.uk/about-us/news/corston-report.

It is useful to be aware of Tracy's aggressive tendencies and as mental health nurses we should seek to understand what motivates her to behave in this way. Women's violence and aggression is no less a threat and reality than men's; however, there are specific gender differences that mental health nurses need to be aware of. You need to consider the context of women's expressions of aggression: while they will direct this at other people, they will also direct this against themselves at times through direct and indirect acts of self-harm. Examples of this may include:

- Gouging – often with sharp objects at pre-existing wounds or scars.
- Cutting – often with sharp objects, which is visible on arms and wrists. However, mental health nurses should also be aware that some women will cut their breasts and buttock areas and other covered areas of the body.
- Inserting – sometimes women will insert items such as razors or broken glass into their orifices (including the genital area).

There is a suggestion that in cases of sexual abuse, women will internalize this damage and turn hatred against their own helplessness into damaging themselves in dangerous acts of self-harm. This fits into notions of self-blaming and re-traumatizing alongside

firmly positioning themselves as victims. Clearly women in the original abusive situation have been disempowered. As humans under perceived threat we will act either to become aggressive (fight) or to become defensive (flight or freeze). There is also a third response and this is to disassociate (Van der Kolk 1996). Kernberg (2001) believes that individuals' self-worth and self-esteem must be restored to prevent aggression and suicide.

Tracy's history and her behaviour are likely to lead to her diagnosis as personality disordered. 'As prevalence rates for personality disorders . . . are very high in forensic populations, it is likely that a considerable proportion of those treated in these settings meet the diagnostic criteria for at least one personality disorder,' according to the British Psychological Society (BPS 2006: 43). BPS (2006: 4) also states that 'Personality disorders are variations or exaggerations of normal personality attributes. Although personality disorder is often associated with antisocial behaviour, the majority of people with a personality disorder do not display antisocial behaviour. Many people with mental health problems also have significant problems of personality.' The DSM-IV (APA 2000) suggests that personality disorders include 'enduring patterns of cognition, affectivity, interpersonal behaviour, and impulse control that are culturally deviant, pervasive and inflexible, and lead to distress or social impairment' (BPS 2006:6).

Student activity 19
To help you gain a basic understanding of what personality disorder means, visit this web link and read through the fact sheets produced by MIND http://www.mind.org.uk.

The DSM-IV groups personality disorder into three clusters:

- In cluster A, which they refer to as the odd/eccentric cluster, they identify three types of disorder: paranoid, schizoid, and schizotypal.
- In cluster B, the dramatic/erratic cluster, there are four types: antisocial, borderline, histrionic, and narcissistic.
- In cluster C, the anxious/fearful cluster, there are also three types: avoidant, dependent, and obsessive-compulsive.

Note that the DSM is currently being reviewed and the next version is due to be published in 2012. The prevalence of personality disorder varies depending

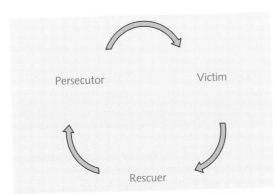

Figure 9.1   Unhelpful responses to 'victims'

upon the population group studied; nationally the figures are around 5–8 per cent of the general population, although this rises to 50 per cent amongst psychiatric inpatients, and as many as 78 per cent of adult prisoners meet the diagnostic criteria for personality disorder (BPS 2006).

The aetiology or causes of personality disorder are multiple and seem to contain bio-psycho-social elements. Just as there is no agreement on a single defining cause, there is also no agreement regarding treatment. Therefore, approaches to Tracy's care will be influenced by what specific model or philosophy informs the practitioner's practice. The BPS (2006: 35) suggests 'that people with personality disorder can be successfully treated using psychological therapies. Treatment benefits appear particularly evident when treatment is intensive, long-term, theoretically coherent, well structured and well integrated with other services and, where treatment has been provided in a residential setting, follow up care is provided.' The National Institute for Clinical Excellence is yet to determine a guideline on the treatment of personality disorders, although some strategies are being worked on. However, in the NIMHE document (2003) there is useful information on best current treatment options. There is considerable interest around the implementation of dialectical behaviour therapy adapted from the work of Linehan (1993). There is also the therapeutic community model; this offers long-term intensive input.

Student activity 20

The web link http://www.therapeuticcommunities.org, can provide you with some valuable resources for further study on this subject. A useful starting point is the frequently asked questions page. We are also learning that in order to improve the services we offer to people with mental health problems, we need to consult them and involve them in the decision-making process.

Student activity 21

Mental health service user groups have contributed to the production of the Personality Disorders Capabilities Framework (2003); within this they specify effective strategies to employ with people with personality disorder. Follow the web link below to the document and compare the examples of both the negative pathway and the positive recovery pathway in relation to the care outlined for Tracy.
http://www.spn.org.uk/fileadmin/SPN_uploads/Documents/Papers/personalitydisorders.pdf

There is ongoing debate over the helpfulness of the diagnosis of personality disorder. Some service user groups have suggested that it would be better to focus on the traumatic experiences that many people diagnosed with personality disorder have undergone. In the next part of this chapter we focus on Feodor and consider further issues around trauma and traumatic experiences in relation to mental health nursing care.

Working with service users who have experienced trauma

In this chapter you have met several people who have mental health problems. The last of these is 'Feodor', who you meet following his arrest and referral to mental health services. It's useful to read the scenario thoroughly first and then access the film, which shows Feodor talking about his situation.

www.oxfordtextbooks.co.uk/orc/clarke

and choose the video link.

Clinical scenario: Feodor

Feodor is a 31-year-old man who was born in the Soviet Russia. Feodor served as a Russian soldier and saw active duty in the 1994–1996 Chechen war, during which time there was indiscriminate bombing and shelling of Chechen towns and villages. According to news sources the Russian soldiers and separatists both used 'dirty war' tactics: kidnappings, contract killings, 'disappearances', torture, and brutality. During this war up to 100 000 civilians were killed, and at least 15 000 Russian soldiers died. Feodor has stated that the Russian people believed what they were told, 'that all Chechens are either criminals or terrorists, and that the Chechens are a big part of the mafia everywhere.'

Feodor has stated that over 250 000 Russians were killed in Chechnya during the collapse of the Soviet Union in 1991: 'That was genocide.' Feodor has referred to hostage situations in both Budennovsk and Beslan when hundreds died. Feodor has quoted the Russian leader Putin as stating 'that the war was over three years ago', but Feodor contends that the brutal conflict goes on unabated. As a soldier he says it is no surprise that they (the Russian army) did what they did; the Chechens gave them no choice. He has come to the UK seeking asylum, work, a better life, a chance to start again, to escape from the nightmares and the fear. He is now opposed to the conflict in Chechnya and has expressed his opposition to many people, some of them with political power and some in senior positions in the Russian army; he believes that he may be at risk of retribution from both the Russians and the Chechens.

He was brought into an acute admission unit by police three weeks ago, in handcuffs, initially on Section 136 of the Mental Health Act 2007. He speaks very good English although on admission he refused to talk for two days. He was subsequently placed on Section 2 of the Mental Health Act 2007. The report by the Police Surgeon (this is usually a doctor with mental health experience and knowledge who works regularly with the police) indicated that Feodor was arrested for public affray but upon being arrested and handcuffed became so distressed both physically and emotionally that the arresting officers felt he needed to be removed to a place of safety and implemented Section 136. Following an interview with the Police Surgeon at the police station he was brought to the admission unit.

During the three weeks Feodor has spent on the unit he has recalled some of his history and informed staff about why he believes he has been admitted. Feodor believes he is in the unit because he disagrees with the Russian involvement with the Chechen conflict. He also believes that he has been admitted to a psychiatric unit because he is a dissident; referring to the previous Soviet policy of incarcerating political dissidents into psychiatric hospitals. He also believes that like Anna Politkovskaya (Russian reporter killed in 2006) and Alexander Litvinenko (also killed in 2006) his life may be in danger.

Feodor has expressed deep sorrow about what happened and his previous life; he would like to move on and start again. Feodor describes how he is feeling now and what he sees his main problems as being. He believes he is unwell because he is unable to sleep properly. He regularly wakes up due to graphic nightmares when he sees badly injured people, children, and his army colleagues, who are covered in blood. He also has problems getting off to sleep initially and does not feel rested after sleep. He is very worried about this as he needs to be very alert at all times because he is in danger.

He feels that his memory plays tricks on him, and at times he experiences very upsetting flashbacks. They come to him when he feels at his most vulnerable and he feels that he is back in the war and it is happening all over again. At times very simple things like a bird flying overhead or the shape of a person's face can make him feel overcome. At these times he shakes, feels as if he cannot breathe, and wants to get away from the area. Sometimes seeing news coverage of war on television can make him feel panicked, especially if it is about Chechnya. Sometimes he can be busy, talking on the telephone, and he will have pictures jump into his head.

He often sees part of a Russian army shirt sleeve in a puddle of muddy water; he doesn't want to look because he knows his friend's arm is still in that sleeve but that his body has gone in the shell fire. He thinks he could have saved his friend's life and blames himself for the death; he believes that it is his fault his friend's children have no father, his wife no husband, and his parents have lost a son.

He tries to keep very busy and avoids everything he can that reminds him of the war, but he struggles to focus and believes that his sleep is so bad that he can no longer concentrate. He doesn't want to get close to anyone, he feels that he is too damaged and has no love or emotions left for normal relationships. Not sleeping and being damaged in this way means that he will sometimes hit people if he feels threatened by them. He suspects that people may be following him and sometimes he will backtrack to deliberately follow them. He believes that he was arrested by the British police on the say-so of the Russian government. Sometimes he will drink to try to sleep and prevent the nightmares but this doesn't really help.

Now watch the video of Feodor.

www.oxfordtextbooks.co.uk/orc/clarke

and choose the video link.

Student activity 22

It is very important that mental health nurses are familiar with mental health law. Feodor has experienced both Section 136 and Section 2 of the Mental Health Act 2007. Visit the web link below and makes notes on both of these sections. Take time out to draw up an information leaflet for service users explaining their rights under both of these sections. You can use this for teaching or information-giving sessions in clinical practice and supporting evidence in your student portfolio

http://www.dh.gov.uk/en/Healthcare/National ServiceFrameworks/Mentalhealth/DH_063423

Assessment by mental health nurse

We are going to provide you with a bio-psycho-social assessment summary that has been collated from the written scenario of Feodor and by directly observing him as he talks about his personal circumstances on film.

Student activity 23

Review the scenario and film:

www.oxfordtextbooks.co.uk/orc/clarke

as you consider the assessment summary and the following questions.

- What do you think is the root cause of Feodor's problems?
- What would you say is the probable diagnosis Feodor will be given by a psychiatrist?
- How would you seek to establish priorities of care for Feodor?

Assessment

The mental health nursing focus should be on the mental health service user's own expressed needs seen from a holistic perspective, considering physical, psychological, and social issues with Feodor.

The priorities that Feodor informs us of are for him to feel safe, to be able to sleep, and to have a normal routine. During the process of telling us about himself and his experiences, Feodor also provides other valuable insights into the way he is feeling and some significant issues for mental health nurses to consider. His reference to 'just stopping' may suggest that he is considering suicide. He says that he thinks about overdosing on alcohol and tablets. He also mentions his anger and his desire to be less angry.

You may have noticed him react rather nervously to a sound outside the door; some people would suggest that this should be considered to be evidence of a startle response. He also talks of dreams that significantly upset him and images, particularly of water, that remind him of distressing experiences. He acknowledges that he would like relationships but has lost so many people he now does not believe in having a future, and we could suggest from this a sense of hopelessness.

He also demonstrates some of the bodily symptoms he experiences, in particular shaking, which is something he feels he has no control over and finds difficult to manage. He also mentions that he has spoken out against Russian military involvement in Chechnya, an action that could quite possibly compromise his safety and result in him seeking asylum in the UK. On the other hand, this type of fear may be associated with paranoia and mental health nurses would need to assess Feodor thoroughly in order to be able to discount this.

Feodor – a service user's perspective

Feodor tells a very poignant story about the trauma of war and the loss of his friends. He really is 'the story behind the headlines' about 'illegal immigrants', 'scrounging asylum seekers', and all the other demeaning and derogatory things we read about. He is obviously a courageous, intelligent, thoughtful, and articulate young man, who speaks excellent English and tells the story in an almost poetic way. He is also quite clear about what would help him to recover.

What he says about officialdom – the filling in of forms and the lack of understanding of his situation – is revealing and says much about the need for basic training in mental health awareness.

Marion Clarke, service user

Assessment summary

Summary of symptoms:

- Evidence of startle response; nightmares and feelings of hopelessness.
- Evidence of suicidal intent and uncontrollable anger.
- Evidence of uncontrollable shaking and possible paranoid ideas.

With this in mind we would need to prioritize Feodor's care. We have identified significant risk factors and these would need to be dealt with urgently, while at the same time we would need to seek to address some of his identified priorities and work in partnership with him.

Identifying needs

In producing a detailed care plan we would need to establish what Feodor's priorities are, but these have to be considered in relation to personal and public safety, government policy, and evidence-based health care.

Risk

In terms of risk we would need to focus on the following: is there evidence of suicidal ideation, and does Feodor have a suicide plan identified? He does express a sense of hopelessness and a lack of future, and while he would like relationships he feels unable to sustain these. Obviously this also links to his social needs.

Social needs

Feodor demonstrates uncontrolled anger and aggressive outbursts. His risk appears to be heightened as he has significant social concerns: a need for a safe environment including a safe place to call home, and support with asylum seeker application.

Physical needs

His obvious biological needs include establishing an appropriate sleep pattern, alcohol intake reduction, and tremor management.

Psychological needs

Psychological issues include a need to establish what is 'wrong' with Feodor. There is a chance of differential diagnosis. Of course there is also the potential for inappropriate treatment as there is a lack of clarity as to what Feodor's mental health problems actually are. We would need to consider thorough and varied assessment strategies to address differential diagnosis.

Feodor is presenting with symptoms from all of the following mental health issues: post-traumatic stress disorder (PTSD); affective disorder; and alcohol-related problems. It is possible to suggest that he is also presenting with symptoms of paranoid schizophrenia.

In light of Feodor's history and the significant issues that he is presenting with, it is appropriate for the mental health nurse to recognize that he is demonstrating the cluster symptoms of PTSD (Box 9.5).

✎Alcohol withdrawal – pharmacist's comment

Mild alcohol dependence may be managed without medication, but if medication is used to reduce the withdrawal symptoms, it should not be given to an intoxicated patient. The first symptoms of alcohol withdrawal occur within hours of the last drink and peak at 24 to 48 hours. These can cover a wide range from tremor, restlessness, sweating, anxiety, nausea, vomiting, and insomnia, to the more serious delirium tremens (DTs) and convulsions. Visual and auditory hallucinations and paranoid ideation may also be seen. Symptoms in those with a mild to moderate dependency usually disappear five to seven days after the last drink.

Chlordiazepoxide and diazepam are the most commonly used drugs to assist withdrawal. The choice is often down to personal preference. They both start with a four times a day dose, and the dose and frequency are reduced over five to seven days. If withdrawal symptoms are problematic, the dose may be temporarily increased back to the previous dose level. Adequate fluid intake must be ensured at this time.

Symptom	Feodor's behaviour
• Intrusive recollections of the trauma.	• Memory 'playing tricks' on him.
	• Graphic images from his conflict experience.
• Avoidance of stimuli associated with the trauma.	• He avoids everything that reminds him of the war.
• Disordered arousal.	• Startle response.
	• Overtly aggressive reactions.

Adapted from Scott and Straddling (2006: 3)

Box 9.5 Cluster symptoms of post-traumatic stress disorder

Student activity 24

In the UK we have established guidelines for the treatment of PTSD. You can access these at the link below. Initially it may be worth looking through the information provided to the public as the complete guidance document is 167 pages long. You can also access a series of slides about PTSD produced by NICE and available at the same link.

http://guidance.nice.org.uk/CG26

Care planning

To give you an idea of what Feodor's care plan might consider we are going to address two issues (see example care plan). What will mental health nurses need to do to ensure goals are met? There should be a prescription of care, detailed enough to enable any nurse to deliver the care safely, effectively, and efficiently. The care plan on pp. 250–2 seeks to provide you

Feodor's care plan

Service User Identified need.	Goals	Prescribed mental health nursing care.
Risk – Feodor feels unsafe, often under threat and menaced, even in his current identified home.	**Short-term goals** • To promote a sense of security. • To reduce aggressive outbursts and violence towards others. **Long-term goals** • To work towards discharging Feodor into a stable identified home environment. • Ensure appropriate support for Feodor's asylum seekers application. • Feodor will feel safe and secure within his new home.	1. Establish a therapeutic relationship, over time. be Be available for Feodor, and seek to develop a rapport with him. Demonstrate cultural understanding and liaise with relevant UK- based support groups for people with common experiences and from a similar cultural background if Feodor is comfortable with this. 2. To offer full explanations of procedures and all activities carried out with Feodor. Check regularly for understanding to avoid misunderstanding or perceived threat and a potentially aggressive response.

Service User Identified need	Goals	Prescribed mental health nursing care.
		3. To discuss stress management and anxiety management strategies as alternatives to aggressive behaviour. Teach Feodor basic relaxation skills, deep muscle tensing relaxation, and breathing techniques. Help him to cognitively reframe situations that he finds threatening by offering an alternative perspective. Encourage him to discuss concerns before taking action.
		4. Liaison with social worker regarding appropriate action. Seek to establish a secure home environment for Feodor, and involve him in choosing area. Contact relevant support agencies, such as specialist legal advisors and asylum seeker support/advice agencies. Useful websites:
		http://www.refugeecouncil.org.uk
		http://www.asylumaid.org.uk
		http://www.asylumsupport.info/nass.htm
		http://www.lag.org.uk
Feodor is unsure why he is reacting the way that he is; he is aware that he is using unhealthy coping strategies to deal with his psychological distress, for example at times drinking excessive amounts of alcohol.	• To determine an appropriate treatment plan for Feodor in discussion with Feodor and the multidisciplinary team. • To reduce, safely, Feodor's alcohol intake. • To educate Feodor on alternative healthy coping strategies. • To reduce Feodor's level of psychological distress.	• Team to meet with Feodor and carry out a range of appropriate assessments to determine specific and appropriate treatment for him. • (If link to PTSD is firmly established, refer promptly to appropriate specialist trauma therapist.) • Carry out specific identification of level of alcohol problem using a specific assessment strategy. Initially working with Feodor to consider the • Antecedents – to his drinking episodes. • Behaviour – what behaviour specifically occurs? Measure this by accurately getting Feodor to record the frequency, intensity, number of alcohol units, and duration of his drinking.

Service User Identified need.	Goals	Prescribed mental health nursing care.
		• Consequences – consider the consequences of his drinking.
		These simple assessment approaches can clearly signify what is leading to these episodes, how serious they are and how Feodor may be reinforcing his behaviour through the end result or consequences of his drinking episodes.
		In liaison with Feodor, medical colleagues, and safe alcohol withdrawal guidelines (http://www.nta.nhs.uk), implement a reduction/withdrawal programme safely. Maintain monitoring of sleep patterns, dietary intake, fluid intake and output, and daily physical observations such as pulse, blood pressure, and respirations.
		Work with Feodor in relation to his psychological distress using stress and anxiety management strategies and cognitive behavioural strategies.
		Refer to specialist trauma therapist if appropriate. The treatment offered by a specialist trauma therapist is likely to include a range of approaches; however, most will discuss in detail the traumatic events, sometimes within a context of the person's resilience and strength of in coping with their reality, which helps to focus on recovery. Alongside this, as the person may become overwhelmed, the therapist may focus on life before the traumatic events to ensure that the person continues in the therapeutic process. They may also help the person write their own biography as a healing process. Over time they will move towards how the person can live now (Scott and Straddling 2006).
		Refer to self-help group and/or culturally appropriate support group.

with an example of a prescription of mental health nursing care.

Rationale

Prescribed care fits comprehensively into both a humanistic psychological framework and the recovery model in its emphasis on relationship forming and valuing the person as their own expert. It is driven by recognized national best practice as advised and established by the NICE guidelines and underpinned by internationally recognized diagnostic measures such as ICD 10 and DSM-IV.

Implementation/evaluation

Cases such as Feodor's are very difficult for mental health nurses to work on effectively. There are issues around language and cultural understanding. Hayward (2007) indicates that the largest numbers of asylum seekers tend to be from Asia, Africa, and Eastern Europe, like Feodor. Hayward (2007: 21) says, 'that many will be working through psychological issues'. Scott and Straddling (2006: 142) recognize that 'before any counselling can begin, the victim of chronic trauma has to feel safe. This is particularly problematic if they are a refugee and their asylum application is still outstanding, and they greatly fear being returned to their homeland in such circumstances'.

Mental health nurses need to be aware that many (already chronically traumatized) asylum seekers have to face what can be a hostile and unwelcoming new country. This alienating and stigmatizing experience, in addition to mental health problems, leads this client group to be amongst the most marginalized of mental health service users. In Feodor's case we have referred to culturally relevant support and self-help groups. Mental health nurses need to be aware that some asylum seekers will avoid this help. Their avoidance can 'extend to other members of their community if they feel they could be betrayed to authorities in their home country, making the provision of social support doubly difficult' (Scott and Straddling 2006: 142).

Our best means of evaluation is seeking to measure in terms understandable by Feodor any improvement in his mental health. We should consider if he has reached the targets identified in his care plan and modify those that have not been attained. In the short term, in partnership with Feodor, we would want to see a significant improvement in his sleeping patterns, his coping strategies, and his feelings of safety. A very simple way to evaluate the effectiveness of our prescribed care is to ask Feodor to rate his feelings of being unsafe, for example, on a scale of 1 to 10, 1 being safe and 10 being totally unsafe. If we get a standard over the first period of implementing the care plan, say within the first week, we can then revisit this measuring tool and subsequent care reviews would indicate that our plan is working or that we need to reassess Feodor's care.

You will have noticed within the rationale provided for the care plan that it is based on evidence-based best practice guidelines, so the care prescribed is believed to be the best and most appropriate for people experiencing Feodor's range of mental health problems. However, it is always worth noting that our job as mental health nurses is to 'individualize' that care plan, to ensure it suits the individual. One suit of clothing will not fit everyone, so we need to be able to adapt and be flexible, innovative, and imaginative in our work with people with mental health problems.

Hopefully this section of this chapter will have enhanced your insight into some of the issues emerging in the UK and internationally as we see globalization, traumatic living conditions, and increased movement of the world's population, and will have raised your awareness of your responsibilities to this potentially vulnerable and growing group of mental health service users. In light of what you have learned in this section of the chapter, the final activity gets you to focus on what other help and support is available for mental health service users like Feodor.

Student activity 25

As Feodor is an asylum seeker, consider what help and advice you would provide in addition to referring him to the following resources:

http://www.refugeecouncil.org.uk
http://www.asylumaid.org.uk
http://www.asylumsupport.info/nass.htm
http://www.lag.org.uk

Summary

In this chapter you have met four individuals, Sarah, Charlie, Tracy, and Feodor, who are all marginalized service users, each with very different nursing needs. We hope that this chapter has provided you with a robust knowledge base to enable you to work with individuals with such differing backgrounds, and allowed you to think about skills of engagement and communication. As a student nurse we would now like you to consider how you can start to help combat discrimination against individuals and groups with mental health problems, and promote their social inclusion (Department of Health 1999), as you move closer to becoming qualified, registered mental health nurses.

References and other sources

References

American Psychiatric Association (2000). **Diagnostic and statistical manual of mental disorders**, 4th edition, text revision. American Psychiatric Association, Washington DC.

Beat (2007). **Something's got to change** [online] <http://www.b-eat.co.uk>.

British Psychological Societ (2006). **Understanding personality disorder: A report by the British Psychological Society**. British Psychological Society, Leicester.

Corston Report (2007) [online] <http://www.homeoffice.gov.uk/aboutus/news/corston-report>.

Crown Copyright (2002). **Updated drugs strategy**. Crown Copyright, UK.

Dawson D (2007). **Eating Disorders**. Channel 4 programme, March 2007.

Department of Health (1999). **National Service Framework for mental health**. DH, London.

Department of Health (2006). **From values to action: The Chief Nursing Officer's review of mental health nursing**. DH, London.

Dryden W (2007). **Dryden's handbook of individual therapy**. Sage, London.

Duker M and Slade R (1994). **Anorexia nervosa and bulimia: How to help**. Open University Press, Buckingham.

Eating Disorders Association (2002). **It's not about food it's about feelings**. EDA, Norwich.

Eating Disorders Association (2006). **Time to tell**. EDA, Norwich.

Garner DM, Rocket W, Olmsted MP, Johnson C, and Coscina DV (1985). Psychoeducational principles in the treatment of bulimia and anorexia nervosa. In D Garner and PE Garfinkel, eds. **Handbook of psychotherapy for anorexia nervosa and bulimia**, pp. 513-72. Guilford Press, New York.

Hayward (2007). Behind the wire. **Nursing Standard**, **21**(33), 21.

Horne T (2004). Prisoners are among the most vulnerable and least well-served of people using mental health services. **Mental Health Today**, September, 20.

Hsu LK (1996). Epidemiology of the eating disorders. **Psychiatric Clinics of North America 19**(4), 681-700.

Johnson ME (2007). **Hope** (unpublished work).

Kendall PC (2000). **Childhood disorders**. Psychology Press, Hove.

Kernberg OF (2001). The suicidal risk of severe personality disorders: differential diagnosis and treatment. **Journal of Personality Disorder, 15**,195-208.

Linehan MM (1993). **Skills training manual for treating borderline personality disorder**. Guildford Press, New York.

Mental Health Act (2007). HMSO, London.

Mental Health Foundation (1999). **Bright futures: Promoting children and young people's mental health**. Mental Health Foundation, London.

Miller WR and Rollnick S (2002). **Motivational interviewing: Preparing people for change**. Guildford Press, New York.

National Institute for Clinical Excellence (2004). **New guidelines to standardise care for adults, adolescents and older children with eating disorders** [online] <http://www.nice.org.uk>

National Institute for Mental Health in England (2003). **Personality disorder: No longer a diagnosis of exclusion**. DH, London.

National Treatment Agency (2002). **The UK drugs strategy**. National Treatment Agency Publications, London.

National Treatment Agency (2006a). **Care planning practice guide**. National Treatment Agency Publications, London.

National Treatment Agency (2006b). **Models of care for the treatment of adult drug misusers: update 2006**. National Treatment Agency Publications, London.

National Treatment Agency (2006c). **Drug Misusers: update 2006**. National Treatment Agency Publications, London.

Palmer (2001). **Understanding eating disorders**. EDA, London.

Rogers CR (1996). **Client-centred therapy: Its current practice, implications and theory.** Constable, London.

Schilder P (1950). **The image and appearance of the human body**. International Universities Press, New York.

Scott MJ and Straddling SG (2006). **Counselling for post-traumatic stress disorder**, 3rd edition. Sage, London.

Selzer R, Hamill C, Bowes G, and Patton G (1996). The Branched Eating Disorders Test: Validity in a nonclinical population. **International Journal of Eating Disorders**, **20**(1), 57-64.

Smolak L, Levine M, and Thompson JK (2001). Body image in adolescent boys and girls as assessed with Sociocultural Attitudes Towards Appearance Scale. **International Journal of Eating Disorders**, **29**, 216-23.

Thambirajah MS (2007). **Case studies in child and adolescent mental health**. Radcliffe Publishing, Abingdon.

Thompson JK and Smolak L, eds (2001). **Body image, eating disorders and obesity in youth: assessment, prevention, and treatment.** American Psychological Association, London.

Tsai G (2000). Eating disorders in the Far East. **Eating and Weight Disorders**, **5**(4), 83-197.

UK Harm Reduction Alliance (2005) [online] <http://www.ukhra.org>.

Van der Kolk BA (1996) The complexity of adaptation to trauma: self regulation, stimulus discrimination, and characterological development. In BA Van der Kolk, AC McFarlane, and L Weisaeth, eds. **Traumatic stress: the effects of overwhelming experience on mind, body and society**, pp. 182-212. Guildford Press, London.

Vostanis P (2007). Mental health and mental disorders. In J Coleman and A Hagell, eds. **Adolescence, risk and resilience: Against the odds**, pp. 89-106. John Wiley and Sons, Chichester.

Wildes JE, Emery RE, and Simons AD (2001). The roles of ethnicity and culture in the development of eating disturbance and body dissatisfaction: A meta-analytic review. **Clinical Psychology Review**, **21**(4), 521-51.

William R and Miller WR (1994). **Motivational enhancement therapy manual**. Diane Publishing, Darby, PA.

World Health Organization (2007). **International classification of diseases and related health problems**, 10th revision. WHO, Geneva.

Young Minds (2007). **Eating problems: Anorexia nervosa** [online] <http://www.youngminds.org.uk/eatingproblems>.

⊘ Online Resource Centre

You may find it helpful to work through our online material, intended to help you to consider and actively work through issues raised by the cases in this chapter:

ⓐ www.oxfordtextbooks.co.uk/orc/clarke

and choose the online resources for this chapter.

☾ Useful links

http://www.Drugscope.org.uk
http://www.talktofrank.com

◯ Further reading

Gega L (2004). Behaviour techniques. In I Norman and I Ryries, eds. **The art and science of mental health nursing**, pp. 679-718. Open University Press, Maidenhead.

Liddle HA (1995). **Troubled teens: Multidimensional family therapy**. WW Norton, New York.

Polivy J and Herman CP (2002). Causes of eating disorders. **Annual Review of Psychology**, **53**,187-213.

Royal College of Psychiatrists (2006). **Eating Disorders** [online] http://www.rcpsych.ac.uk.

Vitousek K, Watson S, and Wilson GT (1998). Enhancing motivation for change in treatment-resistant eating disorders. **Clinical Psychology Review**, **18**, 391-420.

Chapter 10

On becoming a qualified mental health nurse

Victoria Clarke, Linda Playford, Andrew Walsh

Aims

- To provide students with a comprehensive overview of the fundamental skills and knowledge of a qualified mental health nurse.
- To provide students with guidelines for achieving their first qualified mental health nursing post.
- To provide students with relevant information on career development.

Learning outcomes

- Students will be able to complete relevant application forms/CVs for a mental health nursing post.
- Students will demonstrate the ability to present information in a logical and coherent way.
- Students will be able to participate effectively in role play situations.
- Students will demonstrate an awareness of their personal need to receive support through preceptorship after qualifying.
- Students will recognize their own need for effective clinical supervision.
- Students will recognize the need for lifelong learning.
- Students will demonstrate an ability to use personal reflective skills.

Introduction

In this chapter we will consider the knowledge, skills, and attitudes expected of you as a newly qualified mental health nurse, before discussing how to apply for a job and develop your career. To help you consider this we have tried to include contributions from people who have a range of backgrounds and perspectives, who all contribute to mental health services, including a student about to qualify, a modern matron, a clinical manager, a director of nursing, a professor, and service users.

Becoming a staff nurse

To set the scene, our first personal contribution is from Julie Cresswell, a third year student nurse at the Birmingham City University and the Royal College of Nursing's Student Nurse of the Year 2007. We asked Julie a series of questions that we hoped would help you in preparing to become a qualified nurse; these are her answers and thoughts about the future of mental health nursing and her career.

Preparing to qualify: a student's perspective

by Julie Cresswell

Q: What do you think students should be doing to ready themselves for qualifying?

In preparation for qualifying, I am now reflecting upon the experience, knowledge base, and skills that I have developed during my training, along with the transferable skills that I already had before I embarked upon this career. As mental health nursing students, we will all have followed a similar academic course equipping us with a certain level of theory and practical skills. However, what makes us individual is how we intend to use what we have learned throughout our lives and the philosophy that underpins our work. I began this course with the belief that psychiatric nursing was grounded in science. I now feel that while science can hypothesize about the causes of mental illness, understanding and accepting a client's life experience is central to supporting them in times of mental distress. As I progress through my career, my approach may develop or change direction but for the moment, I feel that it will be vital to be able to communicate my own perspective to future employers. Developing your own approach to mental health nursing, along with an audit of what you can offer an employer in terms of practical skills, knowledge, and experience, establishes your own 'unique selling point' in a competitive jobs market.

Q: What are your issues of concern?

I recently shared with a service user that I wanted to work in an acute inpatient setting at the end of my course. She asked me if I was 'mad'. She qualified this with 'You must be, if you think you can pretend to be nice to someone one minute and then inject them when they won't do what you want'. This concerned me. How can we build therapeutic relationships based upon an unequal power base and the ever present threat of coercion? Is it a widely held belief amongst service users that mental health nurses 'pretend' to be nice in order to achieve concordance? What of Carl Rogers's core conditions – warmth, genuineness, empathy? When I chose to pursue this career I knew that I would be working within a powerful legal framework, but this conversation emphasized to me that however good our intentions may be, what is important to service users is how they perceive their experience of the services they receive. When I am more experienced, will I too agree that the area of nursing I have chosen to pursue rightly deserves its reputation amongst some service users as a place of containment and control … and will I have been complicit in it?

Q: How have your values, knowledge, skills, and attitudes changed over the course?

At the outset of this course, I believed that some communication skills were innate. How could you be taught to listen? One of the most valuable lessons I have learned throughout the course has been to employ the skills needed to actively listen to clients and the importance of being able to communicate that you are listening to them. I have realized that you cannot underestimate the power of providing a 'safe' therapeutic environment where clients can express their thoughts and feelings without being judged.

Q: What have been the significant events for you?

While on placement with a community rehabilitation and recovery team, I interviewed, under supervision, a client who experiences continuous persecutory voices. I explained to the client that I wanted to understand her experiences and current coping strategies with a view to exploring further strategies that may help her to live with her 'voices'. She became distressed as she described how her voices had commanded her to harm herself. At the end of the interview, I asked her how she felt. She stated that the interview had made her realize 'what a waste' she had made of her life, but then thanked me for spending time with her. I felt guilty when the client became distressed. I thought that I had caused this reaction by asking her to recount some of the most upsetting episodes in her life. On reflection, I understand that in order to be able to help people regain some control over their lives, we have to be able to work with them to explore how they have come to often very desperate points in their lives. By exploring her voices I had accepted that this was her experience. I am not sure at the time that this was a conscious action, but from this point, I began to realize that this was not simply a client displaying the symptoms of a mental disorder, but a person in mental distress. She had the right to be listened to in a non-judgemental manner; only by understanding and accepting her experiences can we practise empathetically and only then can we work with our clients to help them find ways of coping and hopefully beginning their journey towards recovery.

Q: Any advice you would offer?

Develop a questioning approach to your own practice, the way in which others practice, and towards your client. Such reflection is not always a comfortable experience, but the ability to learn from experience and improve one's future practice is an essential skill.

Q: How would you envisage mental health nursing developing in the twenty-first century?

Mental health nursing will develop in response to and in spite of political, economic, and demographic changes in our society. In the UK, the thrust of consecutive government policy has moved the care of people in mental distress from inpatient units into the community. If amendments to the Mental Health Act 1983 receive support in Parliament, the onus of caring for people who are in mental distress will be further placed upon carers. This factor, considered in conjunction with the major gaps that have been reported in the primary care targets of the *National Service Framework*, will place immense pressure on mental health professionals. It seems that the government has decided that the community is the place to be – but is this realistic? What does this policy say to the service users who are in our inpatient services, and what of the staff who work in acute care? I envisage that unless the emphasis upon care in the community has the necessary resources to provide a comprehensive mental health service, acutely unwell people will be left without the support they need and their families will suffer as a consequence.

In addition, large numbers of political and economic migrants entering the UK, many suffering the trauma of experiences in their war-torn nations, will present mental health services with another challenge.

I feel that closer collaboration with our service users is the most effective way to develop services that most closely match their needs. The movement to challenge psychiatry and the labels that our clients are given is gaining momentum through groups such as the Campaign for the Abolition of the Schizophrenic Label (see the links at end of this chapter). However, I feel that such groups will be limited in their impact unless the psychiatry profession, whose existence is based upon the pathologizing of mental illness, undergoes a revolution! Mental health nurses can strive to challenge the stigma that mental health problems carry with them by supporting our clients in their recovery, looking beyond their diagnosis to understand the person and their experience.

Q: Finally, what is your vision of the future of mental health nursing?

It would be wonderful if there were giant 'ears' on the end of every street corner, in every workplace and in every school. We all want to be listened to. Consecutive service user research reiterates this. This requires investment and planning. We need a mental health service that is properly resourced with experienced, regular staff with an understanding of their clients' needs, instead of the false economy of a workforce made up of temporary staff who require no long-term investment in training or pensions but fulfil the budgetary requirements of their employers. Their transience does not promote the establishment of therapeutic relationships, the basic requirement of any nursing intervention. The future of mental health nursing is dependent upon addressing the question of what keeps the mentally 'well' from becoming 'ill'? There needs to be continued investment in mental health promotion from the antenatal stage, through the education system and in our workplaces. I want a client-centred, responsive service that treats clients holistically, daring to venture outside the framework of the medical model. We need to listen to our clients, to negotiate, not dictate, their care needs.

Getting a job

The next part of this chapter focuses on how you can prepare to get a mental health nursing job. The NHS has been developing a website on which it is intended to host all health care professional vacancies (see the web links on p. 275 for details). You can also look at nursing journals, local health care provider websites, read local and national press adverts, or access careers advice from your university or local employment centre. Many universities offer job fairs to help students find work (a key benchmark for universities is how employable their graduates are).

```
Dear Sir/Madam 1

I am writing to you regarding your recent advert, for a mental health staff nurse. 2

Please could you either send the relevant application form to . . . or email to . . . 3

Many thanks for your help in this matter.

Yours faithfully 4

Name
Notes
1. Use the person's full name if you know it, if not it doesn't hurt to go with a formal
approach such as Dear Sir/Madam.
2. Try to be concise and to the point. Identify any code or reference number associated
with the advert, include the date of any journal in which you saw the advert, and
clearly state what the post is.
3. Make sure you include your full address and ensure that you identify your email
address correctly.
4. Be polite and courteous.
```

Figure 10.1 A sample letter/email

Applying for a qualified nursing post – the first approach

Once you have identified a post to apply for, you will need an application form if required, or to send in your curriculum vitae (CV). You may need to write a letter or email to do this (see Figure 10.1).

Producing a curriculum vitae/ completing your application form

On the website we have provided you with a sample CV and a blank template that you can use in your search for work.

   www.oxfordtextbooks.co.uk/orc/clarke

and choose the online resources for Chapter 10.

Most health care posts would expect you to complete an application form, which is usually very much like a CV. It's well worth photocopying the original form and doing a rough draft before you transfer over the details for the forms that you will send in. It's very

easy to make mistakes and you should ensure that the form they receive is the best it can be.

Remember, you are out to impress a potential employer. It's important that you fully complete the form as required, because if there is competition for a post an incomplete form will go straight into the bin. It is important to be honest and detailed in your application form. Make sure that you include the relevant dates in relation to your history and qualifications; employers like to be able to see that a person has developed and progressed through their careers and education. Your opportunity to impress a potential employer is within the supporting information/ additional information section of the form. It is essential that you target the post you are applying for in this section. If you are going for a job working with older people with mental health problems, you need to not only expand on your experiences of working with this client group, but also demonstrate how your other experiences are transferable to this post.

Student activity 1
You may find it useful to jot down your ideas in relation to the following questions as a way of coming up with your supporting information for an application form.

- *Why do you want this job?*
- *Why do you want to work with this client group?*
- *Why do you want to work for this organization?*
- *What previous experience have you had working in this area?*
- *What other relevant experience have you had that would help you be successful in this post?*
- *What are your relationships like with service users?*
- *What nursing activities did you participate in with mental health service users in this client group in your previous experience?*
- *What are your particular strengths when working with mental health service users?*
- *What are your relationships like with staff?*
- *How do you work in a multi-professional team?*
- *Did you take on particular responsibility for specific activities while working as a student nurse in this area?*
- *Did you make any innovations in practice settings as a student nurse?*
- *What are the personal qualities that you would bring to this post?*
- *What opportunities do you think this post offers to you?*
- *Write about what you would do if successful in getting this job and how you would like to develop it.*

Getting a reference

It is customary when applying for most posts in nursing that you will need to provide at least two references. As a student about to qualify it is usual to ask your personal tutor or university lecturer to provide one of these but it is also important that you ask a clinical nurse you have worked with to provide the other reference. From September 2007 all student nurses commencing their education require a 'sign off mentor', and it may be useful to include this person as your second reference (Nursing and Midwifery Council 2006c). This is a clinician who will sign to say that you are fit for purpose and fit to practise as a qualified nurse.

Getting an interview

Hopefully your hard work and effort in this application will result in you being called for interview. Some organizations will offer a preliminary visit before the interviews take place, and it is well worth taking this opportunity. You can see the services provided, meet staff, and ask questions, all of which can demonstrate a real commitment to getting this post and can be a useful part of preparing for interview.

Preparing for an interview

When you have been offered an interview, you should find out as much as possible about the service (the organization's website is a good place to start). Research both the organization and the specific service you are applying to. Look for the organization's annual report, and their strategic aims, objectives, and mission statement, as these will give an idea of the organization's priorities. You can then refer to this information when it comes to interview. For example if you are asked about how you see the service developing, you can demonstrate that you have done research and mention organizational goals that fit in with your own ideas for the post.

Student activity 2

When attending an interview, remember that how you present yourself will influence the outcome. You may think that the calibre of your work, your ability and references sh ould have the greatest impact and hopefully they do, but people are influenced by how you look, so take this into consideration when attending an interview.

Consider the following questions in your preparation:

- *What is the message I want the panel to get when I first walk in the room?*
- *What do I want people to think of when they look at me?*
- *If I was a mental health service user, or their relative or carer, how would I like the first person I meet on a unit or from a team to look?*
- *If I was a nurse manager, how would I want the team I represented to present themselves? What message would I like them to convey through their appearance?*
- *If I was interviewing someone for a newly qualified nurse's post, how would I expect them to present themselves?*

We asked Rose Cochrane, a modern matron at Birmingham and Solihull Mental Health Trust who is frequently involved in recruitment interviews, to sum up her advice based upon her experience of conducting interviews with newly qualified nurses.

An interviewer's advice for job interviews, by Rose Cochrane

First impressions *are* important and there are things you can do to ensure you are prepared.

- Be on time – if you are unfamiliar with the area where your interview is being held, do a trial run prior to the interview. Arriving at the interview late and looking harassed does not give the best impression.

- Dress smartly – your appearance will give an impression to others about you even before you get the opportunity to speak.

- Prepare for the interview – think about possible questions you will be asked related to the position applied for and practise in role play.

- Research the role and position you are applying for, as this will show the interviewer that you have a real interest in this position rather than just 'getting a job'.

- Preparation prior to the interview will also increase your confidence and help you feel more at ease, resulting in increasing the interviewer's confidence in you.

- As hard as it is, do try to relax and be aware of non-verbal body language. The position you are applying for is likely to include client contact and be dependent on good communication skills, so mumbling throughout the interview or staring at the carpet is not going to impress on the interviewer that you have these skills and abilities.

The points above might appear to be common sense but having experience as an interviewer for recruitment of staff, I can assure you that people attending interviews do not always sell themselves well. I have personal experience of interviewing potential employees who have presented as unmotivated, with no interest in the position they have applied for, and who have shown no evidence that they have even taken the time to look at the job description and person specification. Being asked at the end of the interview what the position is for does not fill the interviewers with confidence, as most people, I think it is fair to say, would expect someone to know what position they are applying for.

Finally, always request feedback. Sometimes we are not aware of things we may do, especially when in situations that are anxiety-provoking such as interviews. If we don't know where we are going wrong, how can we improve? Feedback is not just about identifying things we could improve on, it's also about things we are doing well and can continue to do.

Remember that the interview panel want you to succeed and interview well because they want to feel confident that they are offering the position to the best person for the job. If that's you then you need to do all you can to convince them.

Being successful at interview

Many organizations will have a panel of staff present to interview you. There will often be a representative from Human Resources/Personnel and they are usually there to ensure that equal opportunity and legal requirements are met by the panel. You are also likely to meet members of the team you would be working with if successful, alongside service user and carer representatives. Often the panel will ask you about information you have provided on your application form, specific questions about your employment and educational history, why you want the post, and what you have to offer it. It is also becoming increasingly common for organizations to include an additional two elements in the interviewing process. The first of these is where the applicant is asked to prepare a 10–15 minute presentation on a specific topic. The second element is role play; during an interview someone will ask you specific clinical situation-type questions and then ask you to respond to them as if they were a service user, carer, or colleague.

Presentations

In preparing a presentation for interview, it's useful to start with a structured approach. You may want to consider using the following outline as a starting point.

- Aim: this should state what you intend to do in your presentation.

- Objectives: these should outline how you will achieve your aim, or simply put how you will do this.

- Definition of terms/subject area: it's useful for you to demonstrate your understanding of the topic being presented.
- Development 1: you may go on to provide some views of the topic from others.
- Development 2: you might consider what issues have influenced the subject previously and how it could develop in the future.
- Development 3: you may decide to include professional, carer, and service user perspectives on the subject area.
- Check for understanding.
- Provide a summary of your presentation.
- Conclusion: highlight the main arguments or thrust of your presentation.
- Provide an opportunity for questions and answers.

There are many tools to assist you in presenting your information to the interview panel. You could use paper handouts, overhead transparencies, or PowerPoint as examples, but always check that the interview site has the equipment you need before you commit to one method only.

Role play in an interview

If you are asked to participate in role play, it is important that you are measured in your response. One strategy that may help is to regulate your breathing and work on being relaxed. Once you're put into a situation, take time to decide how best to react and what best to say. Clarify as much as possible to avoid misunderstanding and reflect on your core skills, seeking to demonstrate these (see Chapters 2 and 9). Be prepared to ask questions. Remember, you have support systems to turn to in practice for help; don't be afraid

to indicate that you will check with someone senior if you think this is appropriate. At the same time, you do need to demonstrate an ability to make effective clinical decisions in pressured situations. To establish your priorities in the role play situation, think about what you must, should, and could do. Remember that your interviewers are trying to get an idea about whether you know how to practise safely.

After the interview

If you have been successful, it's a good strategy to ask for post-interview feedback, if available, and use the opportunity to focus on how you could improve and develop your interviewing skills to enhance your career opportunities. Ask what you did well that impressed them but also ask what you could improve upon and how you could enhance your interviewing skills.

Obviously if you weren't successful it's vital to get some feedback on where you didn't succeed and how you could improve your interview skills. Exposing yourself to criticism is never easy but work on trying to manage how you receive the information they give you. Ask them to identify where you went wrong, if there were any specific concerns they had about the content of what you were saying, or any specific attitudinal or presentation aspects about yourself that led to you not getting the job. It is useful to end the feedback session on something positive that you could seek to enhance – perhaps you could ask if they thought you had any particular strengths. You also need to walk away from this feedback with a sense of learning about yourself and how you could develop. Try not to take the feedback personally; rather try to reflect upon what the person tells you and seek to develop your self-awareness and learn positive lessons.

Developing your career

This is an exciting time to enter the profession of mental health nursing, as recent years have been a time of great change (and sometimes challenge!) and this 'revolution' shows little sign of abating. Up until relatively recently the profession was dominated by the influence of institutional attitudes and practices and in many areas associated with a custodial and over-medicalized approach to its clients. As the biggest group in the mental health service workforce, it is certain that nurses will continue to react to and to shape the changes currently taking place (see Box 10.1).

Recent years have seen a change in and a broadening of the career possibilities open to mental health nurses. In the past, mental health nursing careers were largely hospital-based with a move towards management and away from client contact being the main way that people could advance their careers. There is now, however, a greater range of possibilities for people who want to develop their careers, for example nurse consultants were introduced in 1999 as part of an attempt to expand nursing careers. Nurse consultants have become a familiar part of the mental health nursing workforce (if still having a somewhat unclear

- Move from a largely institutionalized service towards a more community-based model of care.
- Mental health nurse training undertaken in academic settings.
- Rise of 'consumerism' generally in health services.
- Rise of Internet and knowledge availability – people able to access information more easily.
- Increasingly vocal resistance and questioning of current service provision by service user-led interest groups.
- Purely medical model approach is increasingly questioned.
- Move towards consideration/adoption of wider range of therapeutic techniques.
- Pressure to adopt more research-based practices.
- Increasing tendency of government to produce guidance about desired standards (i.e. *National Service Framework for mental health*, Department of Health 1999).

Box 10.1 What factors have caused (and will continue to cause) professional change?

role definition) and are generally seen as helping to maintain and promote good quality and standards with both a teaching and a research base to their practice. There has also been a great increase in services provided by the private sector and voluntary groups, all of whom value the skills that mental health nurses can bring to the organization.

Whatever route you have taken to achieve the status of registered mental health nurse, it will have involved a significant personal investment of time and energy. It is understandable that most people reach the end of their training with some feelings of relief that this stage of their lives is over. It would be a mistake, however, to come to the conclusion that there is no further need for development. The Nursing and Midwifery Council (NMC 2001) uses the term 'fitness to practise at the point of registration' to describe the level of competence that should be achieved by a newly qualified practitioner. This is recognition that you will basically be ready for life as a registered nurse; it is categorically not an invitation to stop the development process that you began the day you commenced your nurse training! In fact it would certainly be a mistake to imagine that anyone ever reaches a stage of professional development that could be labelled as 'finished', and the best practitioners understand that mental health nursing is a process of continuing personal and professional development.

It is important that you do not attempt to do anything that you do not feel confident and competent to handle. Often, newly qualified staff find it difficult to admit that they are unsure about areas of knowledge; the NMC advice is quite clear, however:

> You must acknowledge the limits of your professional competence and only undertake practice and accept responsibilities for those activities in which you are competent.
> NMC Code of professional conduct (2008)

When you are delegated duties, it is important that you are assertive enough to make it clear to more senior staff if you do not have sufficient knowledge or experience to carry these out. Most clinical areas and managers recognize that newly qualified staff require a period of greater supervision when first starting out and make some provision for this kind of support. The NMC (2006a) has stated that employers should offer preceptorship support; perhaps this is something that you might ask about at interview?

Preceptorship and supervision

Although you have spent the last few years working towards qualifying as a registered nurse, the idea of finishing your training and accepting this responsibility may feel daunting. You can be assured that you are not alone in feeling this – indeed it might be argued that the caution this should bring to your practice is better than being overconfident.

The NMC (2002) suggests that newly qualified nurses should have approximately four months of formal preceptorship support. You may find that the area you eventually work in has a formalized policy on this and if so you will be allocated a named person who will take a special interest in your development and to whom you can turn for advice. Remember though that every qualified nurse with whom you work is potentially someone you can learn from and don't be too proud to take some advice from experienced care assistants, many of whom have developed excellent interpersonal skills from years spent working closely with clients.

In nursing, a supervisory relationship is different in that this is something that is more closely related to your ongoing professional development. During your training you will have become familiar with the idea of reflection on practice and once qualified this is a good way of thinking about what you need to do. The NMC (2002) recommends that you should have access to a more experienced person who can act as a supervisor but again, how this is handled tends to vary from area to area. If your workplace has a supervision policy in place you should access this, but even if they do not you might want to consider approaching a more experienced nurse and asking them about this (see Box 10.2).

Specialization

One of the reasons that studying to be a nurse is so challenging is the wide range of areas that are touched upon in the training programme. A quick walk around any nursing library should confirm this, as

books from a wide range of subject areas are included – sociology, biology, psychology, psychiatry, pharmacology, etc. Many people find that the eclectic nature of nursing knowledge is one of the attractions of studying it but this can also be a little daunting when one is considering what areas to focus upon. As the extract below from *Alice's adventures in Wonderland* suggests, it is important to have a focal point for your travels.

> 'Would you tell me, please, which way I ought to go from here?'
> 'That depends a good deal on where you want to get to,' said the Cat.
> 'I don't much care where – ' said Alice.
> 'Then it doesn't matter which way you go,' said the Cat.
> '– so long as I get somewhere,' Alice added as an explanation.
> 'Oh, you're sure to do that,' said the Cat, 'if you only walk long enough.'
> Taken from *Alice's adventures in Wonderland* (Lewis Carroll 1865).

Ongoing training offered by employers

Remember that it is in the interest of your new employer to continue to develop staff, as any health care organization needs a constant supply of future leaders as well as experienced practitioners and development is an important part of any staff retention

---

- Clinical supervision supports practice, enabling you to maintain and improve standards of care.
- Clinical supervision is a practice-focused professional relationship, involving a practitioner reflecting on practice guided by a skilled supervisor.
- The process of clinical supervision should be developed by practitioners and managers according to local circumstances. Ground rules should be agreed so that you and your supervisor approach clinical supervision openly and confidently and are both aware of what is involved.
- Every practitioner should have access to clinical supervision. Each supervisor should supervise a realistic number of practitioners.
- Preparation for supervisors should be flexible and sensitive to local circumstances. The principles and relevance of clinical supervision should be included in pre-registration and post-registration education programmes.
- Evaluation of clinical supervision is needed to assess how it influences care and practice standards. Evaluation systems should be determined locally.

Taken from *Supporting nurses and midwives through lifelong learning* (NMC 2002).

Box 10.2 Essential characteristics of clinical supervision

policy. Now you are qualified, you will be starting to discover that sometimes the most difficult things you have to cope with are your fellow staff members (as anyone who ever tried to manage a clinical area will confirm!). For this reason, training offered will often include areas such as how to deal with difficult people and how to positively handle complaints as well as more standard career development issues.

Very often people enter mental health nurse training with a fairly clear idea of the sort of specialist area that they wish to practise in once qualified. Frequently, though, these ideas change as people progress through the course and are exposed to different areas of practice. You may well be surprised at the interests you develop and the directions that these new interests lead you. As mentioned above, managers know that a newly qualified staff member is to some extent 'raw material' and will recognize their responsibility to help in your professional development.

Each different clinical area, as well as sharing core values and skills, will have a further level of more specialist knowledge in which it will be important for you to develop skills. For example if you work with older people then you will need to develop knowledge about dementia care and the physiology of ageing, whereas clearly if you are working with children a different skill set will be required. As mentioned above, mental health nursing is in a state of great change and there is a growing need for people to master skills that previously were less commonly considered by the profession.

There is currently something of a backlash against a purely medical approach, and while medication will continue to be important, there is an increased need for people trained in other therapies, of which cognitive therapy and to some extent brief therapies are receiving a lot of attention (Department of Health 2007).

Most training institutions run more specialist courses for post-registration students and this is a good place to start looking if you want to undertake further education. You are likely to be asked to become a mentor/assessor for current student nurses in your area quite soon and training for such a role will almost certainly be provided by the institution from which they come (remember that it is in the best interests of the training institution to try and improve the quality of student experience in placement).

In recent years there has been an emphasis placed on the importance of research-based practice in health services. The NMC code of conduct (2008) clearly states that your care must be based on the best available evidence, and consequently all nurse training includes an introduction to nursing research. The ability to read research and weigh up the consequences for your practice is important, especially as we and our clients are now exposed to so many sources of information. In the past, knowledge about health care issues was largely confined to professional groups and the public had to rely far more on professionals to access information. Wider access to sources of information via the Internet has changed this situation for ever – understandably, people who are referred to mental health services will often access all manner of information. Unfortunately, the quality and reliability of this information will vary wildly; some will be excellent but some will be poor or potentially dangerous. Increasingly then, the public relies upon us to help differentiate what is useful and what is not.

Most health care trusts employ people who have a research background (certainly this is something you can expect a nurse consultant to be familiar with) and often there will also be research interest groups you can join. Taking an active part in research projects is an excellent way of familiarizing yourself with the research process and from a career development point of view is an attribute valued by employers.

Personal profile development

As you will be aware, you are required to maintain a professional profile (NMC 2006b) in order to be able to demonstrate evidence of your ongoing professional development when you need to re-register with the NMC. The activities you have read about so far in this section on developing your career are aspects of your professional life that you should be recording in your own portfolio. Remember, your portfolio is something that is personal to you; the NMC or your employer does not own it and cannot demand to see it. A fuller description of profile development is beyond the scope of this chapter but you will find guidance on the NMC website (NMC 2006b) or by reading Stuart (2007).

In this, the final chapter, we have sought to encourage you to consider how you can develop your mental health nursing knowledge and skills. In order to support you in this we have asked a range of people to offer you their perspectives on mental health nursing. As an end to this section on career development, Bertha Matunge, who qualified in 2006, writes about her experience of becoming a staff nurse.

My transition from student to staff nurse, by Bertha Matunge

On leaving university I felt confident, motivated, and ready to provide excellent nursing care. Having achieved excellent marks at university and done very well on my placements I felt that becoming a staff nurse would be easy. However, bridging the gap between student and staff nurse was more challenging than I had anticipated.

My first post was a busy 24-bedded adult male acute ward. Not only was the transition to a new environment difficult, the support system I had as a student was no longer there, and I found myself immediately in the role of an accountable and autonomous professional – I had to start thinking and acting like a qualified nurse.

I was allocated to an enthusiastic and knowledgeable mentor. Both my mentor and the rest of the team were quite supportive; however, workload, staff shortages, and pressure of time meant that they could not always provide me with the kind of support I really needed. I had to just jump in and become a member of the team, and although in theory I had a period of supernumerary status, in practice it was not the case. Even when I needed things to be explained it always seemed rushed. I found the reality of practice was nothing compared to the ideal.

Although I did have sufficient knowledge, I lacked experience, and no amount of preparation could have lessened the challenges and stresses that came with the transition. Skills in which I had been confident and practiced as a student, e.g. injection techniques, suddenly I worried about because I did not have the safety net of being a student. I found developing clinical judgement was something that can only come with experience.

Another difficulty was establishing and developing professional relationships, especially with untrained staff. I found delegating to experienced care assistants quite difficult.

What helped me to survive through this transition were the reflective skills I had learned through my time at university. I kept a diary that helped me constantly reflect on my practice, correct mistakes, learn from them, and build on my strengths.

I have learned that no amount of preparation can eradicate the stress that comes with the transition from being a student to a staff nurse, it can only lessen it. Looking back now I can compare the transition period to learning to ride a bicycle. Once the period is over it becomes so much fun and very exciting. Yes, there are still days I meet new challenges, but now I don't feel daunted or overwhelmed. I realize now that reflecting upon the challenges I encountered during my transition actually made me more confident and competent. I am able to work innovatively and I always commit myself to providing holistic care. I am developing clinical judgement and I also appreciate the importance of teamwork, especially working in a busy clinical area.

What will be expected of you as a newly qualified mental health nurse?

Mental health trusts strive to provide high quality, safe services to people with mental health difficulties – at whatever stage of their illness or recovery. The newly qualified mental health nurse will need to ensure they can adapt to a dynamic and evolving NHS. The following is from Ros Alstead, Director of Nursing at Birmingham and Solihull Mental Health Trust, which is the third largest mental health trust in England with a large nursing workforce.

If you had not already noticed it as a student nurse, as a qualified nurse you will become aware that services have to be planned and delivered around the needs of service users and not staff.

Foundation trusts are a new type of NHS organization, called a 'Public Benefit Corporation', answerable to local communities. Foundation trusts remain part of the NHS and continue to follow the principles and standards of the NHS – for example not charging people for their care, not being run for profit, and being subject to regular inspection. The difference is that foundation trusts are able to work more closely with communities to develop services in the way that best suits their needs and also have greater financial freedoms. Put simply, anyone interested in what the trust does can apply to become a member of that trust, and if they want even closer involvement, they

What is expected from newly qualified nurses as professionals,
by Ros Alstead, Director of Nursing

Newly qualified nurses are equipped with a sound knowledge base and come with a fresh perspective and energy into practice. In order to flourish and become confident and capable practitioners, they need to be true to their values and draw on their up-to-date knowledge, and begin to practise in an open, non-discriminatory, and authentic way. Sound supervision to promote this through preceptorship is essential and it is important to be assertive to ensure this is in place.

Newly qualified nurses need curiosity to understand the environment and context they are working in. Forming effective therapeutic relationships with users and carers and learning how to work within integrated multidisciplinary teams are fundamental foundations. Learning on the job from peers and colleagues forms the basis for ongoing professional development, bedding in much of what has been learned at university. This is an exciting and memorable part of our careers as mental health nurses. Being open to ongoing learning opportunities makes us all better practitioners throughout our career; this needs to be established right at the start of becoming a nurse, ruthlessly making time to reflect and improve whatever barriers such as workload are put in your way.

can apply to be elected as a governor. The governors work with the trust's board of directors to agree the future plans of the organization. The governors also have the right to appoint the trust's chairperson and non-executive directors.

The services provided follow the strategic plan of each mental health trust. They are based upon:

- Local needs.
- Health Care Commission requirements, e.g. provision of drug action teams and early intervention services.
- Legislative drivers, e.g. the Mental Health Act.
- Government targets in relation to demographic changes, national reports, and investigations of where things went wrong, and health improvement plans, which target groups and regions to improve health outcomes for vulnerable groups.

Up to 80 per cent of direct NHS care is provided by nurses, working in all settings and across all age ranges. In mental health, nurses are the largest occupational group. Ros Alstead confirms this as she states:

> Mental health nurses form approximately 50 per cent of the Trust workforce with an even greater presence amongst those working clinically. On a daily basis, service users and carers in Birmingham and Solihull depend on the values, knowledge, skills, and expertise of our mental health nurses, who are there either to support people with complex mental health problems in crisis, work with people until they recover, or for others are the lifeline of support throughout their lifetime.

Nurses work across all services provided, giving professional continuity throughout the entire patient

What is expected from newly qualified nurses as employees,
by Elaine Massey, Clinical Manager

Accountability
Gone now are the days when someone was accountable for you – you are now accountable for your own actions or omissions. But remember, even though you are now fully accountable, you are not

strictly on your own – you have a range of resources available:

- An experienced nurse as a mentor.
- Opportunity to discuss clinical practice in clinical supervision.
- Ask about attending preceptorship courses or schemes.

It is normal to be concerned about having so much more responsibility and accountability – but please keep this in perspective.

Day of arrival

On arrival at your first ward, there are several things to remember:

- Dress appropriately. This may seem a trivial issue – but do remember that a nurse who looks neat and tidy is likely to inspire confidence in the team, your clients, and their relatives.

- Always manage a smile, even when the going gets tough, as it helps you remain approachable.

- Show up prepared and ready to contribute to the team.

- Take a notebook to record any important information and don't be afraid to use it.

The first week

No amount of studying can prepare you for actual clinical practice – you can draw on knowledge learned but then you soon realize you still have a lot to learn.

- Ask for help – as a beginner it is usually expected that you will and should ask for help when you need it.

- Ask questions – more experienced staff feel more comfortable when questions are asked of them, rather than them assuming you need to know every minor detail. Be proactive and ask for advice – look for someone who is approachable and works efficiently. When you are feeling overwhelmed and fearful, stay calm and ask questions. Paying attention to answers sends the message that you are trying to learn and develop yourself. A questioning attitude is a positive and healthy approach, and helps create a learning environment. It also keeps the ward staff on their toes!

- Show appreciation to someone who has helped or guided you – they too like to feel valued.

- Start with planning, organizing, and prioritizing your tasks – watch more senior staff organize their shift. The desire to give the very best care can be an enormous burden for a newly trained nurse – so learn to sort out your priorities.

Mistakes

Everyone can make mistakes. Mistakes come in all sizes and shapes; of course it is best to avoid mistakes, especially when they do harm to a patient. The most important thing to remember for the new nurse is to allow a mistake to become an opportunity for learning, so you don't make the same mistake again!

As you progress through your career and with the complexity of your role increasing, mistakes will occur. You should admit to the mistake and take responsibility for it. You need to reflect on how the mistake occurred and ask yourself how you can prevent a mistake reoccurring.

Taking this approach should help you gain some credibility with your colleagues. Promoting an attitude that links mistakes to opportunities for growth helps the nurse feel more relaxed and makes it less likely that the mistake will reoccur.

Client care

The reception given to clients will have an effect on their morale. If you are pleasant and courteous, you are welcomed. Always managing that smile, even when the going gets hard, shows compassion and understanding.

When caring for others, one should consider the total needs of the individual and not just those associated with the reason for admission. It is so important that nurses listen carefully to their clients if they are to have a meaningful relationship.

It is also important to emphasize firstly that you must recognize each person as an individual, and secondly that each individual has their own unique physical, psychological, social, and spiritual needs. You should be conscious that the building and the maintaining of relationships is your responsibility.

Always ensure you ask the client for their consent when undertaking any direct care or have any physical contact. Once consent has been gained for the intervention, you should ensure it is recorded into the client's medical file.

Relatives and carers

The most important thing for relatives and carers is that you are available and approachable to them. It is often necessary to go and meet them and not wait for them to come to you; many relatives are afraid to go and seek information, especially if it means knocking on the office door.

Taking care of yourself

How can you be a good nurse if you don't take care of yourself? Take plenty of exercise, and try and keep fit. Nursing can be a strenuous job.

Always take a snack with you to work, as you never know when you will require a 'pick-me-up'. You don't need to be a nurse long to realize that the demands are high.

pathway. When choosing your employer, remember that mental health nurses play key roles in the non-statutory and independent sectors as well as within the NHS. The newly qualified mental health nurse has a range of clinical settings and roles to choose from, including providing intimate physical care through to formal psychological approaches, and from directly applying constraints under the Mental Health Act to spending extended periods of unstructured time with service users. Additionally, the two-thirds of qualified nurses who work in inpatient care areas also have direct health and safety responsibilities and responsibility for managing the environment.

The mental health nurse as an employee

We asked Elaine Massey, who is a unit manager/carers lead at a mental health trust, for her perspective on what is expected of a newly qualified mental health nurse.

The expectations of the newly qualified mental health nurse as an employee are governed by two forces – the Nursing and Midwifery Council, and their employer trust requirements. Simply speaking, the mental health nurse must work within the code of professional conduct for nurses (NMC 2008) and comply with trust contractual requirements, which includes adherence to local and national polices, procedures, and guidelines. In this section these are explained under the following headings:

- Clinical governance and the newly qualified mental health nurse.
- Continual professional development.
- Policies and procedures.

Clinical governance and the newly qualified mental health nurse

The newly qualified mental health nurse will contribute to the clinical governance of the area in which they are employed. They will:

- Take a proactive role in the management of clinical risk by risk assessments, reporting incidents and near misses (revisit Chapter 5 and look at the examples of good practice around risk management).
- Take all reasonable precautions to ensure a safe and secure environment for themselves and others in accordance with health and safety legislation.
- Ensure compliance with policies, procedures, and clinical guidelines (including NICE guidelines of relevance to your area of work).

- Participate in the setting, maintenance, and improvement of standards of care through participation in clinical supervision, clinical reviews, learning from incidents work, and individual continual professional development.
- Participate in the monitoring of standards and quality of nursing care, through benchmarking, audit, and research.
- Participate in patient and public involvement activities.
- Promote people's equality, diversity, and rights.
- Work collaboratively and cooperatively with others to meet the needs of patients and their families.

Continuing professional development

Your new employer ensures standards are maintained by recruiting, developing, and retaining the best workforce via teaching, research, reputation, and ongoing development programmes. The newly qualified nurse will participate in identifying their own training and development needs on an ongoing basis and annually at their appraisal. Your employer will require you to:

- Attend an induction programme.
- Contribute to the induction and training of new staff members and pre-registration students, acting as a mentor to students as required.
- Develop your own skills and knowledge and seek training where gaps are evident.
- Comply with mandatory training requirements, e.g. basic food hygiene certificate, basic life support, fire update, manual handling, infection prevention and control, etc.

Policies and procedures

The newly appointed mental health nurse should acquaint themselves with key policies and guidelines of their employer, which dictate their practice at a local and national level. Examples of such policies include:

- Management of serious untoward incidents.
- Health and safety at work.
- Management of potential and actual aggression (MAPPA).
- Manual handling.
- Hygiene code.

- Therapeutic observations (including levels of patient observation and what they mean).
- Protection and safeguarding vulnerable adults and children (POVA).
- Clinical supervision.
- Medicines Code.
- Patient leave policy.
- Incident recording.
- Clinical audit.
- Whistleblower policy.

The areas relating to the role of the newly qualified mental health nurse are further explained in terms of how they apply in practice in Box 10.3.

Clinical

- Assessment, planning, implementation, and evaluation of the evidence-based care required, including health promotion for named service users.
- Report and record any changes in the service user's mental/physical/emotional state in the care plan, and to the nurse-in-charge.
- Receive monthly clinical supervision from an identified supervisor.
- Assist in the development of clinical skills within the nursing team to a level of agreed competence, using evidence-based practice.
- Ability to engage, assist, and support carers and family members.
- Establish therapeutic relationships with service users, and implement evidence-based therapeutic interventions with appropriate boundaries.
- Maintain a safe environment and the safety of patients, staff, and visitors. This includes frequently responding to distressed and disturbed behaviour in a way that protects the safety, privacy, and dignity of the individual and others.
- Ensure that patients and carers/relatives are involved in the planning and delivery of care and that they receive a copy of their care plan.
- Participate in carers' assessments when required.
- Ensure patient needs are met by working collaboratively with other professionals and agencies, especially in relation to ongoing care needs.
- Promote good standards of cleanliness of the ward/clinical environment and the control, reduction, and prevention of hospital-acquired infection.

Professional

- Participate in research, service modernization, and clinical governance.
- Ensure confidentiality is maintained at all times in accordance with the data protection act, trust policy, and good practice.
- Conduct yourself in a professional manner towards service users, carers, colleagues, and other agencies.

- Participate in joint working with appropriate experts/agencies.
- Limit your actions to those that you feel competent to undertake.
- Maintain active status on NMC Register.
- Act in accordance with NMC code of conduct and guiding documents.
- Adhere to trust policies and procedures.
- Maintain up-to-date skills and knowledge and awareness of professional issues.
- Maintain a professional portfolio.
- Seek to gain nationally recognized qualifications in psychological therapies relevant to role, e.g. cognitive behavioural therapy, solution focused therapy, dementia care mapping.

Organizational

- Contribute and work towards the service/organizational aims and objectives.
- Understand your responsibility for respecting and promoting issues of spirituality, equality, diversity, and rights.
- Responsible for reading, understanding, and complying with all relevant trust and statutory policies and procedures:
  - A sound knowledge of Care Programme Approach, Health of the Nation Outcome Scale, and risk assessment/management.
  - A sound knowledge of child protection procedures.
- Ability to work over a 24-hour rota.
- Ensure health and safety policies are adhered to.
- Ensure working practices in line with the requirements of the NMC, Mental Health Act, and trust policies and procedures.

Leadership

- Lead by example while being able to acknowledge your own weaknesses and those of others and address them.
- Work within a framework commensurate with your level of knowledge and competence and act accordingly within your sphere of responsibility.
- Ensure you comply with current good practice in informing/updating all members of the multidisciplinary team, colleagues, service users, and appropriate others of changes involving current nursing care plans, progress, mental state, and psychosocial factors in line with best practice.
- Team worker, i.e. ability to develop supportive relationships with colleagues and experience of working collaboratively across professional boundaries.

Box 10.3 Key areas of responsibility for mental health nurses in practice

Mental health nursing – future roles and responsibilities

In the last few years, a number of new roles have been introduced, for example modern matrons and nurse consultants. Also, new skills have been developed, for example nurse prescribing in mental health. In the future, the landscape of mental health nursing is likely to change even more radically with the introduction of New Ways of Working (National Institute for Mental Health in England 2004).

New Ways of Working (NWW) represents a cultural shift in services whereby distributed responsibility is shared amongst team members and is no longer dominated by a single professional group, such as consultant psychiatrists. The principles of NWW lie in how professional groups could extend the boundaries of what they do. NWW describes further opportunities for new roles, such as introduction of advanced practitioners. These changes provide opportunities to make services more service user-centred while delivering high quality care.

In a similar vein, *From values to action: The Chief Nursing Officer's review of mental health nursing* (Department of Health 2006a) made a series of recommendations supporting NWW for mental health nurses. These were developed following a national consultation investigating how mental health nurses could best improve the care provided to service users. A subsequent publication, *Modernising nursing careers* (Department of Health 2006b), provides a broad strategy for the future of nursing across the United Kingdom. It proposes actions that support many of the concepts of NWW and the recommendations of the Chief Nursing Officer's review.

Implications of NWW for mental health nursing practice

Future service providers will need to review nursing roles and evaluate whether they make best use of the range of nursing skills – i.e. ensure that nurses focus on working directly with individuals who have higher levels of need and/or support other workers in meeting less complex needs. Similarly, service providers will develop shared roles between inpatient and crisis home treatment staff. Further development of nurse prescribing roles based on local need and taking into account the potential for service redesign and skill mix review will be undertaken.

Graduate and gateway workers' roles in primary care, supporting the provision of a stepped model of care, will be expanded to allow modernization within secondary mental health services. Reduced caseloads will allow consultant psychiatrists to work in an advisory capacity for the majority of their working week. This will involve them radically streamlining their outpatient clinics and the whole team working together for a common aim and offering a diversely developed skill base. There will also be enhanced and different roles for pharmacists, psychologists, junior doctors, and non-professional staff within community mental health teams.

NWW will also have a significant impact on inpatient care, with each unit having a dedicated inpatient consultant psychiatrist. Care coordinators will regularly visit patients on wards to input into care planning meetings, and multidisciplinary team reviews will be replaced by timetabled sessions when the service users are reviewed at a time convenient to all.

Career paths in mental health nursing, by Professor Mervyn Morris

It is very difficult to predict where your career might take you, because there are so many diverse opportunities, although at the point of qualifying you may feel these are few and far between! When I started training as a nurse 30 years ago I had little idea about my future beyond perhaps aspiring to be a charge nurse one day. I very much looked up to and admired the senior students and qualified nurses I worked with, and feel now as I did then, that no matter what circumstances we work in, we can make an enormous difference to people's lives. My career started in the hospital, where I learned to spend very long periods of time with very distressed people, and this for me is the essence of psychiatric nursing. The most basic of caring skills are the most important: helping people eat, sleep, talk, relax, and feel safe. My mother was also a registered nurse who worked nights, and I learned from her that people in hospital above all else have these most basic needs, often at times when only a nurse is available to meet them. Nurses that I regard as special somehow have developed the ability to give basic care with compassion and communicate a love of people and life, even to someone who feels they are in their darkest and most difficult moment. I know from people who have used services that they remember that 'special' nurse.

Many experiences during my three year nurse training very much shaped my career. First and foremost I was influenced by a placement working on a therapeutic community, which was a ward in the hospital but organized in a completely different way. The day was very much structured around facilitating the residents (patients) to learn about themselves and their relationships through developing a communal environment; people were expected to take a shared responsibility for both the ward and each other. The boundaries between staff and patients were very different, much more open and personal, and yet never compromised our code of professional conduct; and 30 years later I still regularly visit as a friend someone I first met while she was a resident in the community.

I came to believe that all ward environments and time with service users have the opportunity to be therapeutic in this way; that people who have a life of experience that includes mental health problems can understand and help others with similar problems. I have spent much of my career trying to develop an approach to working with people not as patients, but as people with 'lived experience' who have over time developed both wisdom and expertise in living with their difficulties. One example today is my work alongside people who hear voices, a group of people whose experiences I think are generally grossly misunderstood by mental health services. While there are many people who of course struggle to live with these experiences, there are many others who have learned ways of overcoming their voices and other problems, and it is this expertise from experience that I have tried to help capture and pass on to others. 'User involvement' has taken on many meanings in today's health services and, in the way I have come to understand it from my experience, is something I very much believe we as nurses are the most important supporters of.

Psychiatric services began to change dramatically during my first years working as a qualified nurse. The development of community-based mental health services created new career opportunities (and also changed the work of nurses in hospital environments). Working in the community meant spending time with people in very different circumstances, in their own home, no longer trying to look after individuals in the context of managing a ward environment, but instead working with families and the local community as well as the individual. I began to see 'patients' as people in a completely new context, requiring a new set of skills. I had to depend far more on my ability to create a trusting relationship, and came to see myself as someone who could work independently with people's problems. In this respect I undertook additional training in psychotherapy (psychodynamic and systemic family therapy), and then adapted these skills in my work. Part of this training included skills in group work, which (alongside playing football!) helped me to develop my ability to be part of a team and also understand leadership; something that has also been very important in my career.

I have continuously developed myself since qualifying, mostly part-time, often in my own time, and not always by following professional courses. The more I have developed my general interests and grown up as a person – alongside my career focus – the more I have felt confident in being close to people in difficulty. In terms of academic study, the other aspect of my career that I have found very rewarding is research. Understanding research has given me the ability to question and challenge myself and others about practice, and being able to undertake research has given me an opportunity to both better understand and develop nursing and mental health services.

Throughout my career, two themes have been constant: developing new understandings of people and their difficulties, and developing new skills and approaches to offering helpful help. I think finding your own career path as a nurse can be difficult as we often work in organizations that, in a parallel way to what service users often experience, do not see us as individuals. But never have any doubt about your unique potential to give people the strength and opportunity to change their lives and recover from their problems.

The future of mental health nursing

As you contemplate your new career and moving into your first qualified nursing post, it is worth considering what Ros Alstead, Director of Nursing, has to say about the future of mental health nursing.

The future of mental health nursing, by Ros Alstead, Director of Nursing

Mental health nursing has never been a career for the fainthearted. Institutional life in the past had its challenges, accompanied by companionship and the feeling of working together described by some people as 'a big family'. The negative experiences of service users in the old institutional system are hopefully a thing of the past and modern mental health services offer more at an earlier stage to manage and avoid lifelong problems. Service users increasingly are equal partners in deciding options for care and rightly demanding to be fully informed about their condition and treatment. Nurses working within teams work independently more than in the past with regard to decision-making, and increasingly will be refocusing on individuals' physical as well as mental health needs. The development of a range of community services ensures people access services earlier and recover sooner.

Through both genetic and social research we will understand more than we ever have before about the root causes of mental illness. Comprehensively tackling these major public health issues is likely to take much longer and mental health services meanwhile will need to grow, develop, and adapt accordingly. My vision for mental health nurses is to remain adaptable and embrace forthcoming changes, while respecting and never taking for granted the high level of public trust we receive at present. Mental health nurses are highly trusted by the public and this is a privilege we should never take for granted. How we behave and conduct ourselves remains vitally important to the very basis of the therapeutic relationship. This dynamic needs to be nurtured and respected by all or we risk the public losing faith and confidence in what we do and, importantly, the way we do it. My vision for the future involves evolving rather than revolutionizing practice, developing the evidence as well as the art of nursing, always striving to continuously seek the best outcomes for service users and their carers.

A career in mental health nursing

Our next contributor is Professor Mervyn Morris and his contribution demonstrates the potential that mental health nursing offers in terms of a varied and engaging career. Mervyn has strong academic and research ties in both the UK and internationally. Part of his role includes leading the Centre for Community Health Care at Birmingham City University (see http://www.health.bcu.ac.uk/ccmh/index.htm) and working as a Visiting Professor at University College Buskerud in Drammen, Norway, supporting community mental health care developments there. Mervyn also has established links with the World Health Organization in Europe.

His work has a strong emphasis on social perspectives around mental health problems and the recovery approach, as evidenced by his ongoing work with Professor Maris Romme (Romme and Morris 2007). His contribution discusses the importance of valuing people with mental health problems and working with them in mutually respectful learning partnerships.

You may also find it interesting to read a history of mental health nursing by Felicity Stockwell, retired mental health nurse and tutor, which can be found online:

 www.oxfordtextbooks.co.uk/orc/clarke

and choose the online resources for this chapter.

Conclusion by the editors

In this chapter we have sought to provide you with a range of perspectives about mental health nursing. The idea behind this book is to encourage you to develop the fundamental knowledge and skills required in mental health nursing, to think positively about your potential, and hopefully to inspire you to the best possible practice as mental health nurses.

We thought it appropriate that this book should finish as it started by including the opinions of mental health service users. We asked Marion Clarke and Tracey Holley (whose contributions you will have seen throughout the book) to tell us what they think makes a good mental health nurse.

What makes a good mental health nurse – a survivor's perspective

by Tracey Holley

These points are in no particular order, allowing you to reflect upon the importance of each one.

- Emotional intelligence – knowing yourself with all your faults and attributes and being yourself.
- Making a **connection with the person** – and making it on an equal basis.
- Levelling the playing field and knowing there is one – working as a team, knowing me, knowing you, an equal partnership.
- Being able, as far as possible, to put yourself in another's shoes.
- Fostering a relationship which focuses on the commonality of a shared humanness, revealing things about you as a person and not just as a professional in an appropriate and therapeutic way, but at the same time remembering it is not all about you.
- Being self-aware and admitting you are human and that you may not have all the answers as a professional, and sharing this honesty with the person.

- Being empathic, not sympathetic, and knowing the difference.
- Respecting the person's abilities, as well as their vulnerabilities – always ensuring that you tell the person what it is you see in them.
- Facilitating and recognizing potential rather than being too directive; and knowing how to judge when and when not to be directive.
- Realizing that mental distress is not a sign of an unintelligent person; and that mental illness has no boundaries of class or culture.
- Honouring and respecting a person's feelings, emotions, and beliefs, however implausible they seem to you.
- Seeing the person and **not** the illness.
- Believing in someone even when they possess no self-belief of their own.
- Being reassuring with the ability to engender hope – but not false hope – without being patronizing.
- Putting rapport, honesty, and trust before clinical questioning.
- Maintaining a **therapeutic relationship** alongside clinical procedure or questioning as part of your professional responsibility.
- Realizing the need to recap, repeat, reiterate, and reinforce – gently and without fuss, however many times it is needed.
- Displaying patience and understanding at all times, appreciating that mental distress is like a fog, sometimes confusing but often frightening and debilitating.
- Acting as a beacon, a guiding light of **hope** in the darkness of despair of mental illness.
- Understanding the metaphors of describing the indescribable and realizing that for many, their emotional landscape is unchartered territory to them, and that trying to even recognize their emotions let alone to talk about them is seemingly impossible.
- Realizing that mental distress is a very **isolating** experience and thereby making that **connection** and planting that seed of **hope** is vital.

What makes a good mental health nurse – a service user's perspective

by Marion Clarke

The important skills I would highlight are:

- Listening.
- Observation.
- Communication.

All of the above would include the carer as well as the service user.

Knowledge

It is important to know what has been written about mental distress in its various forms, but not to use labels and diagnoses as a dogma, a set of statements and interpretations which are unchangeable.

It is equally important to know about the user/survivor movement and what mental health service users have done for themselves; what they say about their condition and what is needed for recovery. Within this, it needs to be understood that concepts like 'recovery' should not also become dogmatic – 'recovery' means different things to different people and needs to be defined by the person.

Nurses also need an understanding of stages in a process of recovery, and appropriateness – e.g. CBT can be useful at certain times, but not always.

Values

The fundamental one centres on equality and the ability to ask – as well as answer – the question: how would I like to be treated if I were in the other person's place?

The concept of working *with* someone as an equal has to be understood.

Attitudes

Practitioners need to be mature enough to be non-judgemental and to be aware of their own values and attitudes. What prism is being used to view the person in front of them? Which stereotypes are in operation? Does some thinking need to be changed?

This requires practitioners to have not just depth of knowledge around mental distress and mental health, but also to have an open-minded, questioning attitude towards other people and life in general. This doesn't mean that one person should know everything, but that they should be prepared to question and recognize that learning is an ongoing process.

In general, thinking about mental health services, I would say that the most important characteristics should be flexibility and the provision of sanctuary. Flexibility starts at the very beginning when someone asks for help; it means the willingness not to look first for a framework to slot people into, but at what the person is saying or indicating about themselves. What is then offered in terms of services needs to be diverse.

Flexibility would also mean a change in hierarchical ways of working. The fact is that at crucial times nurses spend a lot of time with service users; I feel that their observations and conclusions should carry more weight than they seem to at present. This has implications for research as well.

Sanctuary needs to be provided for people in different ways and at different times: in crisis and for respite and as part of recovery. This also applies to practitioners themselves; mental and emotional distress is exhausting and drains people of energy, both those who are experiencing it as well as those who have committed themselves to working alongside service users.

References and other sources

◯ References

Department of Health (1999). **National Service Framework for mental health**. DH, London.

Department of Health (2006a). **From values to action: The Chief Nursing Officer's review of mental health nursing**. DH, London.

Department of Health (2006b). **Modernising nursing careers**. DH, London.

Department of Health (2007). **Improving access to psychological therapies**. DH, London.

National Institute for Mental Health in England (2004). **Mental health: New Ways of Working**. DH, London.

[online] **http://www.newwaysofworking.org.uk**

Nursing and Midwifery Council (2001). **Fitness for practice and purpose**. NMC, London.

Nursing and Midwifery Council (2002). **Supporting nurses and midwives through lifelong learning**. NMC, London.

Nursing and Midwifery Council (2006a). **Employers' responsibilities**. NMC, London. [online] <http://www.nmc-uk.org/aFrameDisplay.aspx?DocumentID=1567> accessed 09/06/2007.

Nursing and Midwifery Council (2006b). **Personal professional profile**. NMC, London. [online] <http://www.nmc-uk.org/aFrameDisplay.aspx?DocumentID=1583> accessed 02/07/2007.

Nursing and Midwifery Council (2006c). **Standards to support learning and assessment in practice**. NMC, London.

Nursing and Midwifery Council (2008). **The Code: Standards of conduct, performance and ethics for nurses and midwives**. NMC Publications, London.

Romme R and Morris M (2007). The harmful concept of schizophrenia. **Mental Health Nursing**, 27(2), 7-11.

Stuart C (2007). **Assessment, supervision and support in clinical practice: a guide for nurses, midwives and other health professionals**. Churchill Livingstone, Edinburgh.

Useful links

You may find it helpful to work through our online material, intended to help you to consider and actively work through issues raised by the issues in this chapter:

 www.oxfordtextbooks.co.uk/orc/clarke

and choose the online resources for this chapter.

The campaign to abolish the schizophrenia label (CASL):

 http://www.asylumonline.net/index.htm

NHS Careers: England and Wales

http://www.jobs.nhs.uk/

Scotland

http://www.jobs.scot.nhs.uk/version2/byRegion.aspx

Northern Ireland

http://www.hscni.net/index.php?link=jobs

Further reading

Stockwell F (1972). **The unpopular patient**. Royal College of Nursing, London.

Stockwell F (1985). **The nursing process in psychiatric nursing**. Croom Helm, London.

Glossary

a

actualize · The realization that something that exists at a theoretical level may be made real, or substantiated, by acting upon it, e.g. applying anxiety management techniques leading to the successful reduction of anxiety symptoms.

advocacy · This is what someone does when they are speaking up on behalf of another. It may involve pleading a case, or representing the views of someone else who is less able to do this for themselves. It has some of its origins in law and has similarities to pleading a case or defending someone's interests.

affect · If you hear a psychiatrist talking about 'affect' then they are describing a person's apparent mood state.

affective disorder · An affective disorder is one in which a person's mood is considered to be abnormal. An example of this could be seen in the depressed person or in someone whose mood is elated. This term is commonly used in relation to a person who has a manic depressive disorder in which their mood cycles between periods of elation and depression.

akasthisia · A feeling of restlessness and inner tension that may cause the person to pace about and to experience anxiety. It is related to neurological changes brought about by administration of antipsychotic medication.

antibiotics · Substances produced by certain bacteria and fungi that prevent the growth of, or destroy, other bacteria.

antimuscarinic · May also be called anticholinergic and refers to a medication that blocks the activity of acetylcholine (a chemical used by nerves to send signals) in the peripheral nervous system. Some of these drugs are used to reduce extrapyramidal symptoms from antipsychotic medication. Their action results in side effects such as dry mouth, blurred vision, decreased ability to urinate, and constipation.

arrhythmias · In normal functioning, the heart beats at a steady rate, which slows or increases to match the demand being placed upon it (i.e. when resting or exercising). An arrhythmia is a condition in which the normal heart rhythm becomes too fast, too slow, or irregular. Hypokalaemia (see below) is one of a number of conditions that can cause this.

assertive outreach · An intense model of case management providing frequent team support in the community.

assistive technology · The use of technological aids to help a person with memory problems. Aids can include devices that help with safety, such as giving warnings if gas is left turned on, or sounding an alarm if the person wanders away from the house at night.

avoidant · Feeling of inadequacy; socially inhibited with a fear of negative evaluation of self.

b

barrier cream · A medicated cream applied topically (i.e. to the skin) as a protective covering to the skin.

benzodiazepines · Drugs used for their therapeutic effects on anxiety while also promoting sleeping, e.g. diazepam, temazepam, and nitrazepam (see also Chapter 8).

biomedical model · This model exclusively considers pathology, biochemistry, and physiology of disease in diagnosis and treatment.

bio-psycho-social · An approach to the understanding of a person's problems that takes into account a range of possible influences. 'Bio' refers to possible underlying physical causes of problems; 'psycho' relates to the possibility of a psychological cause to problems; 'social' acknowledges the effect that our environment and relationships with others may have.

blunted affect · A term you may hear in practice – what it means is that the person seems apathetic and unresponsive, indifferent to their surroundings and circumstances.

(Note: Critics of psychiatric practice would say that psyshiatric medication has a tendency to produce such behaviour in a person.)

c

capacity · The mental ability to understand information that allows an individual to make their own informed decisions about different aspects of their care and treatment.

Care Programme Approach · A systematic procedure (introduced in 1991) for the delivery of care reflected in and recorded on structured documentation, relating to all the stages of an adult's care and treatment while in the care of the mental health service. This documentation should contain information about all health and social care needs and includes monitoring and review systems to ensure the service user receives the appropriate care and treatment from a multidisciplinary team.

case management · A single or multidisciplinary approach to coordinating care that involves a whole system approach, including bio-psycho-social needs.

clinical supervision · Clinical supervision helps the practitioner develop their practice within a supportive relationship with a clinical colleague.

CMHN · Community mental health nurse, sometimes called community psychiatric nurse (CPN). A person who holds appropriate qualification(s) in mental health or allied studies, is registered with a professional body, and practices in this field.

coerce · To compel or pressure someone to do certain things, sometimes using physical or psychological pressure to get them to agree to things they do not voluntarily want to do.

complex needs · The *National Service Framework for mental health* (Department of Health 1999) states that 'complex needs' is a term that may be used to describe a person who has two or more disorders and/or medical needs.

compulsory detention · When a service user is detained in a psychiatric hospital, without their agreement/consent, under mental health legislation because they are considered to be suffering from mental illness and to be in need of care and/or treatment.

confusion · Disturbed orientation with regard to time, place, and person, sometimes accompanied by disordered consciousness.

constipation · Incomplete or infrequent action of the bowels, with consequent filling of the rectum with hard faeces.

d

delusional ideas · A delusion is usually described as being a false and fixed idea that does not correspond to the person's usual belief system and is held despite evidence to the contrary.

dependent · Requires constant reassurance and feedback from others while not taking responsibility for their own actions.

depot injection · A medication injected into muscle tissue that is slowly absorbed over a period of time.

diabetes mellitus · A disease resulting from a disturbance in the oxidation and utilization of glucose, which is secondary to a malfunction of the beta cells of the pancreas, whose function is the production and release of insulin. Note that because insulin is involved in the metabolism of carbohydrates, proteins, and fats, diabetes is not limited to a disturbance of glucose metabolism.

type 1 diabetes
A form of diabetes that is usually due to autoimmune destruction of the pancreatic beta cells that produce insulin. This type is treatable only with injected or inhaled insulin.

type 2 diabetes
A form of diabetes characterized by insulin resistance in target tissues with some impairment of beta cell functioning. Can be treated by diet, tablets, or injections of insulin, depending on the severity of the condition.

differential diagnosis · This is a medical term used to describe the consideration of alternative diagnoses that may fit with the person's symptoms.

deliberate self-harm · The intentional or purposeful act of causing oneself personal harm or injury.

disassociate · The mental behavioural process is separated from the conscious identity of the individual.

disorientation · The loss of proper bearings, or a state of mental confusion with regard to time, place, or identity.

diuretics · Drugs used to increase the output of urine. Usually used to treat heart failure and hypertension, they also have the effect of temporarily appearing to reduce weight. This weight 'loss' is actually due to the body having less fluid – it is a dangerous practice that should be firmly discouraged.

diversity · In a population context it refers to a varied range of people who may differ from each other on the basis of gender, sexuality, race, beliefs (including religious beliefs), language, and customs. This will mean there are varied needs/requirements on this basis, as well as some universal needs and characteristics.

dystonia · Involuntary spasm and repetitive contraction of muscles causing abnormal movements. It can appear without apparent cause in some people but is often associated with antipsychotic medication.

e

echolalia · The repetition of words spoken by another person.

electrocardiograph (ECG) · This is a test that measures the electrical activity of the heart. Heartbeats are controlled by a wave of electrical impulses and these are represented in graph form by the ECG machine. Problems in heart function can be identified from this.

electro-convulsive therapy (ECT) · This treatment is not as widely used as it used to be and is now generally only used when individuals have been unresponsive to other forms of treatment. It is most commonly used in severe depression but is still sometimes used to treat other illnesses such as bipolar disorder. The treatment involves passing an electrical current through the brain to produce an epileptiform fit. Research suggests that it is the fit rather than the current that produces the therapeutic effect.

electrolyte disturbance · In human physiology an electrolyte is a salt that is dissolved in bodily fluid and that conducts an electric current. This is essential to the functioning of the nerves, heart, and muscle tissue. Examples of electrolytes include calcium, chloride, magnesium, phosphate, potassium, and sodium. An imbalance in these substances in the body can be caused by diuretics (see above), as the body loses too much fluid. This is a medical emergency as it is potentially fatal.

empirical · Something based upon experience and observation, as opposed to systematic logic (source: *Webster's New World Medical Dictionary*).

euthymic · A psychological state that is neither elated nor depressed. A reasonably positive mood.

evidence-based · Practice based upon the process of using best available research and clinical expertise; the use of an approach proven to work.

extrapyramidal symptoms · The extrapyramidal system is a network of nervous tissue in the brain that is involved in coordination of movement. This system is damaged by repeated use of common antipsychotic medications, and resulting problems include akasthisia, dystonias, and tardive dyskinesia (all defined in this Glossary).

f

functionality · In the context of deliberate self-harm, the action or behaviour that serves a function or purpose such as help-seeking or alleviating difficult emotions.

g

gait · The manner of walking.

Glasgow coma scale · A standardized system for quickly evaluating the level of consciousness in the critically ill. Measures include: eye opening according to four criteria; verbal response against five criteria; and motor response using six criteria. Scores of seven or less qualify as 'coma'. Coma is defined as no response and no eye opening.

h

hallucinations · Usually described as being 'sensory perception in the absence of sensory stimuli', or in plainer English this is when a person may see, hear, feel, smell, or taste something that is not really there.
visual hallucination – seeing things that are not there.
auditory hallucination – hearing strange things (usually voices).

holistic · In nursing this word refers to a model of assessing and delivering care needs. It involves seeing the person as a whole and taking into account their physical, spiritual, emotional, social, economic, and educational needs. Another use of the word is when referring to alternative therapies.

homeostasis · The state in which the body attempts to maintain a constant level of optimal intenal functioning. This requires the ability to constantly monitor and adjust bodily symptoms (such as cardiac and respiratory functioning) to maintain equilibrium.

humanism · A branch of psychotherapy concerned with the uniqueness of the individual and the individual's natural tendency towards growth.

humanistic · An approach that values and privileges the human person and their thoughts, feelings, and interests as paramount.

hyperglycaemia · An excess of sugar in the blood. The normal fasting range is 2.5–4.7 mmol/litre. Hypoglycaemia is a sign of diabetes mellitus.

hypoglycaemia · A condition in which blood sugar level is less than normal. Usually arising in diabetic patients as a result of insulin overdosage, delay in eating, or a rapid combustion of carbohydrate due to, for example, rapid exercise.

hypokalaemia · Also known as potassium deficiency. Potassium is essential to the normal functioning of the heart and muscles and an imbalance of this causes very serious complications.

hyponatraemia · A condition in which the concentration of sodium in the body is too low.

i

incontinence · An inability to control natural functions or discharges. Urinary incontinence is an inability to control the outflow of urine; faecal incontinence is an inability to control the movements of the bowel.

insight · The ability to recognize one's own thoughts, ideas, and beliefs as out of proportion, or not in touch with reality, or as being an aspect of a mental illness. It is similar to self-awareness but is specifically used in connection with recognizing what is illness and what is not in this context.

intuitive · An immediate understanding, knowledge, or truth about something without obvious reasoning or logic.

l

labile/lability · Instability or lability of mood is the tendency to sudden changes of mood of short duration.

lithium · A drug that is used as a mood stabilizer in disorders of mood. It requires regular blood tests to monitor the blood levels, as the therapeutic range is critical.

n

narcissistic · Lacking empathy for others; arrogance; grandiose ideas about self with the need to be admired.

nursing process · This is a structured process by which nurses deliver care to patients, supported by nursing models or philosophies. The nursing process shows how nurses identify and problem-solve service users' health and social care needs based on their own contribution to care.

o

obsessive-compulsive · An obsessive-compulsive disorder is an anxiety state in which a person experiences obsessive thoughts. Very often, as a way of coping, the person feels driven towards repetitive actions such as hand washing, repetitively checking things, or having to perform rituals before doing certain things.

p

palpitations · This is a term used to describe the experience of being aware of one's own heartbeat. Normally, of course, we do not notice this, but at times this can become apparent. Often this is associated with anxiety. In some cases, however, it can be a symptom of heart disorder and it is important that this possibility is not overlooked – a physical check-up would be safe practice.

paresthesia · This is a term that describes a sensation of tingling in the fingers. It is caused by the hyperventilation that may occur when a person becomes anxious. When we breathe too quickly it causes blood oxygen levels to rise and carbon dioxide levels to fall – this causes a change in the blood's pH (acidity) and it is this that is associated with the tingling feeling in the fingers.

Parvolex (acetylcystenie) · A drug that can protect the liver from damage following an overdose of paracetamol.

peristalsis · A wave-like contraction, preceded by a wave of dilatation, which travels along the walls of a tubular organ such as the alimentary canal, tending to press its contents onwards.

person-centred nursing · The design of care with the individual's thoughts, feelings, and beliefs at its core.

philosophy · A particular set of ideas, beliefs, or laws relating to the truth or rules about something. The principles or reasoning of an approach or idea, which explains or gives reasons for the way something is or occurs.

polypharmacy · This is a term often (but not exclusively) applied to the care of older people. It is when a person has been prescribed a range of different medications. Sometimes too many medicines are prescribed by different doctors and there has been insufficient coordination of this prescribing. The result may be that the person has either too many medicines to take and/or that these medications are contra-indicated and may cause further health problems.

positive risk · Empowers the person to decide the level of risk (where possible) to be taken with their health needs.

post-traumatic stress disorder (PTSD) · This is a term used to describe the psychological disturbance experienced by people who have undergone a traumatic event. These disturbances can include intrusive thoughts, nightmares, and flashbacks to the original trauma.

PRN · Pro re nata – whenever necessary. Note that good prescribing practice should indicate a maximum number of administrations in a given time period.

psyche · Often taken to refer to the human mind in terms of emotional and cognitive processes. In Freudian theory it is composed of three elements: the Id, the Ego, and the Superego.

psychodynamic model · This describes the idea that our past/childhood experiences and the hidden conflicts these cause have an influence upon our future behaviour. Freud was mainly responsible for the development of this theory.

psycho-social interventions · Based upon the stress vulnerability diathesis, requiring coordinated care that involves psychological, spiritual, and sociological interventions, as well as medication.

r

reality orientation · An approach in which the person with memory problems is reminded about the date, time etc. with memory prompts such as notice boards, as well as with sessions in which these things are discussed.

recovery · Recovery from mental illness requires a person to develop the skills to overcome or manage the impairment that the illness creates, in order to live as normal a life as possible by their own standards.

recovery approach · This is an approach to a person's problems that does not imply that a 'cure' will be found. Instead, a person's individual response to coping with possibly long-term mental health problems is emphasized (see Chapter 6 for more discussion of this concept).

reflexive · A process where thoughts and ideas keep going back and forth between people, being shaped and developed as ideas are shared and reflected upon.

relapse signature · The unique combination of factors relating to an individual service user, put together in a systemic way, which identify predictors and patterns of relapse.

relapse triggers · Any factors that are known to contribute to the deterioration of a service user's mental state and negatively affect recovery and wellness.

re-traumatizing · Reliving a past experience that has a negative impact.

S

schizoid (personality) · Detachment from social relationships with a limited range of emotions in interpersonal settings.

schizophrenia · A major psychotic illness that may affect a person's perceptions, cognition, behaviour, and emotions.

schizotypal · Inability to form close relationships with a deficit in social and interpersonal skills.

self-actualization · This is the concept of individuals reaching their optimum potential, making the most of their abilities and becoming the best they can be.

self-blaming · When a person takes on responsibility for things that have gone wrong in their life, when usually they are not to blame.

serious mental illness (SMI) · Applies to the situation where people have a diagnosed mental illness that is affecting multiple areas of their life, requiring frequent and prolonged support from mental health services.

somatization · In psychology, this is a term that describes physical symptoms experienced by a person which seem to have no obvious physiological cause. The physical symptoms are thought to be a manifestation of underlying psychological distress.

stress · This might be defined as how you feel when you are under pressure. It is perfectly normal (and even desirable) to experience a little stress as we work towards achieving our goals in life. However, there is a lot of evidence that chronic levels of stress have a harmful effect upon a person's mental and physical health and it is important that nurses should consider the effect of this both on the people we see in clinical practice and on our own lives.

subdural haematoma · A blood clot between the arachnoid and dura mater. It may be acute or arise slowly from a minor injury.

suicide · The act of intentionally taking one's life.

supervised discharge · Introduced to reduce risk of relapse in the community by providing comprehensive care planning for recovery and fast access back to hospital if required.

t

tardive dyskinesia · A neurological disorder that causes abnormal movements. These can include facial movements involving the lips and tongue. Movements in the arms and legs can also be experienced. This is most often caused by repeated administration of antipsychotic medication and is mostly irreversible.

termination · The end stage and formal ending of a therapeutic/professional working relationship with a service user.

therapeutic communities · Living in a community with the emphasis focusing on the individual's interaction and interpersonal skills in order to bring about change.

thought echo · The person may experience an auditory hallucination in which they hear their thoughts as if being spoken aloud.

thought insertion/withdrawal · These terms describe characteristic problems with thinking that people may complain of. In thought insertion, the person perceives thoughts as seeming to have come from an external source. With thought withdrawal, thoughts seem to have been taken out of one's head.

transference · Unconscious response in which the person experiences feelings/attitudes associated with another individual, usually in their past.

counter-transference
The above, but this time the response is coming from the nurse towards the client.

u

unconditional positive regard · This was a term used by Carl Rogers, an important psychological theorist. When we treat people with unconditional positive regard, we indicate to them (even when they may not feel this about themselves) that we regard them as being capable and of worth. This belief is one of the necessary conditions that will allow a person to make changes in their lives.

urinary tract infection (UTI) · An infection of the tract that conducts urine from the kidneys to the exterior, including the ureters, the bladder, and the urethra.

Index